BIOACTIVE COMPOUNDS IN PHYTOMEDICINE

Edited by **Iraj Rasooli**

Bioactive Compounds in Phytomedicine
Edited by Iraj Rasooli

Published by InTech

Janeza Trdine 9, 51000 Rijeka, Croatia

Publishing Process Manager Masa Vidovic

Technical Editor Teodora Smiljanic

Cover Designer InTech Design Team

Additional hard copies can be obtained from orders@intechopen.com

Bioactive Compounds in Phytomedicine, Edited by Iraj Rasooli
p. cm.
ISBN 978-953-307-805-2

For EU product safety concerns:
IN TECH d.o.o., Prolaz Marije Krucifikse Kozulić 3, 51000 Rijeka, Croatia,
info@intechopen.com or visit our website at intechopen.com.

Meet the editor

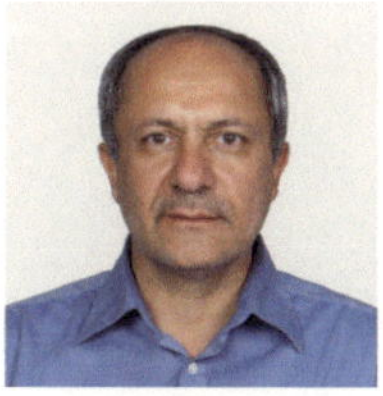

Dr. Iraj Rasooli was born in 1960 in Ahar, Iran. He received his BSc in Microbiology from Shivaji University (India) before obtaining his MSc and PhD in 1992 and 1998 respectively in Microbiology from Bombay University (India). He joined Shahed University in 1993 as an assistant professor where his focus has been on research activities on biological properties of essential oils from medicinal plants and he has published a number of papers in a number of notable national and international journals. He was awarded Razi festival prize by the president of Islamic Republic of Iran in 2002. Professor Rasooli went to the University of Calgary (Canada) in 2002 for his sabbatical where he accelerated his level of knowledge of molecular biology at Prof. Anthony Schryver's laboratory. To date he has published 86 full length papers on bioactivities of essential oils and molecular microbiology. He continues teaching and researching in his current role as Dean of Science faculty at Shahed University, Tehran, Iran.

Contents

Preface

Individuals are increasingly taking personal responsibility over their health, both in the prevention and treatment of disease. This is particularly true for a wide variety of chronic or incurable diseases such as cancer, diabetes, arthritis or acute illnesses readily treated at home like common cold. During the last fifty years the practice of herbalism has become mainstream throughout the world. This is due in part to the recognition of the value of traditional medical systems, particularly of Asian origin, and the identification of medicinal plants from indigenous pharmacopeias that have been shown to have significant healing power, either in their natural state or as the source of new pharmaceuticals. When mixtures of several crude extracts are used in formulations, enhancement of the beneficial effects or greater toxicity is expected through either synergistic amplification or diminishment of possible adverse side effects. It is also presumed that their combination could prevent the gradual decline in efficacy that is frequently observed when single drugs are given over long periods of time. Nowadays such remedies can still be found in ethnic and health food stores, but are also available in pharmacies and grocery stores. Unfortunately there is no universal regulatory system that ensures that these remedies are what they say they are, do what is claimed, or most importantly, are safe. Many patients with chronic allergic conditions seek complementary and alternative medicine therapies. This trend has begun to attract interest from mainstream health care providers and scientific investigators and has stimulated government agencies to provide support and guidance for the scientific investigation of complementary and alternative medicine. This effort may lead to improved therapies and better health care/patient outcomes. This book presents an update on the most promising herbal remedies. The objectives of this book were to determine the bioactivities of herbal medicines by giving some examples of recent research outputs. Results of this study are aimed toward helping avoid potential drug-herb interactions; helping decision makers to decide on the proper policies in the medical and the non-medical fields concerning herbal remedies and other types of complementary and alternative medicine.

Prof. Iraj Rasooli
Department of Biology,
Shahed University,
Tehran-Qom Express way,
Iran

Part 1

Herbal Therapy

1

Selecting Medicinal Plants for Development of Phytomedicine and Use in Primary Health Care

Wagner Luiz Ramos Barbosa[1] et al.*
[1]*Universidade Federal do Pará*
Brazil

1. Introduction

The world market for herbal medicines is around US$ 40 billion, whereas in Brazil it is estimated to be around US$ 1 billion. Data from the World Health Organization (WHO) shows that more than a half of the world population makes use of some type of medicinal herb searching for relief for painful or unpleasant symptoms. From that total at least 30% are provided by medical prescription (WHO, 1978).

The application of traditional or popular knowledge about the use of healing plants, in the development of herbal drugs proves to be a fairly consequent and consistent strategy, as it can generate employment and income from the participation of the organized community in the process of development, production and insertion of the so developed product in the pharmaceutical market. It still may be appropriate from an ecological standpoint, when the botanical raw material for the production of this herbal medicine is obtained from specimens grown in deforested areas. When a project with this design is originated and developed in the scope of Pharmaceutical Sciences it is called an Ethnopharmaceutical study (BARBOSA, 1998).

Since 2006, the Popular Phytotherapy became a therapeutical option supported by the Brazilian government, through the National Policy on Integrative and Complementary Practices (BRAZIL, 2006). After that, new regulatory documents have been promulgated to standardize the use of medicinal herbs. The National Policy on Phytopharmaceuticals and Medicinal Plants in its guidelines, establishes that a list of regional plants is to be defined, representing the Regional Popular Phytotherapy (BRAZIL, 2006b). These policies advocate the inclusion of the use of medicinal plants in primary health care, which shall be employed with highest efficacy and safety and must be object of the actions of Pharmaceutical Services, which are also to be applied to manufactured drugs (BARBOSA & PINTO, 2005).

* Myrth Soares do Nascimento[1], Lucianna do Nascimento Pinto[1], Fernando Luiz Costa Maia[1], Antonio Jorge Ataíde Sousa[1], José Otávio Carréra Silva Júnior[1], Maurícia Melo Monteiro[2] and Danilo Ribeiro de Oliveira[3]
[2]*Universidade do Estado do Pará, Brazil*
[3]*Universidade Federal do Rio de Janeiro, Brazil*

The National Policy on Phytopharmaceuticals and Medicinal Plants (BRAZIL, 2006b) has the overall objective "to ensure the Brazilian population the safe access and rational use of medicinal plants and herbal medicines." The Pharmaceutical Sciences can contribute strongly to this purpose, attending the first specific objective of the document, "expand the therapeutic options for users with guaranteed access to medicinal plants, herbal medicines and services related to herbal medicine, with safety, efficacy and quality regarding the integrality of health care, considering the traditional knowledge about medicinal plants." Achieving this goal requires the combination of elements of Pharmaceutical Sciences such as Pharmaceutical Care and Quality Control, with traditional knowledge.

This concern of the regulatory agency promotes the standardization of herbal medicines facilitates the evaluation of important aspects such as efficacy and safety in the use of these medications, as the difficulties to standardize the active pharmaceutical ingredient and the formulation development of phytomedicines from medicinal plants of popular use represent the major challenge in the country.

Phytomedicines must contain as active ingredients exclusively plant material derivatives. The addition of an isolated substance from any source eliminates this characteristic of the product. Apart from the methodology chosen for processing the plant material, one must consider the seasonality of its biochemistry, the soil and climate characteristics of its growing place or occurrence and the popular and scientific names of the plant (MACIEL, 2002). Studies show that the secondary metabolism of the plant can vary considerably depending on factors such as: seasonality, temperature, water availability, UV radiation, nutrients, altitude, air pollution, and even induction by mechanic stimuli or attack by pathogens (GOBBO-NETO, 2007). Thus, for developing a phytomedicine it is determining to have a well defined plant species, including the unambiguous botanical characterization.

How to define from which plant species an herbaceous medicine can be developed?

There are some strategies to reach this definition and here we will discuss about some of them which are well known and a new one will be introduced, where therapeutic products are directly handled, and which was born within the Pharmaceutical Science.

The WHO has recommended that member countries, especially the developing ones, shall seek to expand their therapeutic arsenal for public health through the use of medical home practices employed by the people. These recommendations are summarized in the four items mentioned below (MATOS, 2000):

- Undertake regional surveys of plants used in the practice of people's or traditional medicine and scientifically identify them;
- Support the use of useful practices selected by their efficacy and safety;
- Suppress the use of practices considered useless or harmful;
- Develop governmental programs that allow the cultivation and use of the selected plants.

The scientific research on medicinal plants generally originates medicines in shoter time, often with lower costs and therefore more accessible to the population, which in different places on the planet, can't afford the high costs of medicines used to face the primary needs in health care, especially because in most cases the raw materials used in manufacturing these products are imported. For these reasons or deficiency of the public primary health care in Brazil, about 80% of the population lacks access to essential medicines (TOLEDO et. al., 2003).

From a socioeconomic perspective, it is necessary to highlight some aspects such as the demand for phytotherapy and the cost of the medicines, the potential for generating occupation and income in the phytopharmaceuticals productive arrangement, especially under the social economy, the efforts of research that prove, scientifically, the medicinal properties of plants, and the need for restructuring the health care system, including the preparation of professionals working in this area (NUNES et. al., 2003).

The recovery and revaluation of the use of medicinal herbs in Brazil today are demanding a certain worry since many medicinal plants of high value may disappear from the forests and scrub lands, even before scientists can discover their properties, and turn them into medicines. The main step that must be taken is to develop techniques for cultivation and harvesting without compromising the reproduction of these species. Another measure is to prevent urban sprawl from causing the destruction of peripheral green areas which are rich in medicinal herbs (ADEODATO et. al., 1996).

Medicinal plants, which have assessed their therapeutic efficacy and toxicology, or safety of use evaluated, among other properties, are scientifically approved to be used by people in their basic health needs, according to the ease of access, low cost and compatibility with cultural traditions. Since medicinal plants can be classified as natural products safe to use, the law allows them to be marketed by notification to the health regulatory agencies (BRAZIL, 2010), and they can be cultivated by those who follows agronomical good practices. So, the assisted self-medication is practiced in cases of health problems that might be considered simpler and more commonplace within a community. This practice tends to reduce the demand for health care professionals, rationalising and reducing the cost of Public Health Service (LORENZI & MATOS, 2002).

Despite these recommendations, it seems that the use of medicinal plants in public health service is still not a reality in different localities in Brazil and, by extension, in the American Continent. This fact can be explained by the lack of scientific data on native species or the lack of systematization of the existing data. The lack of political interest signals that this issue is not a priority for many governments in different parts of the world. As long as the practice of phytotherapy does not bring financial rewards, private capital will not feel encouraged to invest in this niche of market, which meanwhile is interested in more profitable and less regulated activities.

1.1 Techniques and methods for selecting medicinal plants

In the investigation of medicinal plants, a relevant moment, which can set the course of the work and its impact on all points of view, is the criterion used for the selection of the plant species to study. Cuéllar and Guirado (2008) refer to genomics, metabolomics and ecological, botanical taxonomic and epidemiological based studies. On the other hand Albuquerque and Hanazaki (2006) point out other ways to study the medicinal plants, among which we highlight five basic types of approaches: the randomized, the ethological, the chemotaxonomic (also known as phylogenetic or chemosystematic), the ethnodirected (or ethno-oriented) and finally, the exploration of promising biological test results (ELIZABETSKY; SHANLEY, 1994).

Some of these options are analyzed below.

1.2 The randomized approach

Several important authors, here mentioned, recognize the randomized approach as an approach without criteria. Calderon (2000) and others who worked with forest plots, do not identify this form of selecting plants for research, as random. So, the question here to be discussed is whether it is a type of random selection criterion or whether it should be identified separately as another type of approach?

The randomized investigations consist in random selection and collection of plant species for study, according to the plant availability. When carried out in regions with high diversity and endemism the probability of finding novel substances, bioactive or not, is certainly higher in this type of selection (MACIEL et al., 2002, OLIVEIRA et al., 2010). It is an indispensable approach, once it can demonstrate the potential of different plant species that had never been investigated. According to Souza Brito (1996), this type of selection provides an endless source of new structures, since nature is a vast chemical laboratory. However, there are many mistaken views and criticisms about this approach due to its randomness, which does not mean the absence of criteria (ALBUQUERQUE, HANAZAKI, 2006).

1.3 The ecological approach

The ecological approach, also known as *field observations*, consists in observations of interactions between organisms in their ecological environment, inducing to potential biological activity (antibacterial, antifungal, agrotoxic, pesticide) (GUIRA; CUÉLLAR, 2008). This approach searches for secondary metabolites and biological activities and it may be performed by the selection of young leaves x mature leaves for a given species, or between different species that are shadow resistant and not shadow resistant, among other characteristics (COLEY et al., 2003), though little explored, it has achieved excellent results.

Briskin (2000) states that secondary metabolites present in plant species have ecological functions which can justify their use for application in the development of therapeutic resources for humans. For example, metabolites involved in plant defense against microbial pathogens may be useful as antimicrobial drugs in humans, since they are not very toxic. Likewise, secondary products with repellent action (e.g. unpleasant flavor or odour) against herbivores by neurotoxic activity could have beneficial effects in humans such as antidepressants, sedatives, muscle relaxants or anesthetics, through their action on the CNS. Therefore, the observation of these ecological relationships is a useful tool in the selection of plant species.

According to Albuquerque and Hanazaki (2008) this approach intends to evaluate the use of secondary metabolites by animals or other non-nutritional substances from plants, aiming to combat diseases or controlling them, as it can be seen in the works developed by Carrai (2003) and Krief (2004). In the latter, it was observed that leaves of *Trichilia rubescens* Oliv. eaten by chimpanzees in Uganda showed antimalarial activity. This result shows the importance of the ethological approach in the discovery of useful plant species of medical and pharmaceutical interest.

A variation of the ecological approach is zoopharmacognosy, also called animal self-medication (self-medication in animals), which proposes the selection of species regularly ingested by animals, especially primates; to reduce microbial infestation, pain (BERRY;

MCFERREN; RODRIGUEZ, 1995. In: BIRD; BRIJESH; DASWANI, 2007). To the selection criterion based on the observation of the relationship between animals and plants, Albuquerque and Hanazaki (2008) attribute the term "ethological approach" based on the habits of animals, how they behave in their natural environment.

1.4 The chemosystematic approach

When the definition of a plant species, which will be source of a phytomedicine, is based on the structural analogy of the substances present in this plant material, with other known active substances present in different botanical family, genus or even species, we can infer that this strategy is based on chemosystematics, a system created by Professor Otto Richard Gottlieb (1982) to organize and understand the plants. This system consists in identifying groups of chemicals present in plants, considering the taxonomic organization of these plants. To illustrate this topic, consider the use of a plant species containing antiplasmodic indol derivatives as active principle in the development of an antimalarial phytomedicine.

Would a plant species from a different genus, containing such substances, give origin to the same phytomedicine?

Depending on the results the later plant produces in *in vitro* biological tests, it may be true. On the other hand, *Mikania* species (Asteraceae) which contain coumarin in their composition, exhibit different pharmacological activities and alleged popular use, including antimalarial properties. Therefore, the strategy based on chemosystematics can bring in it some uncertainty, once the chemical composition, which can explain the relationship between botanical species, genera and even families, is not decisive enough to guide the development of a phytomedicinal product and to validate the alleged use, as well as it does not confirm the safety and efficacy of the derivative proposed for the development of the product, requiring indeed the realization of a pharmacological prospection in order to characterize the wanted activity for the phytomedicine. The contribution of chemosystematics is to offer to the phytochemical analyst a range of possible chemical structures to be searched in the preparations obtained from the plant material.

The chemosystematic approach, also called phylogenetic, consists of selecting a species from a family or genus, for which some phytochemical knowledge of at least one species of the group is known (ALBUQUERQUE, HANAZAKI, 2006). The presence of different compounds, which can be used as biosynthetic markers, is used by botanists in taxonomy studies and the chemosystematic approach is used as a successful tool in the selection of families, subfamilies and genera to be investigated in terms of produced metabolites (BASSO et al. 2005). That is, through the chemotaxonomy, one can select plants from known families and genera to produce certain classes of substances (e.g. alkaloids, flavonoids, steroids, etc.), especially those recognized by their biological activities and therapeutic applications, preferably associated to these metabolites. As an example we can cite the case of galantamine, used in the treatment of Alzheimer's disease, first isolated from the species *Galanthus nivalis*, Amaryllidaceae family. Since then, numerous chemosystematic studies verified the presence of galantamine and acetylcholinesterase inhibitory activity in several species of the genus *Galanthus* (MARSTON; KISSLING; HOSTETTMANN, 2002). Following the same line, Ronsted et al. (2008) continued searching for alkaloids with acetylcholinesterase inhibitory activity in several species of other genera of Amaryllidaceae family, especially *Narcisus*, obtaining excellent results.

Considering that in this case we deal with the selection of plant species for the development of herbal medicines or for direct use in primary health care, this feature of the method, enabling the discovery of molecules, does not influence the discussion and treatment of the theme in this chapter, without, however, making value judgments on this important application. Even within the pre-formulation studies carried out during the experimental stage of drug development it is an advantage for researchers to know in advance which class of metabolites to prospect in order to develop detection, characterization and quantification of markers of the active pharmaceutical ingredients and the final product, and with these data to establish their quality control process. This step of the process is determining for the registration of an herbal medicine in Brazil.

2. The ethnoguided approach

The ethnoguided approach consists of selecting plant species in accordance to the indication of specific population groups in certain contexts of use, emphasizing the search for the locally built knowledge regarding their natural resources and their application in their health systems (GUIRA; CUÉLLAR, 2008). Plant species are raised by a quali-quantitative survey. This survey usually relates symptoms, signs and diagnosis of low-gravity diseases to medicinal plants that the respondents know about and their use according to the cultural elements that characterize the ethnicity or human group to which they belong, considering the territory as the basis for this characterization.

In this type of approach the ethnobotany, ethnopharmacology and ethnomedicine can be highlighted. Recently ethnopharmacy has been structured to provide an interface between Pharmaceutical Science and Popular Phytotherapy where medicinal plant species can be selected for the development of phytomedicines and for use in primary health care, in compliance with the requirements of safety and efficacy (BARBOSA, 2008).

Below we schematically present the key steps for developing an herbal medicine considering as a starting point the selection of a medicinal plant according to the ethno-oriented method. Note that the remaining steps of the process do not allow a review of the plant identity, once they are irreversible and consume the collected and processed plant material, making its selection and identification a crucial step of the process as a whole. In Figure 1 below, Material Plant, Crude Extract and Standardized Extract, direct derivatives of the medicinal plant, are shown in the purple sequence. The procedures to which these materials are subjected are in green and the blue area shows the pharmacological assays. Note that both standardized extracts as well as fractions of these extracts can be pharmacologically evaluated and taken to the formulation step where the composition of the active pharmaceutical ingredient will determine the pharmaceutical form to be developed and the experiments required for this procedure.

See below a schematic sequence of processes for developing phytomedicine (Fig.1).

In Brazil, the National Health Surveillance Agency accepts ethno-oriented surveys as the basis for the registration of plant species which are used for the development of herbal medicines (BRAZIL, 2010) or for use in primary health care (BRAZIL, 2010b). The methods applied in these surveys produces plant species lists and information that provide the starting point for developing a formulation, when their allegation of use are already available. It is also associated with a historical use of the plant, often for a long period,

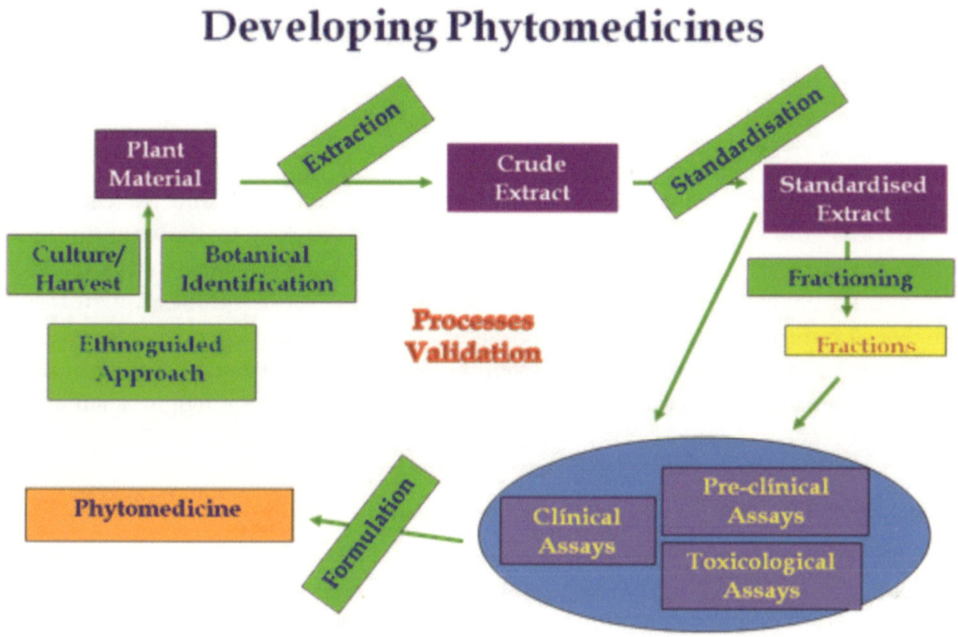

Fig. 1. Schematic sequence of the steps in developing phytomedicines, starting from an ethnoguided survey.

which being documented by scientific literature can contribute to validate its safe use based on official resolution. These requirements serve as the basis for the necessary experiments for pre-formulation studies.

2.1 Ethnobotany

Defining a medicinal plant for developing a phytomedicine under the vision of Ethnobotany, a survey of plant species used by a particular human group, certainly ensures botanical classification of the plant, since the core activities of Botany is to determine the taxa of a botanical sample. Moreover, important information for the production of plant material for the development process could also be provided by this approach. However, information like remedies preparation, allegations of use, including dosage, and evaluation of the remedy use and the relationship between user and derivatives prepared with plant material, are not part of the necessary instrumental for the practice of Ethnobotany.

In order to introduce a discussion on the survey of medicinal plants which are traditionally or popularly used for medicinal purposes, and within a historical perspective, this is what the Ethnobotany is about, a term coined by Harschberger and, which according to Schultes, pointed out ways that could serve to the scientific research (SCHULTE, 1962). Amorozo & Gely (1988) complement that ethnobotany, when applied to medicinal plants, acts in complicity with ethnopharmacology and medical anthropology, as it contextualizes the use of these plants in a treatment system peculiar to a specific human group.

According to Heinrich and Bremner (2006), the ethnobotany investigates the relationship between humans and plants in all its complexity, and is usually based on a detailed observation and study of the plants used by a society, including all its cultural beliefs and practices associated with that use. For such research, the ethnobotanists use a complex set of methods derived from the social and cultural sciences, including the taking of detailed field notes and the carefully documented collection of plant samples that allow a precise determination of the corresponding species.

Regarding the ethnobotanical approach method, Elisabetsky (1987) and De La Cruz Mota (1997) advocate the devolution or the return of prepared data to the communities and Martin (1986), supports the inclusion of the communities in the research so that the constant ethnobotanical making will promote the development and preservation of plant resources, knowledge of nature, the restoration of ecological balance with improved life quality. One must still think about the profits arising from the business performance of the technological development, which starts with the study of the ethnobotanical knowledge, whether in form of royalties or compensation to the communities participating in the research.

2.2 Ethnopharmacology

The relationship with the environment makes different human cultures absorb a wide variety of customs and knowledge from this environment in which they live. This knowledge evolves and over time is incorporated into the patterns of each population group across generations. The most representative and discussed case at a global level is the use of natural products arising from the knowledge of traditional peoples as Indians or riverbank people. In this case, a greater attention is given to those people who live in tropical regions where the natural range of options is presented in higher proportions, as in the Brazilian Amazon (PINTO & MADURO, 2003).

The most accepted definition of *Ethnopharmacology* is "multidisciplinary scientific exploration of biologically active agents traditionally employed or observed by man" (SOUZA et al. 2004). Another useful definition was proposed by Dos Santos & Fleurentin (1990) as an "interdisciplinary scientific study of materials from animal, vegetable or mineral origin and related knowledge and practices that different cultures use to modify the state of a living organism by therapeutic (curative/prophylactic) or diagnostic purposes". According to Bourdy (2008), many ethnopharmacological studies seek to correlate pharmacological activities found in a traditional remedy with active pharmaceutical ingredients through natural products chemistry. Ethnopharmacology, therefore, in its interdisciplinary nature, attempts to associate at least three points of view, a cultural, a biological and a chemical ones in a complementary approach.

The Ethnopharmacology seeks to know the illnesses that lead particular human groups to practice Herbalism; it discusses symptoms and signs, as well as, experimentally, applies pharmacological models to elucidate the action mechanism of phytoderivatives. This information is also very important for the development of herbal medicines, but the evaluation of the original form of use is decisive for the elaboration of the phytopharmaceutical formulation, moreover, it allows the use of medicinal plant *in natura* or in magistral or officinal formulations, after pharmaceutical manipulation in pharmacies.

The ethnopharmacological method combines the study of popular knowledge with chemical and pharmacological techniques. Allegations of popular therapeutic use of a particular plant species are important for the investigation of its pharmacological and toxicological effects (ELISABETSKY, 2003).

Albuquerque and Hanazaki (2006) claim that the ethnopharmacological approach is the study of traditional preparations used in health systems and disease, which include, isolated or combined, plants, animals, fungi or minerals. According to Maciel et al. (2002), on this approach the selection of species is carried out according to the therapeutic use evidenced by a particular ethnic group and it most likely favors the discovery of bioactive substances, the development of herbal medicines and the introduction of medicinal plants in primary health care. Many studies based on ethnopharmacological approach, report results that range from strictly botanical information, such as plant taxonomy, to general information such as part of the plant used and alleged use (UBOM, 2010; GIUSTI & PTERONI , 2009; IGNACIMUTHU et al ., 2006; GIDAY,. 2001).

Ethnopharmacological strategies have been widely used to conduct biological screening in various therapeutic areas such as cancer, immunomodulatory drugs, allergy drugs, analgesics, contraceptives, antimalarial, anti-diarrhea, antimicrobial, antiviral, etc. (ELIZABETSKY; SHANLEY , 1994).

Ethnopharmacology, an important methodology for the study of plants used in folk medicine, is characterized as a strategy for the investigation of medicinal plants that combines information acquired from users of medicinal plants with chemical and pharmacological studies. This method, still according to Elisabetsky, allows the formulation of hypotheses about the pharmacological activity and the compound responsible for the reported therapeutic action. Elisabetsky says "Ethnopharmacology is not about superstitions, but of popular knowledge related to traditional medicine systems" (ELISABETSKY, 2003).

2.3 The ethnomedical approach

The Ethnomedicine refers to the study of diseases, their causes and therapeutic measures taken by the various societies of primitive peoples as well as by popular social communities. It deals with natural and ancient therapies used to combat diseases and emphasizes the relationship between the patient and caregiver, between the patient and society. Ethnomedical studies contribute to the knowledge of the techniques used by many ancient peoples with regard to the treatment and knowledge of diseases (BENSON, 1980).

Since ancient times people treated their body and soul illnesses by asking for help to the supernatural. Certain peoples of northern Asia, where the tribal priest was called the shaman, used magical means, rites and knowledge of nature to heal health problems, associating them, among others, with knowledge about healing plants and connecting with their gods. So, they antagonized the disease with the active ingredient of the plant and with the ritualistic method, they incited the faith, the confidence in the procedure and in the shaman, who, in Brazilian Amazon, is called "pajé" or "benzedor" (shaman healer), according to more or less intimacy with the "enchanted" and the "forest spirits" (MAUES & VILLACORTA, 2008).

A significant part of what today is therapeutically used, started from information obtained from traditional communities that use natural products in their practices to survive and handle the environment. According to Guirado and Cuellar (2008) the ethnomedical approach consists in investigating the plant species on the basis of traditional use by different peoples, providing an interface between modern clinical medicine and folk medicine.

2.4 Ethnopharmacy

The strategy that can gather more information directly linked to the galenic development of a phytotherapeutical formulation is the ethnopharmaceutical approach of medicinal plants. Here, the semi-structured interviews script allows assessing, among other, the nosological profile of the approached human group and the medicinal plants used to treat the signals and symptoms mentioned by the interviewers. The method also evaluates the utilization of synthetic and herbal medicine by the group, and proposes the participatory observation of the remedies preparation using the most promising plant and finally observes aspects related to the plant itself. In this way it is possible to characterize the needs of this human group in terms of products which solve most of its health problems, this can be seen as a market analysis under the pharmacoeconomics point of view; also under this perspective, it is possible to determine the scale of this demand, verifying which synthetic medicines are not accessible to users and which herbal remedies they prepare to meet the lack of those products which are not distributed by the market (open or State), and also by observing the preparation of remedies by the community, a pharmacist can deduce a pharmaceutical form for the product under development and discover new procedures, as well as new pharmaceutical adjuvant.

For Heinrich (2001), the Ethnopharmacy is the interdisciplinary science that deals with the study of pharmaceutical resources considered in relation to cultural determinants that characterize the use of these resources in a particular human group. It involves studies on the identification, classification and cognitive categorization of plant material from which the drug will be produced (Ethnobiology), preparation of dosage forms (ethnopharmaceutics), allegation of the effects associated with the preparation (ethnopharmacology) and socio-medical aspects implied in these uses (ethnomedicine) (PIERONI et al., 2002).

Heinrich (2007) returns to the subject stating that ethnopharmacy includes pharmacognosy, pharmacology, galenic, and also the pharmaceutical practice and clinical pharmacy, thus allowing the utilization of local resources in the primary health care, and therefore it provides an interface to the Pharmaceutical Assistance necessary to the implementation of Phytotherapy in Primary Health Care.

The ethnopharmacy was introduced in Brazil in 1995 with the publication of the article "Ethnopharmaceutics: an approach to medicinal plants from the perspective of Pharmaceutical Sciences" (BARBOSA, SILVA, SOLER, 1996). The inventory of data from a group or local community on therapeutic resources shows itself as an adequate tool to document important information to design actions in the Pharmaceutical Sciences area, both from a technological standpoint as for healthcare, since it allows to obtain information about infectious diseases, the appropriate medicinal plants indicated for their treatment and it infers the most suitable methods for their preparation and use (PINTO, 2008).

In Brazil, Ethnopharmacy is defined as an interdisciplinary science that investigates the perception and use of traditional remedies, within a human group. It deals with the study of pharmaceutical resources considering the relations with the cultural context of its use, or the study of cultural determinants that characterize the uses of these resources in this culture. This study involves plant ethnotaxonomy, by which the drug is produced; the preparation of popular use form (ethnopharmaceutics); the biological evaluation of the pharmacological activity of such preparations (ethnopharmacology); clinic ethnopharmacy; medical anthropology or ethnomedicine; pharmacotherapeutic follow up and pharmacosurvaillance.

As a set of materials and practices used to maintain and restore health within a regional cultural context, several papers have been published; Bulus (2003) reported the ethnopharmacy of malaria in Nigeria; Pieroni (2005), the therapeutic resources of a community rooted in the northern Albanian Alps; he has raised about 70 taxa and 160 preparations; Thabrew (1991) described three species used as immunomodulators in liver disorders, in traditional herbal medicine in Sri Lanka. These papers report surveys conducted according to the ethnopharmaceutical methodology.

The ethnopharmaceutical method was developed by integrating environmental and cultural elements, thereby becoming a strategy for preserving the cultural heritage of human groups and actions for recovering deforested areas (BARBOSA, 1998).

Souza (2011) proposes the Ethnopharmacy as a science that permeates across the ethnosciences related to medicinal plants, especially regarding their use, articulating it with those belonging to the identities and cultural imagery of the focused human groups. Ethnopharmaceutical science seeks to understand the use of medicinal plants through the social representations of communities based on the oral diffusion of knowledge about the community's relationship with the environment, availability of medicinal plants, as these representations are keys to the establishment of the safety validation process and rational use of medicinal plants

Thus, we propose two strands to the ethnopharmaceutical methodology: as a science (where there is an object, methodology and production of knowledge) and as a social technology where it develops products, methods and services together with communities, replicable in other communities, aimed in improving their life quality and favoring their social inclusion.

To illustrate the proposal presented above, we show the figure 2 below that tries to characterize the composition and the insertion of Ethnopharmacy in the science and technology fields and thereby demonstrate the breadth and scope of its instruments when applied in Popular Phytotherapy survey, with the aim of pointing out plant species for phytomedicine development and their use in primary health care.

The ethnopharmaceutical survey is an instrument of the quantitative research advocated by the social technology Ethnopharmacy, which brings together a methodology and a theoretical basis to leverage the popular herbal medicine as a basis for Pharmaceutical Attention in medicinal plants, after processing of the collected data by the Pharmaceutical Science.

The contribution of accessed human groups is significant, as well as the participation of the academy and the public sector; the participation of the private productive sector is still lacking, which, in Brazil, needs to adequate its action and thought to the national sanitary surveillance rules in order to contribute in building this important economic and social sector that is the market for herbal medicines.

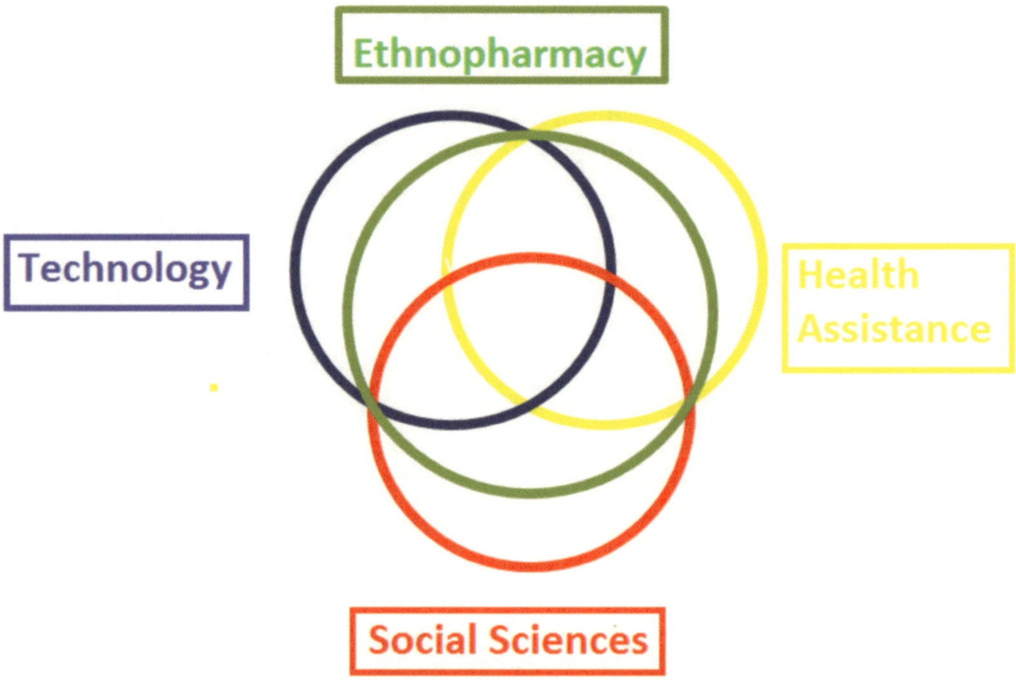

Fig. 2. Representative diagram of the interdisciplinarity of Ethnopharmacy.

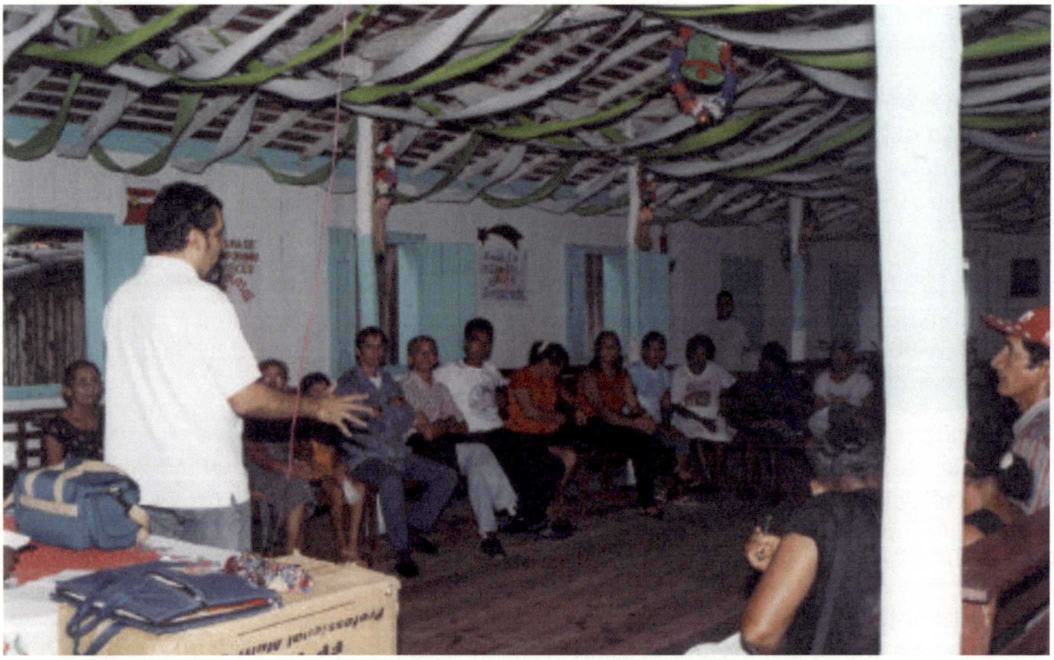

Fig. 3. Meeting of researchers in Ethnopharmacy of Para Federal University with members of local collectivities, including traditional specialists, discussing the local phytotherapy (Igarapé Miri, Para, BR)

2.4.1 The ethnopharmaceutical approach and the use of flora

Different methodologies have taken into account the human and cultural component in their survey and approach of plant species with therapeutical popular use. The ethnobotany and ethnopharmacology dispute the antiquity: there are still ethnomedicine, the ethnobiology and there are others emerging.

In the development of herbal medicine, ethnobotany and ethnopharmacology play an important role towards this approach when aiming the popular information retrieval, the empirical knowledge which has been transmitted from generation to generation by shamans and healers in all cultures and traditions. The ethno-oriented survey puts the popular information as an important reference for the experiments both with regards to the exploitation and use of herbal drugs and phytomedicines, as well as for the development of new remedies.

Following this track, the instrumentation of methods and techniques has been established in the pursuit of a unique language that features not only recognition but also the application of traditional knowledge about plants and/or healing practices. One should also take into account the idea that the notion of illness and healing practices are understood through cultural references. In this context it is assumed that there are subjective factors related to the values and traditions of individuals and cultures that influence the formation of symptoms and how to treat them. This is therefore, the track that leads to the concept of the ethnopharmaceutical approach, demarcated on its roles and joints to other research areas by the objectives (BARBOSA, 1996):

- To understand the cultural meaning of a given disease and its healing process in a given community;
- To raise the traditional use of plant species in these communities while observing the social anthropological view, the inter-relationship of possible medicinal effects, their use in food and involved ritual habits as therapeutic tools for treatment of diseases;
- To recognize the plant species used, their botanical and popular nomenclature;
- To recognize in the traditional remedy the pharmaceutical form involved in its preparation;
- To prepare, in an interdisciplinary way, a method to exploit the species involving from cultivation to marketing;
- To propose, based on the plant investigation, from the scientific point of view, new applications for the species, either through pharmacological, biological and/or suitable technological approaches in the Pharmaceutical Sciences field;
- To standardize the pharmacognostic, phytochemical and pharmacotechnical protocols for regulation and quality control in the marketing and use of herbal medicine, among others;
- To produce knowledge from the results obtained during the development and use of the investigated medicinal plant.

The cultural elements of the community, related to fundamental traditional healing practices regarding the use of plant species, have been undergoing a process of devaluation, even discredit, due to the scrapping of medical care, caused by political and economic reasons. Moreover, the easy access to the allopathic medicine, encouraged by official policies of distribution of these drugs without proper pharmaceutical care, has led, even in communities with ancient traditions, such as indigenous peoples, a depreciation of the traditional healing practices, so that the only alternative that remains to the ordinary member of the community is to ingest the industrial drug according to color or flavor, with the (dis) orientation of hardworking, but unprepared people for this important task.

In this context, briefly exposed, because it is matter for reflection in a specific chapter, the ethnopharmaceutical approach comes as an element of preservation and appreciation of traditional therapeutic practices, since all the experimental work is based on valuable information gathered from the plant user. This information is firstly systematized and documented, making it possible to provide a memory of the practices and the empirical knowledge of people about the plants used therapeutically.

The empirical statements, allegations of a plant use, refer to symptoms that correspond to a pharmacological test model, which can validate the indication of the preparation traditionally used obtained according to pharmaceutical techniques properly deduced from the popular mode of preparation. These data, together with those obtained from the chemical analysis of the plant, will enable to propose a defined therapeutic formulation containing a biologically active extract or an active fraction of this extract, ingredient that may be monitored for quality because it was chemically analyzed and presents the original activity properly quantified (effective dose and "toxic" or lethal dose) indicated by the community.

Among the information collected from communities, one should consider and seek to interpret the apparently unimportant data related to the symptoms described, to the collection of plant material, to the preparation of the medicine and to the usage of this drug. These data may be critical to the success of the experimental work. Details concerning these apparently mystical aspects of the plant use may indicate some procedures to be followed when preparing the material for testing and analysis, so it should not be seen merely as superstition.

2.4.2 Data produced from selected species according to the ethnopharmaceutical method

An ethnopharmaceutical survey conducted in 2008 in the State of Pará, Amazonia, Brazil showed that an Iridaceae (*marupazinho*) was indicated to treat diarrhoea, anaemia and abdominal pain.

Alleged use	Medicinal Plant	RAUPF
Anaemia	*Pariri*	100%
Verminoses	*Caxinguba*	100%
Flu	*Lemon*	88%
Diarrhoea	*Marupazinho*	79%
Rheumatisms	*Ginger*	75%
Headache	*Rue*	70%
High blood pressure	*Garlic*	67%
Gastritis	*Pirarucu*	50%
Fever	*Catinga de Mulata*	42%

Source: from Pinto, 2008, (yet unpublished data).

Table 1. The alleged medicinal uses of plants according to the relative frequency of alleged use (RFAU) calculated according to Amorozo & Gely (1988).

Combining these symptoms and adding information obtained from a traditional specialist we can infer that this plant could be used to treat amoebiasis (yet unpublished data). Indeed, in the Amazon region this plant is an important therapeutic option, used in primary health care. Jardim et al (2007) had demonstrated the use of a tea from the bulbs of this plant in the popular phytotherapy, to treat diarrhoea. The here mentioned ethnopharmaceutical survey discloses a convergence of popular use (AMOROSO; GELY, 1988) of about 80% for diarrhoea (Table 2), which rises to about 100% when other symptoms of amoebiasis are associated. These surveys were carried out in different cities of the state of Pará. Additional phytochemical and galenic studies were performed and a formulation will soon be developed; furthermore, the data already obtained can indicate the plant to be accepted as a medicinal plant of interest to the Brazilian primary health care system (BRASIL, 2010).

An ethnopharmaceutical approach started a multidisciplinary study on a Piperaceae and an Euphorbiaceae and enabled the development of formulations to control arterial hypertension and to treat bacterial skin affections, whose patenting processes are in course.

A Bignoniaceae mentioned by virtually all respondents, more than 1,200 people (Table 1), as having anti-anaemic activity, also shows important antifungal activity on skin affections (BARBOSA, 2008) among others. After the extract administration in animals, the haematological parameters were evaluated in their collected blood samples. The extract did not affect the following parameters: leukocytes, red blood cells, haematocrit, haemoglobin, MCV, MCH and MCHC, however, a significant increase in platelet counts for the experimental group could be observed, what can indicate that the aqueous extract stimulates the production of platelets (yet unpublished data) (Table 2).

Haematimetric Index	*Control group n=20*	*Experimental group n=20*	*P* value*
Haemocyte (/mm^3)	5.7±1.6	6.2±0.9	0.6423
Haematocrit (%)	41.3±9.2	41.5±3.7	0.4525
Haemoglobin (g/dL)	13.8±2.7	13.7±1.1	0.4275
MCV (fL)	50.2±2.7	51.6±1.9	0.1555
MCH (pgL)	16.5±0.7	16.9±0.7	0.2164
MCHC (g/dL)	33.1±1.2	33.09±1.6	0.9427
Platelets (mm^3)	702±244	888±201	0.0498

Table 2. Haematimetric indices and platelet counts of animals exposed to plant extract and the control group. Hematologic parameters of control group are similar to other studies in which the same strain of mice was used, and corroborate the study by Pessoa et al. (2008) that observed the lack of significance between hematological parameters of *Rattus norvegicus* treated with plant extract.

The approximation of ethnopharmacy with pharmaceutical care provided the establishment of a new attribution to the ethnopharmaceutical method, namely: the selection of popular medicinal herbs for introduction in primary health care. *Eleuthrine plicata* (BRAZIL, 2009), *Arrabidea chica* (BRAZIL, 2011) and *Zingiber officinalis* (BRAZIL, 2010B), are species listed in official documents that have been related in ethnopharmaceutical surveys conducted in different localities in the Amazonian state of Pará.

3. Comparison between the randomized and ethnoguided approach

It is expected that the traditional knowledge about medicinal plants indicates the presence of biologically active substances. The collection of plants traditionally used for biological assessment can be a great advantage, or a shortcut, increasing the chances of discovering new drugs (ELIZABETSKY & SHANLEY, 1994). Table 3 shows the enormous potential of the ethnopharmacological approach found in several studies, compared with the randomized approach.

Some studies have compared the results obtained by the random selection of plants with the ethnopharmacological approach, also called ethnoguided approach. In Rwanda, Africa, 100 medicinal plants were tested for antimicrobial activity. From these, 68 were referred for infectious diseases, 37% of which were active, whereas for the 36 medicinal plants that were included by the random approach only 22% showed activity (VAN PUYVELDE & BOILY, 1986). In another study conducted at Sinai (Egypt) for plants with antimicrobial activity, 83.3% of the species obtained positive results by the ethnoguided approach against 41.7% in the randomized approach (KHAFAGI & DEWED, 2000). In Brazil, a study of antimalarial activity performed with extracts from 295 plant species, 273 were tested by a randomized approach with only 0.7% of positive results, whereas for the 22 medicinal plants with indications for fever and malaria the positive results represented a total of 18% (CARVALHO & KRETTLI, 1991). In Belize, Central America, random collections of plants sent to the National Cancer Institute (NCI, USA) for anti-HIV activity resulted in 6% of active samples. However, with ethnopharmacologically selected samples, from a healer in a small village in Belize, an activity of 25% was obtained, showing a percentage four times higher (GUIRA & CUELLAR, 2008).

BIOLOGICAL ACTIVITIES	RANDOM (%)	ETHNO (%)
Antineoplasic	6	25
Antihypertensive	31	44
Anthelmintica	9.8	29.3
Ichthyotoxicity	9.6	38.6
Toxic/venoms	10.5	52.2
Anti-HIV	8.5	71.4
Antimicrobial	22	37
Antiplasmodial	0.7	18
Acetylcholinesterase inhibition	8	42.3

Source: from Oliveira et al.

Table 3. Comparison between the numbers of hits achieved by Ethnopharmacological x Random approaches in the search for different biological activities (OLIVEIRA *et al.* 2011).

Slish and colleagues (1999), when evaluating plant extracts obtained by the ethnoguided method (n = 31) for the relaxation effect in rat aortic smooth muscle, had a score of 12.9% active species, whereas by the random approach (n =32) no active species were observed. In an assessment with 80 traditional medicine plants from Reunion Islands for angiotensin-converting enzyme inhibitory activity, which plays an important role in blood pressure regulation and diuresis, 44% of the species indicated by their antihypertensive or diuretic effect were active against 31% of the species without such indications (ADSERSEN & ADSERSEN, 1997).

The selection of plants for use in primary health care should be based on the nosology of the region, referred to in the Brazilian Policy for Phytomedicine and Medicinal Plants (BRAZIL, 2006), which is determined by an interview survey conducted among local experts in the communities . The nosological map obtained, defines the range of plants that are then selected according to technical criteria, considering their agronomic and pharmaceutical aspects. The list of the plants used to treat diseases that compose the nosological profile emerges from the treatment of the information provided by the respondents, applying the programming rule of the Pharmaceutical Assistance (BARBOSA, 2008).

4. Possible innovations in phytomedicine development from the ethnoguided surveys

The development of herbal medicines, as they need to generate specific parameters for each formulation, is more productive in terms of knowledge than in terms of the synthetic analogue, once the constitution of each species that gives rise to herbal medicines varies from one species to another. Compatibility studies of adjuvant in relation to the components of plant extracts, the need to characterize quality markers, pharmacologically active or not, all this set induces a creative process marked by strong innovative character. Some topics are presented below:

- Regulation of pre-products and insumes; in the legal-administrative sphere, the phytomedicines bring and impose the need to develop regulatory frameworks that do not exist in many countries.
- Documentation of traditional knowledge in the form of a regionalized National Plant Pharmacopoeia; in continental countries like Brazil, or which have microclimates with different biomes, this is a remarkable feature, and the existence of national human groups with appropriate cultural heritage, possessing their own herbal knowledge also influences.
- Development of products to attend the national nosology; as a result of the ethno-oriented surveys which, besides the list of plants can generate a regionalized nosological profile; this profile guides the development of therapeutical formulations to treat local diseases, often neglected by large laboratories .
- Using the production of medicinal plants to recover degraded areas; to meet the national and local demands for plant material both for herbal medicines production as for use in primary health care, it is necessary to cultivate selected species, which can be intercropped and would not make sense to grow them in forested areas, but in areas that could be recovered.
- Involving the communities in the production projects; since it is an ethno-oriented process, it involves communities *per se*; in the case of Ethnopharmacy, a social technology, the involvement of organized human groups is higher and can trigger initiatives.

- Applying new methods for development; the partnership of the academy in the development of phytomedicines, required due to the low participation of the pharmaceutical productive sector in this process, induces the application of modern techniques, as the academy, apart from contributing to the process still needs to produce knowledge in accordance to the regulatory sector.

5. Medicinal plants in the basic health care from ethnoguided approach

In Brazil the traditional use of medicinal plants was recognized by the public health administration and was integrated into the official health system through the National Policy of Complementary and Integrative Practices (BRASIL, 2006b).

To support this therapeutical option available to the general population that uses the Integrated Brazilian Health System (SUS), regulatory documents were elaborated and promulgated which present a list of medicinal plant species of popular or traditional use, selected on basis of a set of information that indicates and supports the alleged use of these plants, its form of use and the cares to be taken in the preparation and the administration of the therapeutical product.

The information that substantiates the inclusion of a given medicinal plant species into the primary health care is carefully conferred in the scientific literature. Data on botanical, agronomical, pharmacognostic and chemical characteristics are checked for the unequivocal description of the plant material to be considered as a potential source for an officialised phytotherapeutical. Results concerning the effectiveness and security of the herbal drug or its derivatives as well as information about toxicological, pre-clinical and clinical investigation of the plant species, herbal drug or preparations obtained from them, complete the set of data. So, in this way, medicinal plant species are inserted into the list of phytotherapeutical for use in the basic health attention. Nowadays vegetal species and derivatives species are available as therapeutic resource in the basic pharmaceutical assistance program.

Since information about a given medicinal plant species is still to be produced, the plant is inserted in the national Relation of Medicinal Plants of Interest for the Integrated Brazilian Health System (RENISUS), where the medicinal plants species that present good potential to generate products of interest to the SUS, or plant species that can be incorporated into the Live Pharmacies (an official program of medicinal herbal gardens cultivated in units of basic health assistance) or generate phytotherapeutical (teas, tinctures, pomades or other simple pharmaceutical forms) are inserted.

The purpose of this list is to guide studies and research that can support the elaboration of a relation of available phytotherapeuticals for safe and effective use by the population, to treat some mild illnesses. Currently, "espinheira santa"and "guaco"phytotherapeutic derivatives are offered, respectively, for gastritis and ulcer, and for cough and influenza (BRAZIL, 2009).

In RENISUS there are 71 medicinal plant species with therapeutical potential to induce the development of research projects and to motivate organization of productive arrangements; which are disclosed by the National Programme of Medicinal Plants and Phytomedicines of the Health Ministry. Amongst these medicinal plant species *Cynara scolymus* (artichoke), *Schinus terebenthifolius* (aroeira da praia) and *Uncaria tomentosa* (cats claw) can be found, which are used, according to the popular knowledge, to treat digestive disorder, vaginal inflammation and articulation pains, respectively, and whose indications are scientifically confirmed (BRAZIL, 2009).

6. References

Adeodato, S., Oliveira, L., Oliveira, V. 1996. Uma farmácia no fundo do quintal. Globo Ciência, 6(64): 44-49.

Adsersen A, Adsersen H 1997. Plants from Réunion Island with alleged antihypertensive and diuretic effects -an experimental and ethnobotanical evaluation. *J Ethnopharmacol 58*: 189-206.

Albuquerque NP, Hanazaki N. 2006. As pesquisas etnodirigidas na descoberta de novos fármacos de interesse médico e farmacêutico: fragilidades e perspectivas. Brazilian Journal of Pharmacognosy, 16 (Supl.): 678-689.

Amorozo MCM, Gely A. 1988. Uso de plantas medicinais por caboclos do Baixo Amazonas, Barcarena, Pará, Brasil. Belém, PA: Boletim do Museu Paraense Emílio Goeldi. Série Botânica. 4: 1, 47-131.

Barbosa WLR (Org.), 2008. Etnofarmácia: Fitoterapia Popular e Ciência Farmacêutica, UFPA, 150pp.

Barbosa WLR, 1998. Aproveitamento Farmacêutico da Flora Como Instrumento de Preservação Cultural e Ambiental. Poematropic. , 01, 43 - 45.

Barbosa WLR, Silva WB, Soler O. 1996. Etnofarmacêutica: uma abordagem em plantas medicinais pela perspectiva das Ciências Farmacêuticas. Rev. Bras. Farm. 77, 82 - 84.

Barbosa, WLR *et al.* 2008. *Arrabidaea chica* (HBK) Verlot: phytochemical approach, antifungal and trypanocidal activities. Rev. Bras. Farmacogn., 18, 4, 544-548.

Barbosa, WLR, Pinto, LN (2005) Semeando saúde - Uma proposta de orientação para o uso adequado de plantas medicinais nas comunidades do entorno da Universidade Federal do Pará, Belém-PA. V Simpósio Brasileiro de Farmacognosia, Recife-PE.

Basso LA, *et al.* 2005. The use of biodiversity as source of new chemical entities against defined molecular targets for treatment of malaria, tuberculosis, and T-cell mediated diseases. Mem Inst Oswaldo Cruz, 100 (6).

Benson, H. 1980. Medicina Humanista (the mid body effect). São Paulo: Editora Brasiliense.

Berry JP, *et al.* 2007. Approaches towards the preclinical testing and standardization of medicinal. Foundation for Medical Research 106-122.

Boily Y, Van Puyvelde L, 1986. Screening of medicinal plants of Rwanda (Central Africa) for antimicrobial activity. J Ethnopharmacol 16: 1-13.

Bourdy G, *et al.* 2008. Ethnopharmacology and malaria: New hypothetical leads or old efficient antimalarials? *Int. J. Parasitol.* 30:1, 33-41.

Brasil, 2006. Ministério da Saúde. Decreto nº 5813 de 22 de junho de 2006. Aprova a Política Nacional de Plantas Medicinais e Fitoterápicos. Diário Oficial da República Federativa do Brasil. Brasília, DF, 23 jun. 2006. N. 119, SeçãoI.

Brasil, 2006b. Ministério da Saúde. Portaria nº 971 de 3 de maio de 2006. Aprova a Política Nacional de Práticas Integrativas e Complementares. Diário Oficial da República Federativa do Brasil. Brasília, DF, 04 maio 2006.

Brasil, 2009. RENISUS - Relação Nacional de Plantas Medicinais de Interesse ao SUS; DAF/SCTIE/MS - RENISUS; Ministério da Saúde. Brasília, DF. Available at:

http://portal.saude.gov.br/portal/arquivos/pdf/RENISUS.pdf.

Brasil, 2010a, Ministry of Health, Sanitary Surveillance Agency (ANVISA), RDC 14/2010.

Brasil, 2010b, Ministry of Health, Sanitary Surveillance Agency (ANVISA), RDC 10/2010.

Brasil, 2010c. Ministry of Health, Sanitary Surveillance Agency (ANVISA), Farmacopeia Brasileira 5th. Edition.

Briskin DP 2000. Medicinal plants and phytomedicines. Linking plant biochemistry and physiology to human health. *Plant Physiology* 124: 507–514.

Bulus, A et al.. 2003. Studies on the use of Cassia singueana in malaria ethnopharmacy. J. Ethnopharmacol.. 88 (2-3):261-267.

Calderón AI, Angerhofer CK, Pezzuto JM 2000. Forest plot as a tool to demonstrate the pharmaceutical potential of plants in a tropical forest of Panama. *Econ Bot*, 54: 278-294.

Carrai V, *et al* 2003. Increase in tannin consumption by sifaka (*Propithecus verreauxi verreauxi*) females during the birth season: a case for self medication in prosimians? *Primates* 44: 61-66.

Coley PD, *et al.* 2003. Using ecological criteria to design plant collection strategies for drug discovery. *Front Ecol Environ* 1, 421–428.

de la Cruz-Mota MG. 1997. Plantas medicinais utilizadas por raizeiros. Uma abordagem etnobotânica no contexto da saúde e da doença. Dissertação de mestrado, Universidade Federal de Mato Grosso, Cuiabá.

dos Santos JR, Fleurentin J. 1990. L'ethnopharmacologie, une approche pluridisciplinaire in Ethnopharmacologie : sources, méthodes, objectifs. Actes Du 1er Colloque Européen d'Ethnoparcologie, Metz, 22-25 mai. Ed. ORSTOM, pp 26-39.

Elisabetsky, E. 2003. Etnofarmacologia, São Paulo: Ciência e Cultura. 55: 3, 35-36.

Elizabetsky E, Shanley P. 1994. Ethnopharmacology in the Brasilian Amazon. Pharmacology and Therapeutics, 64, p.201-214.

Elizabetsky, E. 1987.Pesquisa em plantas medicinais. *Cien. Cult.*, v.39, p.697-702.

Giday M. 2001. An etnhobotanical study of medicinal plants used by de Zay people in Ethiopia. CBM:s Skriftserie 3: 81-99.

Gottlieb, OR., Micromolecular Evolution, Systematics and Ecology. An Essay into a Novel Botanical Discipline, Springer-Verlag: Heidelberg, 1982; p 170.

Guirado OAA, Cuéllar AC. 2008. Strategies for the selection of medicinal plants to be studied. Revista Cubana de Plantas Medicinales, 13 (3).

Heinrich M, Bremner P. 2006. Ethnobotany and Ethnopharmacy - Their Role for Anti-Cancer Drug Development. Current Drug Targets, 7: 239-245.

Heinrich M. 2001. Ethnopharmazie und Ethnobotanik. Eine Einf¨uhrung. Stuttgart Germany.: Wissenschaftliche Verlagsgesellschaft.

Heinrich, M. 2007. Ethnopharmacy and natural product research - Multidisciplinary opportunities for research in the metabolomic age. Phytochemistry Letters,. 1, 1-5.

Ignacimuthu S, Ayyanar M, Sankara Sivaraman K. 2006. Ethnobotanical investigations among tribes in Madurai District of Tamil Nadu (India). Journal of Ethnobiology and Ethnomedicine 2:25.

Jardim, MAG; Ferreira, MR; Leão, RBA, 2007. Levantamento de plantas de uso terapêutico no município de Santa Bárbara do Pará, estado do Pará, Brasil. Rev. Bras. Farm., 88:1, 21-25.

Khafagi I, Dewedar A, 2000. The efficiency of random versus ethno-directed research in the evaluation of Sinai medicinal plants for bioactive compounds. J. Ethnopharmacol. 71:3, 365-376.

Krief S, *et al.* 2004. Novel antimalarial compounds isolated in a survey of self-medicative behavior of wild chimpanzees in Uganda. *Antimicrob Agents Ch* 48: 3196-3199.

Lorenzi, H., e Matos, F. J. A. 2002. Plantas medicinais no Brasil: nativas e exóticas. Nova Odessa. Instituto Plantarum. 512p.

Maciel MAM, *et al.*. 2002. Plantas medicinais: a necessidade de estudos multidisciplinares. Quimica Nova, 25 (3): 429-438.

Marston A, Kissling J, Hostettmann K, 2002. A rapid TLC bioautographic method for the detection of acetylcholinesterase and butyrylcholinesterase inhibitors in plants. *Phytochem. Anal.*, 13:1, 51-54.

Martin GJ. 1986. El papel de la etnobotânica en el resgate ecológico y cultural de America Latina. Congresso Latino Americano de Botánica. 40 Simpósio de Etnobotânica. Medelin. 67-77.

Matos FJA. 2000. Plantas Medicinais: Guia de seleção e emprego de plantas usadas em fitoterapia no nordeste do Brasil. 2ª Ed. Fortaleza: Imprensa Universitaria/UFC,. 232p.

Maués, RH; Villacorta, GM (Org.) 2008. Pajelanças e religiões na Amazônia. Belém:EDUFPA.

Nunes, G.P., *et al.* 2003. Plantas medicinais comercializadas por raizeiros no Centro de Campo Grande, Mato Grosso do Sul. Revista. Brasileira de Farmacognosia, 13(2).

Oliveira DR, *et al.* 2011. Ethnopharmacological versus random plant selection methods for the evaluation of the antimycobacterial activity. Rev. Bras. Farmacogn. ahead of print Epub May 20, 2011.

Oliveira DR, *et al.* 2010. Authorization of the traditional knowledge associated access for bioprospecting purposes: The case of UFRJ and the Association of the Oriximiná Quilombola Communities - ARQMO. *Rev Fitos 5*: 59-76.

Organização Mundial de Saúde. International Conference on Primary Health Care, Alma-Ata, USSR, 1978. Disponível em: <http://www.who.int/hpr/NPH/docs/ declaration_almaata.pdf>. Acesso em: 08 novembro 2009.

Pessoa DLR, *et al.* 2008. Avaliação pré-clínica dos parâmetros hematológicos após tratamento agudo com *Arrabidaea chica* Verlot (Pariri) em Rattus norvegícus. I oficina FNEPAS do Estado do Maranhão, I amostra maranhense de experiências multidisciplinares de integração ensino-serviço-comunidade nos cursos de graduação da área de saúde. Universidade Federal do Maranhão. São Luiz, Brasil.

Pieroni A, Giusti ME. 2009. Alpine ethnobotany in Italy: traditional knowledge of gastronomic and medicinal plants among the Occitans of the upper Varaita valley, Piedmont. Journal of Ethnobiology and Ethnomedicine 5:32.

Pieroni A, *et al.* 2002. Ethnopharmacy of the ethnic Albanians (Arbëreshë) of northern Basilicata, Italy. Fitoterapia, 73: 217-241.

Pieroni, A. *et al.* 2005. Traditional phytotherapy of the Albanians of Lepushe, Northern Albanian Alps. Italy: Fitoterapia.. 76 (3-4), 379-399.

Pinto LN, 2008. Plantas medicinais utilizadas em comunidades do município de Igarapé Mirí, PA - Etnofarmácia do município de Igarapé Mirí, PA. Dissertação (Ciências Farmacêuticas) - Universidade Federal do Pará.

Pinto, A.A.C e Maduro, C.B. Produtos e subprodutos da medicina popular comercializados na cidade de Boa Vista, Roraima. Acta Amazônica, 2003, 33(2), 281-290.

Ronsted N, *et al.* 2008. Phylogenetic selection of Narcissus species for drug discovery. *Biochem. System. Ecol.* 36, 417-422.

Schultes RE. 1962. The role of the ethnobotanist in the search for new medicinal plants. Lloydia, 25: 4, 257-266.

Sousa AJA, 2009. Etnofarmácia de Benevides-PA: Uma oficina para produção e dispensação de fitoterápicos. Dissertação (Gestão de Recursos Naturais e Desenvolvimento Local) - Universidade Federal do Pará.

Souza Brito ARM, Souza Brito AA. (1996). Medicinal plant research in Brazil: Data from regional and national meetings. In: *Medicinal Resources of the Tropical Forest - Biodiversity and its importance to human health* (Cap. 28, 386-401). Ed. by M.J. Balick, E. Elisabetsky and S.A. Laird. Columbia University Press, 440pp.

Thabrew, M. I et al. 1991. Immunomodulatory activity of three Sri-Lankan medicinal plants used in hepatic disorders. J. Ethnopharmacol. 33:1-2, 63-6.

Ubom RM. 2010. Ethnobotany and biodiversity conservation in the Niger Delta, Nigeria. Internetional Journal of Botany, 6 (3): 310-322.

Toledo, ACO, *et al.* 2003. Fitoterápicos: uma abordagem farmacotécnica. Revista Lecta, 21(1/2):7-13.

2

Hepatoprotective Effect of *Zanthoxylum armatum* DC

Nitin Verma[1] and Rattan Lal Khosa[2]
[1]*Institute of Pharmacy and Emerging Science (IPES), Baddi University of Emerging Science and Technology, Makhunmajara, Baddi,*
[2]*School of Pharmacy, BIT, Meerut, U.P., India*

1. Introduction

The liver is the prime organ concerned with various states of metabolic and physiologic homeostasis of organism and is a key organ of metabolism and excretion playing an important role in the maintenance of internal environment of the body through its multiple and diverse functions. It is continuously exposed to a variety of xenobiotics and therapeutic agents exposing the organ to numerous and varied disorders. There is a progressive increase in the incidence of hepatic damage mainly due to the viral infection, hepatotoxic chemicals (alcohol), toxin in food (especially aflotoxins), peroxides (particularly peroxidized edible oil), pharmaceuticals (antibiotics, chemotherapeutics, and CNS active agents), environment pollutants and xenobiotics *(Hikino et al 1988).*

Though liver disease are among the most important disease affecting mankind , no remedy is available at present in the modern system of medicine which include corticosteroids and immunosuppressive agents which bring about symptomatic relief supporting only the process of healing of liver regeneration and in most cases have no influence on the disease process. Further, their use is associated with the risk of relapses and danger of side effects. An actual curative therapeutic agent has not yet been found and thus management of liver disease is still a challenge to the modern scientific community. Hence increasing attention is being given to plants recommended for the treatment of hepatic disorders in traditional system of medicine. A number of medicinal preparations have been advocated especially in Ayurvedic system of Indian medicine, for the treatment of liver disorders. Their usage is in vogue since centuries and are quite often claimed to offer significant relief. In addition, the use of many folklore remedies mainly plant products are also common throughout India.

About 600 commercial preparations with claimed liver protecting activity are available all over the globe. In India about 33 patent herbal formulations are available for liver ailments and these preparations are a variety of combinations out of 100 Indian medicinal plants belonging to about 40 families *(Handa et al 1986).* Only a few scientific data with regard to their hepatoprotective action are on record. Phytoconstituents remains to be a major contributor in the treatment of liver disorders. The growing concern for the identification of novel hepatoprotective agents from natural sources is evident from literature available on the same.

1.1 Free radicals in hepatic disease

The role of free radicals in the hepatic disorder is being suggested because of the fact that the detoxification of xenobiotics and toxic substances, an important function of liver, leads to the generation of large amounts of reactive oxygen intermediates. Though liver is one of the organs best supplied with antioxidant, chronic exposure to such substances overpowers the antioxidant defense system and cause hepatic damage. The role of lipid peroxidation (LPO) induced damage in the pathogenesis of chronic liver disease based on enzymatic studies (lysosomal enzyme in the serum), has been suggested. Pathological free radical reactions probably play a role in the hepatotoxicity of halothane, hydrazine, acetaminophen, carbon disulphide and α-methyl dopa. Free radical reactions participate secondarily in the development of organ damage in Wilson's disease, haemochromatosis and secondary haemosiderosis. The majority of drugs used in the treatment of liver diseases are antioxidants (Vitamin E, lipoic acid, methionine etc.) *(Feher, et al 1986)* .The injurious roles played by the free radicals have brought in to use the antioxidants obtained from the plants for alleviating the severity of liver disorders *(Meyer, et al 1990)*. Some plants which exhibit hepatoprotective and antioxidant activities are give belows:

Silymarin (Silybum marianum) *(Romellini, et al 1976)*; schizandrins wuweizischun (Schizandra chinensis) *(Handa, et al 1986)*; Saikosaponin (Bupleurum falcatum) *(Hikino, et al 1988)*; glycyrrhizin , glycyrrhetic acid (Glycyrrhiza glabra) *(Handa, et al 1986)*; catechin (Uncaria gambir)*(Handa, et al 1986, Galvez, et al 1995 & Ubeda et al 1995)*; epicatechin (Acacia catechin) *(Handa, et al 1986)*; andrographolide, andrographoside, neoandrographolides (Andrographis panicles) *(Handa, et al 1986 & Kaul, et al 1994)*; picroside (Picrorrhiza kurrao) *(Handa, et al 1986)*; acicubin (Plantago asiatica) *(Handa, et al 1986)*; ginsenosides (Panax ginseng) *(Handa, et al 1986)*; piceid and resveratrol (Polygonum cuspidatum) *(Handa, et al 1986)*; arcapallin (Artemisia capillaris) *(Handa, et al 1986)*; Sb-1 (Scutellaria baicabensis); α-tocopherol (embryos of cereals, vegetable oil, fresh vegetables) *(Handa, et al 1986)*; curcuminoid (Curcuma longa)*(Ravishankar, et al 1993)*; oil (Bunium persicum); quercetin , kaempferol naringenin (Helichrysum arenarium) *(Handa, et al 1986)*; kaempferol 3-rhamnoglucoside, quercetin 3- rhamnoglucoside, stepposide (Euphorbia palustris and E. stepposa) *(Handa, et al 1986, Galvez, et al 1995 & Ubeda, et al 1995)*; mixed flavonoids (Mentha arvensis, Stachy neglecta, Colinicum coggyria, Anemone hepatria, Convallaria majalis , Ononis arvensis) *(Handa, et al 1986, Galvez, et al 1995 & Ubeda, et al 1995)*; brevifolin hyperin, ellagic acid (E. nematocypha) *(Handa, et al 1986, Galvez, et al 1995 & Ubeda, et al 1995)*; Costus speciosus *(Verma & Khosa 2009)* and Zanthoxylum armatum *(Verma & Khosa 2010)*.

2. *Zanthoxylum armatum* DC

Synonyms: *Zanthoxylum alatum* Roxb.
Family: Rutaceae

2.1 Common (Indian) name

Hindi - Darmar, nepali dhaniya, tejphal, tumuru
Bengali - Gaira, tambul,
Oriya - Tundopoda
Sanskrit - Tumburu, dhiva, gandhalu

2.2 Distribution

A large genus of aromatic, prickly, dioecious or rarely monoecious tree or shrubs, mainly pantropical, through also distributed in the subtropics. The genus as dealt with in the article includes species of *Fagara,* through some authors treat them as two distinct genera. About 13 species are recorded from India.

Zanthoxylum armatum DC found in the hot valleys of the Himalayas from Jammu to Bhutan at altitudes of 1,000-2100 m and in Eastern Ghats in Orissa and Andhra Pradesh at 1,200 m., in India. It is also sometimes planted for hedges in Assam.

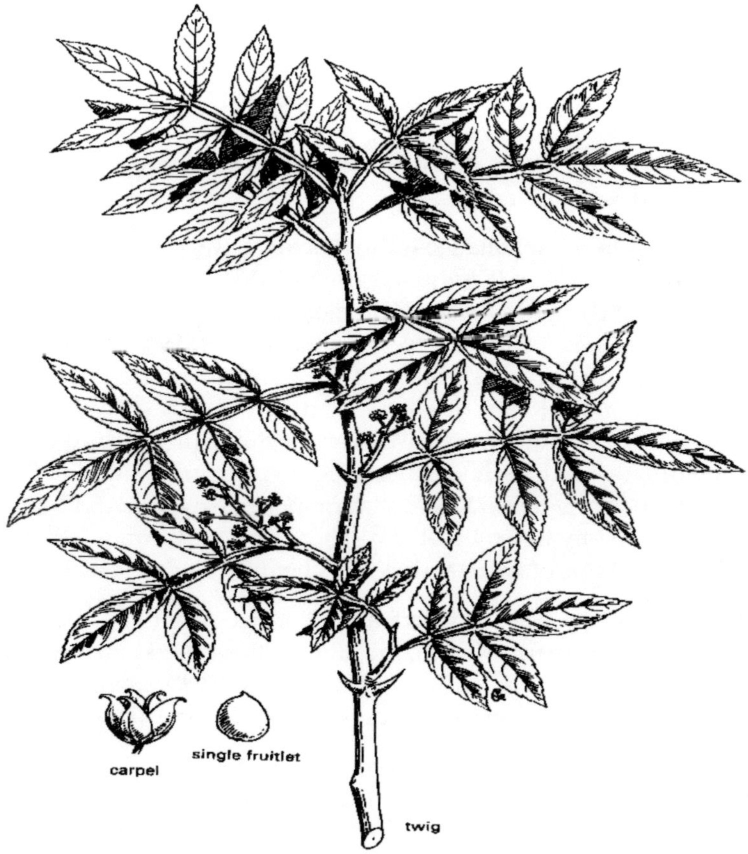

Fig. 1. Zanthoxylum armatum

2.3 Description

Zanthoxylum armatum DC, is an armed scandent or erect shrub or a small tree , 6 m tall or more with dense foliage, branches armed, the prickles flattened, up to 2 cm. long, bark pale brown, deep-furrowed, leaves imparipinnate or trifoliolate, 5-23 cm. long, often with flattened prickles , leaflets up to 5 pairs, opposite, ovate to lanceolate , entire to glandular crenate, acute to obtusely acuminate, flower green or yellow, in dense terminal, and occasionally axillary sparse panicles, follicles generally reddish, sub-globose, glabrous, seeds solitary in a fruit, globose, shining black. *(Kirti & Basu 1975).*

2.4 Phytochemical review

Several alkaloids have been isolated from the stem-bark and root-bark. The fruits of a number of species yielded essential oils. The oils from Z. *acanthopodium,* Z. *armatum,* and Z. *nitidum* are potential source of linalool, an important perfumery material; the first two species are also employed on a limited scale for the production of wartara oil. Z. *americanum* Mill. , a shrub of eastern North America, is used in its native country for toothache and rheumatism.

The stems and roots contain β-amyrin, β- sitosterol, L-asarinin, L-planinin, and zanthobungeanine.

The fruits contain 3.5% oil. The characteristics and constituents of the oil are summarized in Table. The fruit oil contains the rare monoterpine triol, 3, 7-dimethyl-1-octane-3, 6, 7-triol. It contains: limonene **(I)**, linalool **(II)**, methyl cinnamate **(III)**, myrcene and α-thujene **(IV)** as the main constituents. The oil also contains 1, 8-cineol, *p*-cymene **(V)**, cis-ocimene **(VI)**, γ-terpinene, camphor **(VII)**, α-fenchol **(VIII)**, carvone **(IX)**, tagetonol and alloaromadendrene, besides α-terpeniol and β-caryophyllene.

The seeds contains 6-hydroxynonadec-(4Z)-enoic acid ($C_{19}H_{36}O_3$, m. p. 40-42°C) **(X),** 8-hydroxy pentadec-(4Z)-enoic acid ($C_{15}H_{28}O_3$) (viscous) **(XI),** 7-hydroxy-7-vinylhexadec-(4Z)-enoic acid ($C_{18}H_{32}O_3$) **(XII)** and hexadec-(4Z)-enoic acid ($C_{16}H_{30}O_2$, m. p. 49-50°C) **(XIII)** along with *cis*-9-hexadecenoic, eicosenoic, palmitic acid **(XIV),** tambuletin and methyl cinnamate has been reported in seeds *(Ahmad et al 1993).* Further the chemical studies on the seeds of *Zanthoxylum alatum* Roxb. (Rutaceae) led to the isolation of two new phenolic constituents characterized as 3-methoxy-11-hydroxy-6,8-dimethylcarboxylate biphenyl **(XV)** and 3,5,6,7-tetrahydroxy-3',4'-dimethoxyflavone-5-β-d-xylopyranoside **(XVI)** along with the five known compounds, 1-methoxy-1,6,3-anthraquinone, 1-hydroxy-6,13-anthraquinone, 2-hydroxybenzoic acid, 2-hydroxy-4-methoxy benzoic acid, and stigmasta-5-en-3β-d-glucopyranoside, on the basis of spectral data and chemical analyse *(Akhtar et al 2009).*

A number of alkaloids has been isolated and reported from the various parts of the *Zanthoxylum armatum* Dc. berberine (bark), dictamnine (stem-bark), magnofluorine(0.02% as picrate), xanthoplanine (0.01% as picrate) (wood and bark), magnofluorine (0.17% as picrate), xanthoplanine, skimmianine, dictamnine and γ-fagarine *(Wealth of India 2005).*

A new amide designated as armatamide along with two lignans, asarinin and fargesin, α- and β-amyrins, lupeol, and β-sitosterol-β-D-glucoside - has been isolated from the bark of *Zanthoxylum armatum.* The structure of the new compound was deduced by spectral and chemical analysis as N-(4′-methoxyphenyl ethyl)-3, 4-methylenedioxy cinnamoyl amide *(Kalia et al 1999).*

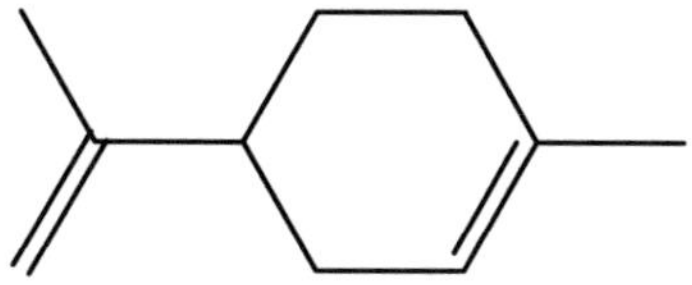

limonene
(I)

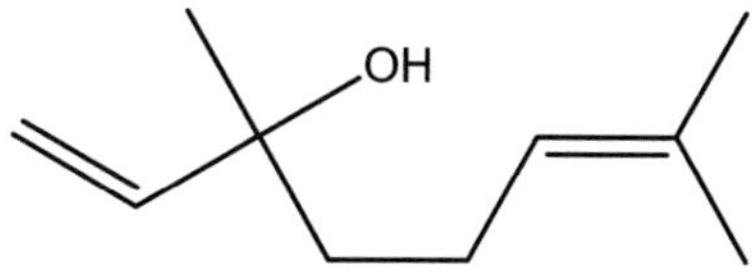

linalool
(II)

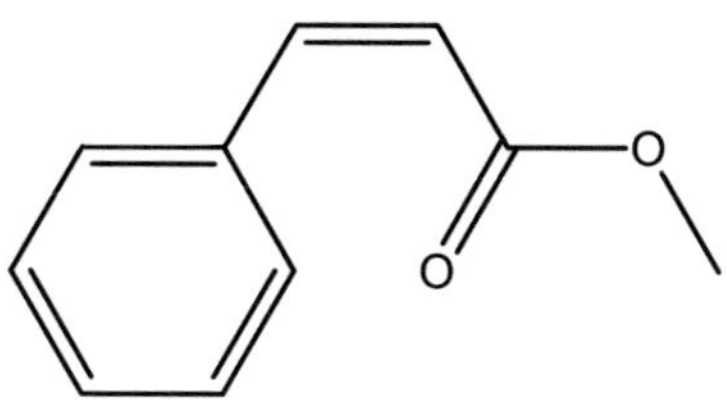

methyl cinnamate
(III)

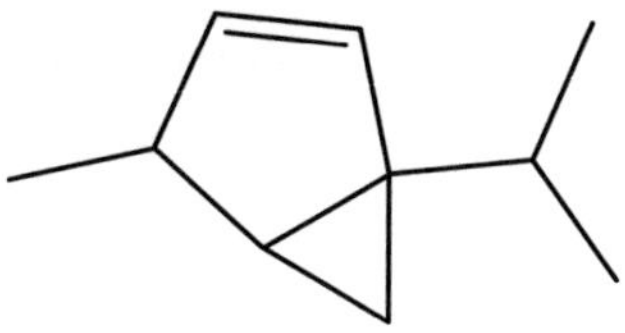

thujene
(IV)

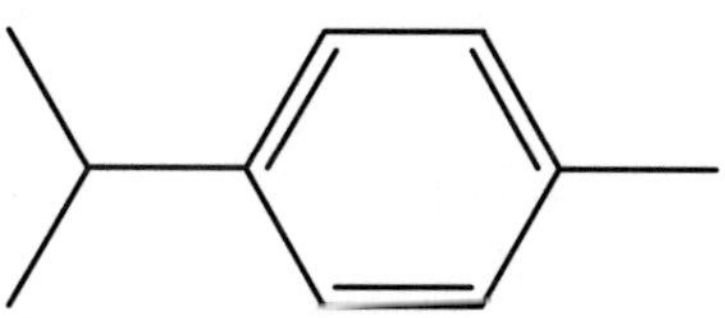

***p*-cymene**
(V)

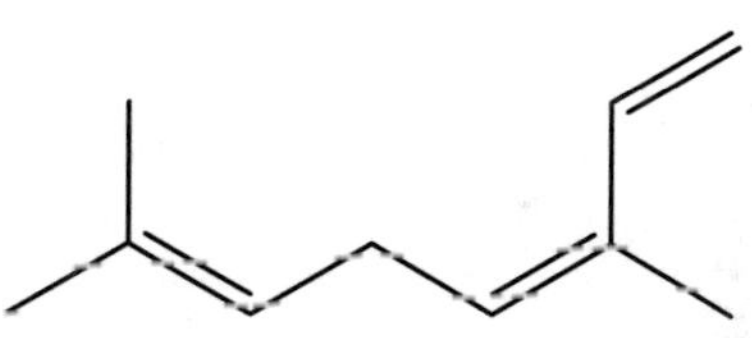

***cis*-ocimene**
(VI)

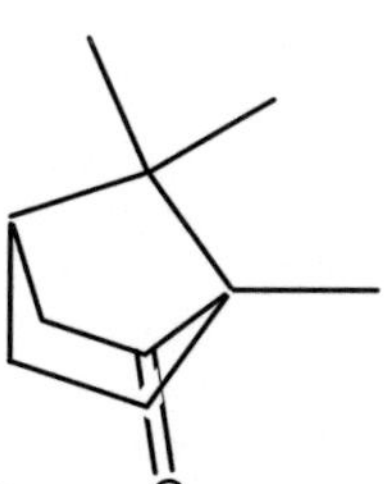

camphor
(VII)

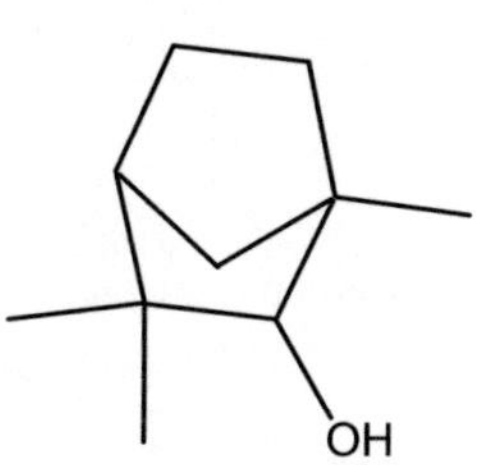

alpha-fenchol
(VIII)

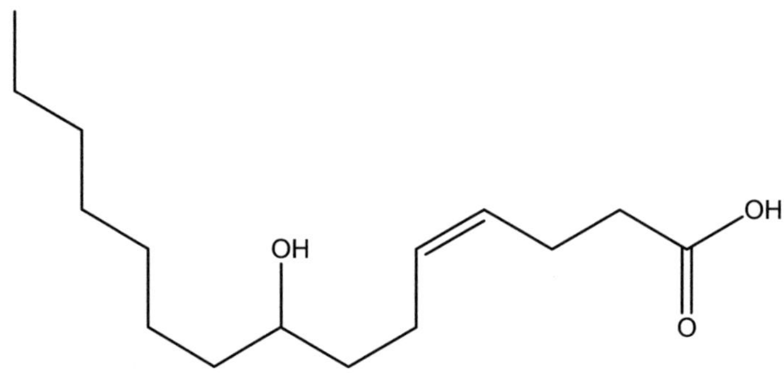

8-hydroxy pentadec-(4Z)-enoic acid (XI)

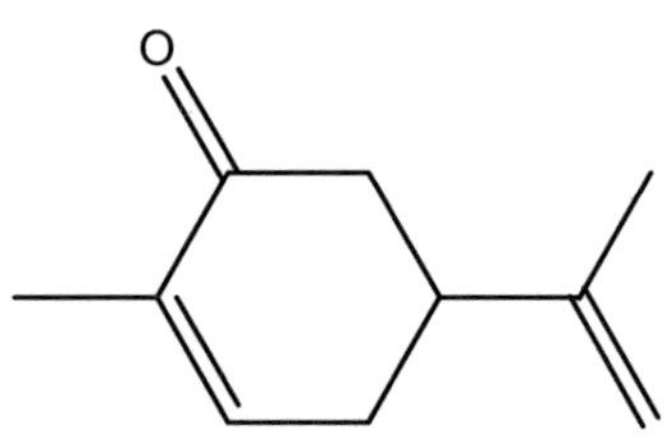

carvone
(IX)

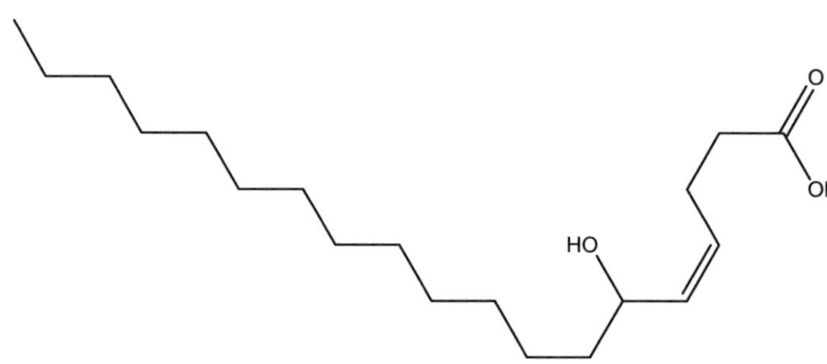

6-hydroxynonadec-(4Z)-enoic acid
(X)

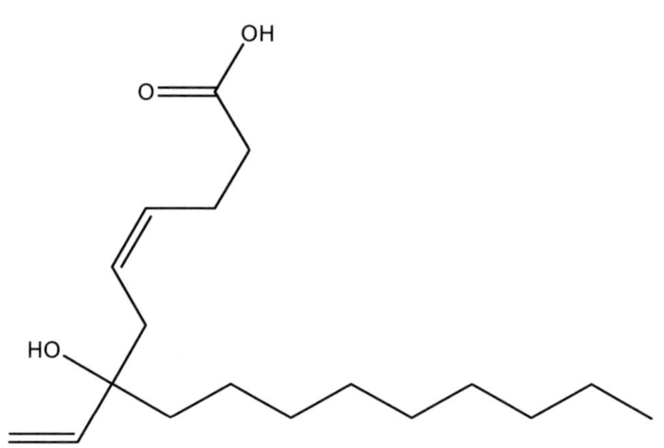

7-hydroxy-7-vinylhexadec-(4Z)-enoic acid
(XII)

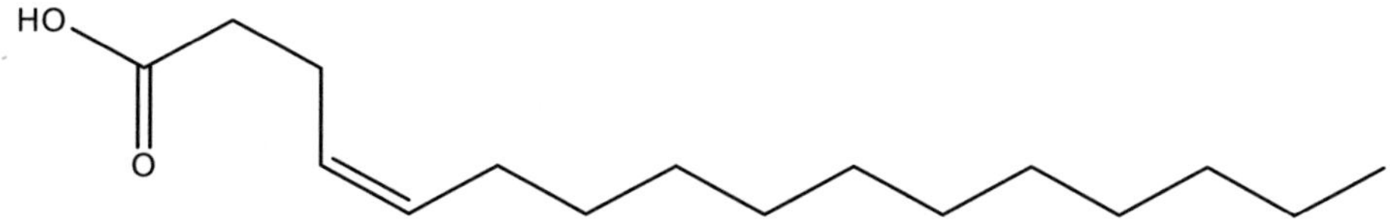

hexadec-(4Z)-enoic acid
(XIII)

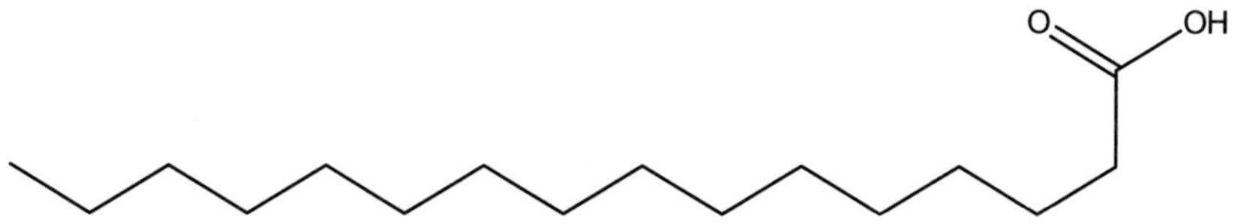

palmitic acid
(XIV)

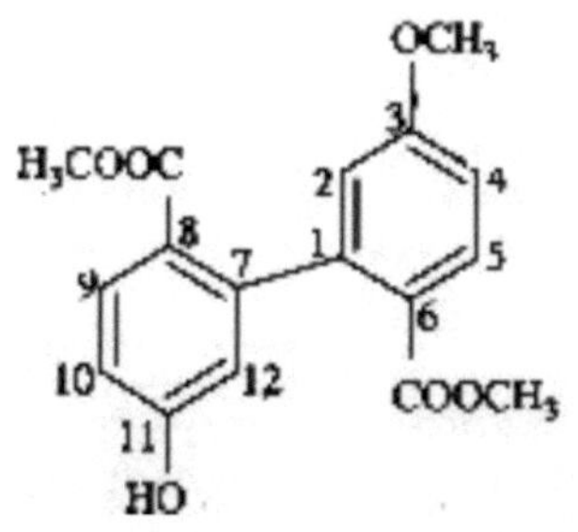

3-methoxy-11-hydroxy-6,8-dimethylcarboxylate biphenyl (XV)

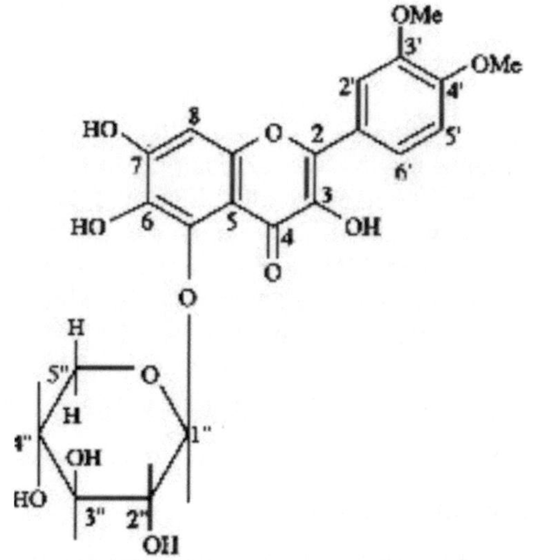

3, 5, 6, 7-tetrahydroxy-3', 4'-dimethoxyflavone-5-β-d-xylopyranoside (XVI)

2.5 Pharmacological review

The bark, fruits, and seeds of Z. *armatum* are extensively used in indigenous system of medicine as a carminative, stomachic and anthelmintic. The stem has exhibited hypoglycemic activity in the preliminary trials. The bark is pungent and used to clean teeth. The fruits and seeds are employed as an aromatic tonic in fever and dyspepsia. An extract of the fruits is reported to be effective in expelling round worms. Because of their deodorant, disinfectant and antiseptic properties, the fruits are used in dental troubles, and their lotion for scabies.

Zanthobungeanine, found in stems and roots shows inhibitory activity to platelet aggregation, L-plananin is the most active compound.

The bark is used in India, for treating diarrhea and cholera. The fruits are analgesic and anodyne and used in tooth powder.

The bark of several Indian species of *Zanthoxylum* is medicinally active and noted for febrifugal, sudorific and diuretic properties *(Wealth of India 2005).*

The essential oil is said to possess antiseptic, disinfectant and deodorant properties. The freshly distilled essential oil from the seeds exhibited strong antibacterial activity against *Escherichia coli, Vibro cholera, Micrococcus pyrogens* var. *aureus, Shigella dysenteriae* and *Salmonella typhi.* The seed oil possesses ascaricidal, antibacterial, anthelmintic and antifungal properties. The oil on account of high percentage of linalool is highly fragrant and attractive and can be commercialized on this account.

The oil obtained by steam-distillation of the fresh plant showed antifungal activity against a number of fungi.

It is established that plants which having antioxidant property also exert hepatoprotective action *(Fehar et al 1986).* As Z. *armatum* has shown significant antioxidant activity *(Verma et al 2008)* and also contain phenolic compounds, therefore, we have to investigate the hepatoprotective activity of ethanolic extract of Z. *armatum* in rats.

3. Experimental

3.1 Plant material

The *Zanthoxylum armatum* were procured from the Plant Physiology Division, Jawaharlal Nehru Krishi Vishwa Vidyalaya, Krishi Nagar, Jabalpur, M.P. (India) and authenticated by the taxonomic division, National Herbarium of Cultivated Plants, National Bureau of Plant Genetic and Resources, New Delhi. A voucher specimen **(vide accession no. NHCP/NBPGR/2007/100/2225 dated 22/08/2007**) was retained in our laboratory. The plant material was dried under shade at room temperature, reduced to moderately coarse powder and extracted successively with petroleum ether (60-80°C) and 95% ethanol using soxhlet apparatus. The ethanolic extract was dried under vacuum (yield, 6.67%). The defatted ethanolic extract of *Zanthoxylum armatum* (EEZA) was used for the preliminary phytochemical screening and hepatoprotective studies.

3.2 Preliminary phytochemical screening

A preliminary phytochemical screening was carried out for the extracts employing the standard procedure revealed the presence of various phytoconstituents *viz.* alkaloids, steroids, terpenes, flavonoids, saponins, tannins, glycosides, carbohydrates and proteins *(Harborne 1998).*

3.3 Chromatographic studies

Thin layer chromatography (TLC) and High Performance Thin Layer Chromatography (HPTLC), of the alcoholic extract of *Costus speciosus* was done.

3.4 Animals

The Institutional Animal Ethics Committee, (IAEC) review the protocol and approved the use of animals for the studies**, (Ethical clearance number: 711/02/a/CPCSEA).**

Wistar albino rats of both sexes (weighing 130–170 g) were used in the present study. They were housed in clean polypropylene cages (38X23X10 cm) with not more than three animals per cage and maintained under standard laboratory condition (temperature 25 ± 2°C) with dark and light cycle (12/12 h) and provided standard pellet diet (Hindustan Lever, Kolkata, India) and water *ad libidum.*

3.5 Acute toxicity studies

Acute toxicity study was performed for the extract according to the acute toxic classic methods as per OECD guidelines *(OECD Guidelines 1996).* Wister albino rats were used for acute toxicity study. The animals were kept fasting for overnight providing only water, after which the extract was administered orally 500 mg/kg b. w. and observed for 14 days. The animals were observed If mortality was observed in 2 out of 3 animals, then the dose administered was assigned as toxic dose. If mortality was observed in 1 animal, then the dose administered was repeated again to confirm the toxic dose. If mortility was not observed, the procedure was repeated for further higher dose i.e. 2000 mg/kg.

3.6 Assessment of hepatoprotective activity

The rats were divided in to four groups of six rats each. The animals of group A and group B served as control and carbon tetrachloride (CCl_4) control received vehicle (0.1% tween 80, 10 ml/kg b. w.). Group C served as standard and received silymarin (100 mg/kg b. w. in 0.1% tween 80), and group D was given EEZA (500 mg/kg b. w. in 0.1% tween 80). All administration of doses was made by gastric intubations once daily for 7 days.

On the 8th day 1 h after the administration of last dose, the animals of group B; C and D were given an intraperitoneal injection of CCl_4 with an equal quantity of liquid paraffin (0.5 ml/kg b. w.). All the animals were then fasted for 24 h and anaesthetized and the blood was collected by cardiac puncture. The liver was quickly dissected, washed with ice-cold saline and stored in freezer. The blood samples were allowed to coagulate at room temperature for 1 h. Serum was separated by centrifugation at 12,000 rpm at 4^{0}C for 5 min *(Verma et al 2007).*

3.6.1 Biochemical estimation

Serum was analyzed for various biochemical parameters, i.e. serum glutamyl oxalacetic acid transaminase (SGOT, AST), serum glutamyl pyruvate transaminases (SGPT, ALT) *(Reitman et al 1957)*, alkaline phosphatase (ALKP) *(Bessey et al 1946)* and for serum bilurubin (SBLN) *(Malloy et al 1937).*

3.6.2 Histopathological studies

The hepatoprotective activity was confirmed through histopathological studies on liver of rats. Slices of liver were cut and washed in Ringer's solution soaked with filter paper for 1.5 min, then liver slices were fixed in Carnay's fluid I (Ethanol: chloroform: Glacial acetic acid- 6:3:1) and processed for paraffin embedding following the standard microtechniques. Sections of liver, stained with aqueous haematoxylein and alcoholic eosin were observed microscopically for histopathological changes *(Galigher et al 1971).*

3.6.3 Statistical analysis

The data represent *M ± S.E.M.* Results were analyzed statistically by one-way ANOVA, followed by Students'*t'* test. The minimum level of significance was set at $P<0.001$ compared to control. The entire statistics were estimated by using **Sigma Stat 3.5™**, statistical software.

4. Result & discussion

4.1 Phytochemical screening

Phytochemical screening for the ethanolic extract of *Zanthoxylum armatum* revealed the presence of phytoconstituents like sterols, alkaloids, phenolic, flavonoids and reducing sugars. The ethanolic extract did not cause any mortality up to 2000 mg/kg and considered as safe.

4.2 CCl_4 induced Hepatotoxicity

The results of CCl_4-induced hepatotoxicity are represented in Table 1. CCl_4 intoxication in normal rats elevated the levels of SGOT, SGPT, ALKP, SBLN and liver inflammation were observed significantly indicating acute hepatocellular damage and billiary obstruction. The rats that received 500 mg/kg of EEZA showed a significant ($P<0.001$) decrease in all the SGOT, SGPT, ALKP, SBLN levels and liver inflammation, compared to induced control group.

Normal histology of rat liver showed sinusoidal degeneration (Fig. 2a). The liver sections of the rats treated with CCl_4 showed cellular degeneration hydropic changes which were more around the central vein and fatty changes with wide spread hepatocellular necrosis and centrolobular necrosis (Fig. 2b). The liver section of EEZA treated showed micro fatty changes with dense collection of lymphoid cells, suggesting evidence of very little necrosis or degeneration. There was no hepatocellular damage, except small arrears of focal degeneration and sinusoidal dilation in treated rat livers (Fig. 2c and d).

CCl_4 is biotransformed in to cytochrome P450 in the liver endoplasmic reticulum to the highly reactive trichloromethyl free radical which in turn reacts with oxygen to form a trichloromethyl peroxyradical, which may attack lipids on the membrane of endoplasmic

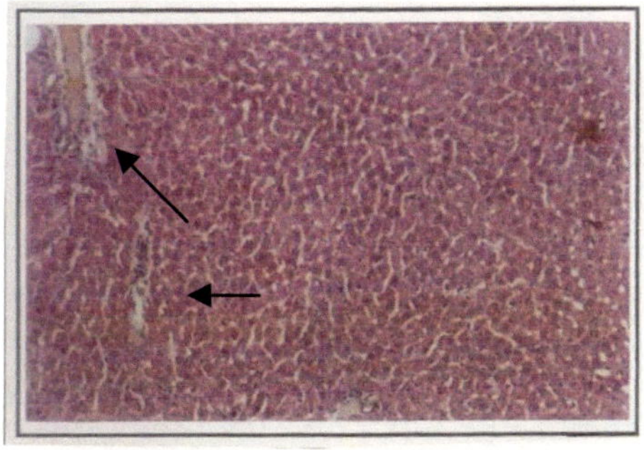

(a) Group I (control) - section shows central vein surrounded by hepatic cord of cells (normal architecture).

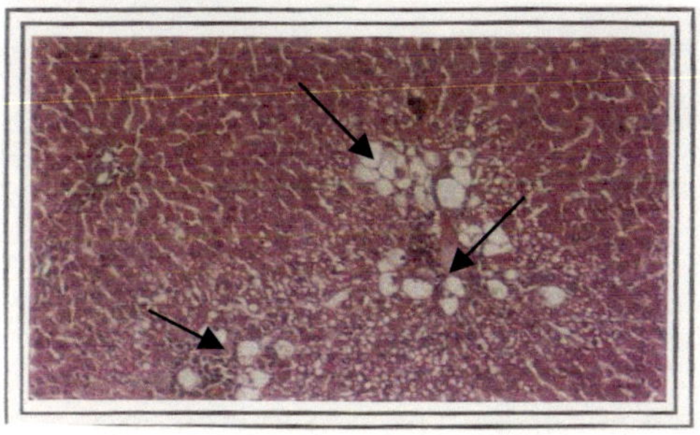

(b) Group II (CCl_4 treated) - section shows patches of liver cell necroses, inflammatory collections and accumulation of fatty lobules around central vein.

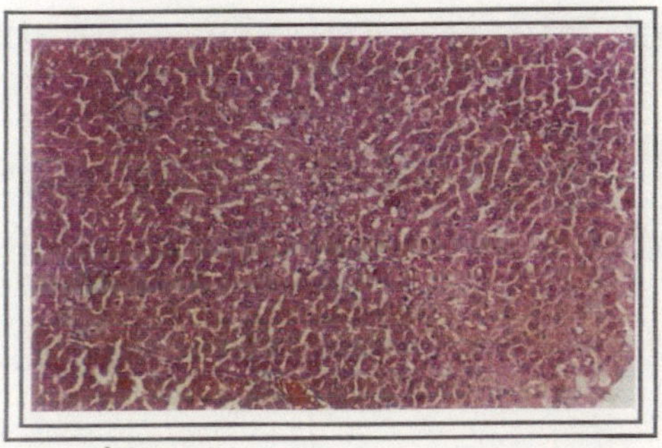

(c) Group III (Standard silymarin treated) almost near normal.

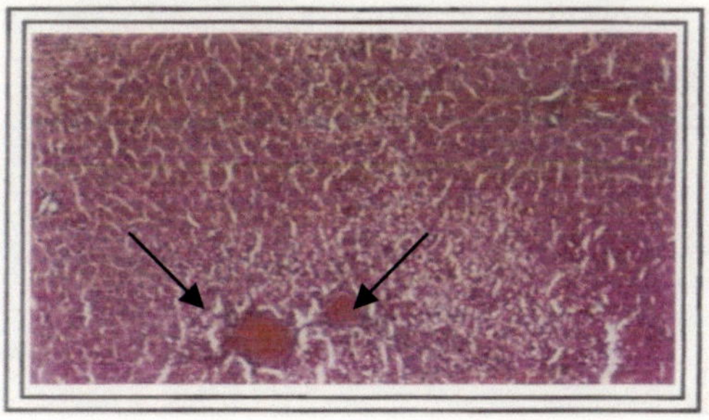

(d) Group IV (treated with ethanolic extract of *Z. armatum*) **-** minimal inflammatory cellular infiltration. Almost near normal liver architecture. Regeneration of hepatocytes around central vein.

Fig. 2. Histopathology of liver tissues at X 400 magnification

reticulum more readily than trichloromethyl free radical. The trichloromethylperoxy radical leads to elicit lipid peroxidation, the disruption of Ca^{2+} homeostasis, elevation of hepatic enzymes and finally results in cell death *(Clawson et al 1989).*

The results obtained from the present study indicated that the EEZA exhibited hepatoprotective effect against CCl_4-induced liver damage by normalizing the elevated levels of the hepatic enzymes. This suggested the possibility that EEZA is able to condition the hepatocytes, so as to cause accelerated regeneration of parenchyma cells, thus protecting against membrane fragility and decreases of leakage of the marker enzymes into the circulation as compared to silymarin, reported to have protective effect on the plasma membrane of hepatocytes *(Ramellini et al 1976).* The results supported the use of this plant for the treatment of hepatitis in oriental traditional medicine.

Parameters	**Biochemical Parameters**					
	SGPT(IU/L)	**SGOT(IU/L)**	**SALP(IU/L)**	**Bilirubin(mg/dl)**		**Liver weight (gm)**
Groups				**Total**	**Direct**	
Group A Control	53.25±3.83	382.50±21.32	196.68±1.09	0.93±0.03	0.17±0.08	3.21±0.22
Group B Toxicant (Induction control)	268.32±23.04***	702.45±6.6***	489.23±5.7***	3.14±0.24 ***	1.29±0.25***	3.38±0.24**
Group C Standard (Silymarin 100mg/kg b.w.)	78.67±7.33	408.29±4.68	213.55±4.27	1.64±0.82	0.19±0.0 3	3.22±0.01
Group D EEZA (500mg/kg b.w.)	104±9.75*	438.00±7.0**	249.59±6.07*	1.82±0.38**	0.24±0.88*	3.32±0.10**

Note: n= six animals in each group
EEZA= Ethanolic extract of Zanthoxylum armatum
Values are expressed as Mean ± SEM
* $p<0.05$ compared to control.
** $p<0.02$ compared to control.
*** $p<0.001$ compared to control.

Table 1. Effect of Ethanolic Extract of *Zanthoxylum armatum* on CCl_4 Induced Hepatotoxicity in Rats.

Flavonoids have been reported as active substances for the treatment of hepatitis induced by chemicals *(Khalid et al 2002)* and virus *(Kang et al 2006) in vitro* and *in vivo*. Ethanolic extract of *Z. armatum* showed positive results for the presence of phenolics and flavonoids during preliminary phytochemical screening. The possible mechanism may be that the antioxidant potentiality of flavonoids can scavenge free radicals and protect the cell membrane from destruction. Hence, the transaminases (ALT/AST) may not leak into blood from the necrotic hepatocytes.

5. References

[1] Hikino, H. and Kiso, Y., In: *Economic and Medicinal Plant Research,* Eds: Wagner, H., Hikino, H. and Farnsworth, N. R., (Academic Press, London), vol.2, 39, 1988.

[2] Handa, S.S., Sharma, A. and Chakraboti, K.K., *Fitoterapia,* Vol. LVII, 307, 1986.

[3] Feher, J., Csomos, G. and Vereckei, A. (Eds), *Free Radical reaction in Medicine,* Springer-Verlag, Berlin, 107, 1986.

[4] Meyer, B. and Elstner, E. F., *Planta Med.,* 56, 666, 1990.

[5] Romellini, G. and Meldolesi, J., *Arzneim Forsch, (Drug Res.),* 26, 69, 1976.

[6] Galvez, J., DeCruz, J. P., Zarzuelo, A. and DeLacuesta, F.S., *Pharmaco.,* 51,127, 1995.

[7] Ubeda, A., Esteve, M.L., Alcarz, K.H., Cheeseman, T.F. and Slater, T.F., *Phytother. Res.,* 9, 416, 1995.

[8] Kaul, I.B. and Kapil, A., *Indian J. Pharmaco.,* 26, 297, 1994.

[9] De, S., Ravishankar, B. and Bhavsar, G.C., *Indian J. Pharmaco.,* 26, 297, 1994.

[10] Verma, N. and Khosa, R.L., *Nat. Prod. Rad.,* 8, 123, 2009.

[11] Verma, N. and Khosa, R.L., *J. Biochemistry & Biophysics,* 47, 124, *2010.*

[12] Kirtikar, K.R. and Basu, B. D., *Indian Medicinal Plants,* Lalit Mohan Basu, 4, Leaders Road, Allahabad., 461, 1975.

[13] Verma, N. and Khosa, R. L., *Indian J. Nat. Prod.,* 24, 3, 2008.

[14] Verma, N. and Khosa, R. L., *Naresuan Phayao Journal,* 1, 99, 2008.

[15] Akhtar, N., Ali, M., and Alam, M.S., *J. Asian Natural Prod. Res.,* 11, 91, 2009.

[16] Anonymous, *The Wealth of India-A Dictionary of Indian Raw Materials & Industrial Products,* Vol. XI (X-Z) Publication and Information Directorate, CSIR, New Delhi. 568, 2005.

[17] Kalia, N.K., Singh, B., and Sood, R. P,. J. Nat. Prod., 62, 311 *1999.*

[18] Harborne, J. B., *Phytochemical Methods: A Guide to Modern Techniques of Plant Analysis,* Chapman & Hall, 1998.

[19] Guidance document on acute oral toxicity testing, Series on testing and assessment No. 24, Organization for economic co-operation and development, OECD Environment, health and safety publications, Paris, 1996.

[20] Verma, N., Khosa, R. L., & Pathak, A. K., *Indian J. Nat. Prod.,* 23, 2007.

[21] Reitman, S., & Frankel, S. A., *American J. Clinical Pathology,* 28, 1957.

[22] Bessey, O. A., Lowery, O. H., & Bros, M. J., *J Biological Chemistry,* 164, 321, 1946.

[23] Malloy, H. T., & Evelyn, K. A., *Journal of Biology chemistry,* 119, 481, 1937.

[24] Galigher, A. E., & Kozloff, E. N., *Essential of Practical Microtechnique,* 2nd Edition, Lea and Febiger, Philadelphia, 77, 1971.

[25] Clawson, G. A., *Pathology and Immunopathology Research,* 8, 104, 1989.

[26] Ramellini, G., & Meldolesi, J., Arzneim *Forsch (Drug Research),* 26, 69, 1976.
[27] Khalid, H. J., Sheikh, A. S., & Anwar, H. G., *Fitoterapia,* 73 , 557, 2002.
[28] Kang, E. H., Kown, T.Y., Oh, W.F., Park, S.I., Lee, Y. I., *Antiviral Research*, 72, 100, 2006.

3

Current Status: Mexican Medicinal Plants with Insecticidal Potential

Ludmila Elisa Guzmán-Pantoja, Laura P. Lina-García, Graciela Bustos-Zagal and Víctor M. Hernández-Velázquez
Laboratorio de Control Biológico, Centro de Investigación en Biotecnología, Universidad Autónoma del Estado de Morelos, Morelos, Mexico

1. Introduction

Plants have been used for thousand of year as a source of bioactive substances for therapeutic, agricultural and industrial purpose; in this regard the search for compounds active on these sources is an alternative for development of agrochemicals (Dayane et al., 2009). The plans, their derivatives or extracts have been studied for different biological activities in economically important pests, assessing their toxic effects lethal, antifeedant, repellent, fumigant, growth regulation and deterrent to oviposition, among other (Isman, 2006; Singh and Saratchandra, 2005).

The ecological balance and the organisms of various ecosystems are vulnerable by excessive or careless use of pesticides in agricultural or urban system. In theory, through using these products is to provide enough food and pest control, in contrast, often cause undesirable and dangerous environmental situations. Therefore, before to take a decision on the use of any pesticide, you should be aware that if the use of these substances is performed under controlled conditions and with full knowledge of its adverse properties, the survival of living things and balance of nature can become seriously affected (SEMARNAT, 2011).

The use of plants as a source of active compounds emerged as friendly alternative the indiscriminate use of synthetic products for pest control, which has causes toxicity to human health, biodiversity impoverishment, damage to beneficial organisms and favor the emergence of strains of pests resistant to these product, so it is common to increase the application rate risk to public health and the environment (Siqueira et al., 2000).

The rescue of rudimentary practices used by farmers in pest management is one of the options to find alternatives to the frequent use of synthetic pesticides. This report compiles information about the use of Mexican medicinal plants, native and introduced in the pest control mainly of the system agriculture and livestock primarily, and report an analysis of current status and recommendations for use botanical insecticides.

Currently investigations are conducted to determine the potential pesticide plant (used in herbal medicinal) , its derivatives or extracts, such as several spices of the family Asteraceae, Euphorbiaceae, Solanaceae, Meliaceae,Convolvulaceae, Lauraceae, Piperinaceae, and Anonaceae, among other (López-Olguín et al., 2002; Pereda-Miranda & Bah, 2003; Prakash &

Rao, 1997; Ramos, 2010; Rodríguez et al., 1982). For instance in the family Convolvulaceae, some species of the genus *Ipomoea* such as *I. tricolor*, *I. batata* and *I. murucoides* are traditionally used as nutricional, emetic, diuretic, diaphoretic, purgative (Pereda and Bah, 2003) and pesticidal agents (nematodes, insects, and weeds) (Jackson & Peterson, 2000; Vera et al., 2009; Vyvyan, 2002).

2. Botanic pesticide

In ancient culture and in different parts of the world has existed for thousands of years (~1500 before J. C.) empirical knowledge of the use of plants for pest control, for example, the neem in India, rotenone in East Asia and South America, pyrethrin in Persia (Iran) and sabadilla in Central and South America later botanical insecticides were introduced in Europe and Unite States (Weinzierl, 2000). Since the late 1800s to the 1940s, these products were widely used to protect crops and stored products. It was in the early 1940s and the 1950s which the development and commercial success of synthetic insecticides led to the abandonment of botanical insecticide in agriculture of the industrialized countries, as they won space on the market as products cheaper, effective, long-lasting and readily available. Only the botanical insecticides which remained in use in the Unite States after 1950, were pyrethrins (such aerosol spray and in home and industry) and nicotine (used primarily in the gardens). Already in the 1990s renewed interest stems from the use of botanical pesticides, because it is recognizes the impact on health and environmental that the synthetic insecticides cause, and their presence in food (Weinzierl, 2000).

Botanical pesticides are formulations of organic solvents and aqueous based on different parts of plants (crude extracts) or derivatives thereof, are prepared in powder or liquid concentrates that can be incorporated into talc or clay for application either concentrated or diluted in a solvent such as water, ethanol and petroleum ether, among others (Isman, 2008). These products consist of a group of active ingredients of different chemical nature (Isman, 1997). Preparations from plants such as pyrethroid, rotenone, neem, and citronella, commonly are formulated as liquid concentrates or extracts. The processed form of these products, are purified and isolated substances from plants through a series of extraction and distillation (Weinzierl, 2000).

Through different studies have found that the biological activity of botanical extracts pesticides it is different significantly depending on the species of plants, plant parts used for the preparation of the extracts, the physiological state of the part used, of the solvent extraction, and the insect species under study (Shaalan et al., 2005). Although these products are of natural origin cannot be assumed to be completely safe, some plant-derived compounds, such as nicotine are extremely toxic to humans, or when used several times in continuous time, can affect the natural biotic control of pests by their natural enemies. Therefore, it is important to use correctly the technique and safety equipment when working on the preparation and application of botanical extracts, and recognize the appropriate dose formulation and its use in a program of integrated pest management, which will help efficiently to obtain the benefits of these products. Despite there are many plants and chemical constituents known to have insecticidal properties or insectistatic, few have been used for commercial production. Issue that has been reviewed by several researchers as Graiger and Amhed (1988) and Isman (2008). The Use large-scale commercial of the plant extracts as insecticides began in the 1950s with the introduction of nicotine from *Nicotiana tabacum*, rotenone from *Lonchocarpus* sp, derris from *Derris elliptica*, and pyrethrum from flowers of *Chrysanthemum cinerariaefolium* (Isman, 2008).

Gaugler (1997), mentioned concerning this that the inconvenient of these products are offset by its lower toxicity, higher levels of security and in addition to generally exhibit lower accumulation in the environment, characteristics that should be used to promote their sales (Silva et al., 2002). These products have the advantage of being generally compatible with other programs acceptable alternative integrated pest management, such as practices, cultivation of plants resistant to pests, pheromone oils, soaps, entomopathogenic, predators and parasitoids, among others (Brechelt, 2008). Botanical pesticides already registered and approved are promoted for organic crop production especially in industrialized countries and for production and postharvest food protection in developed countries (Rodriguez, 1997).

Actually in the Unite States the registration of the botanical insecticides request few requirements, for that reason allows a wide range of these products, including pyretrins, neem, rotenone, sabadilla, ryania, and nicotine. Essential oils are also sold although several of them do not have a complete record (Isman, 2006). In Latin America, it is common that the production of oil and botanical extracts for pest control is done without regulatory system and small scale for local use in low-income populations. As in all developing countries, lack of training of relevant legislations to regulate these products has complicated the registration process, this is the case of Mexico with the insecticide Biocrack® (garlic extract) Berni Labs who have gave the record seven year after starting its activities (Silva *et al.*, 2002). On the other hand, Mexico allows the use of many products sold in the Unite States as the PHC™ NEEEM™ (31.2 g i.a. L^{-1} azadirachtin) and NEEMIX® 4.5 (47.6 g i.a. L^{-1} azadirachtin) and the insecticides approved for their use are pyrethrum, rotenone, nicotine, garlic and capsicum extract and powder the mixture of neem leaf and seed (Grain Protector®, Mexican Fitorganic) (Isman, 2006).

In Mexico, Ultraquimia Group S.A. de C.V., manufactures organic and agrochemicals products used in the control of plant health problems and carry out coordinated studies with researchers from the National Research Institute Forestry, Agriculture and Livestock (INIFAP) to determine the biological effectiveness of botanical insecticides produced, such as BIODI®e, PROGRANIC® CinnAcar and PROGRANIC® Nimicide 80 among others, recommended for control of Diaforina (*Diaphorina citri*), mealybug (*Planococcus citri*), whitefly (*Bemisia tabaci, Trialeurodes vaporariorum*), aphids diver *(Paratrioza cockerelli)*, bold *(Phyllocoptruta oleivora)*, asian citrus psyllid *(Diaphorina citri)*, diamond back moth *(Plutella xylostella)*, worm looper *(Trichoplusia ni)*, thrips *(Thrips spp., Frankliniella spp., Caliothrips phaseoli, Heliothrips sp.)* and aphids *(Aphis spp, Myzus persicae, Brevicoryne brassicae, Toxoptera spp.)*.

Isman (1999) indicated that within 10 to 15 years, specifically the botanical insecticides probably represent about 50% of the total insecticide market. However, the current availability of biopesticides market comprises a small portion of the total volume of pesticides available. According to FAO data, world consumption of bioinsecticides for 2009 represented 0.2 % of the total consumption of insecticides (FAO, 2009). Nevertheless, these products remain important in the insect pest management for the reasons mentioned above.

FAO (1999) indicated that little information exist about the use of botanical pesticide on the crop protection or stored food, also have been few evaluation of the effectiveness of these materials under real conditions of use on field. Currently plant species more recognized and evaluated under laboratory conditions belong to the genus *Azadirachta, Piper, Chenopodium, Ipomoea, Mentha, Annona,* and *Tanacetum*. However, the use of most of these plants has not been divulged due to lack of appropriate programs and properly established of outreach and training. Multinational corporations in western Mexico are implementing alternative pest management in tobacco-growing areas, to try to reduce the amount of synthetic pesticides used; in this sense, botanists become an effective and attractive alternative (Isman, 2008). Several traditionally used plant preparations have found local commercial markets, for example *Ryania speciosa* (Ryania) (Flacourtiaceae) which contains an insecticidal alkaloid, and *Haplophyton* spp. (Apocynaceae) have been used in the West Indies and Mexico for crop protection (FAO, 1999), situation depicted a growing and progressive interest in the use of this alternative in pest management, however the situation is confused, because sometimes ambiguous recommendations are made about the local use of these products without having been previously validated by field investigations and biosecurity. In Mexico and throughout Latin America, this is common, and is manifested in the publication of manuals that describe and encourage the use of botanical pesticides, which usually collect basis of partial observations and reviews established by the people that have empirically determined the effectiveness of certain plants and their formulated in the pest management.

Undoubtedly, it is not strange that in the short term register new plants and compounds with potential usefulness pesticide or plaguistatic with novel modes and sites of action to ensure their gradual distinctiveness in the market and enabling to increase the range of low-risk alternatives for pest management.

3. Modes and sites of action

In the current development of botanical insecticides has increased interest in the characterization of the active compounds. Secondary metabolites of plants with insecticidal or insectistatic properties cause alterations in biochemical and physiological insects (hormonal, neurological, nutritional or enzymatic) when operating with repellent, antifeedant, growth regulation, oviposition deterrent and lethal toxicity, among other activities (Isman, 2006; Singh & Saratchandra, 2005).

Different modes of action are described for many active compounds, for example, when are applied on the crop to be protected, they can act systemically in the plant by penetrating through the stomata and transported through the vascular system, altering its enzymatic complex, transpiration and changes in the composition of sap; other phytocompounds increase plant's energy, promote the synthesis of sucrose to help strengthen your metabolism and immune defense system. In many cases induce repellency and excitement of the nervous system from insect pests hindering the flight and oviposition therefore decrease the populations of insect pests.

The mechanism of action and target sites of the active phytochemicals on insects is diverse. Some cause effects by contact or ingestion being generally difficult their detoxification. The extracts or phytocompounds that acting through contact can penetrate and dissolve the lipoprotein matrix of the cuticle and cell membranes of insects destroying the exoskeleton, disrupting permeability and cellular physiology, causing dehydration and consequently death or reduce the oxygen consumption of nymphs, larvae and adults killing them by asphyxiation, affect the peripheral and central nervous system causing hyperexcitation, hypersensitivity, to external stimuli, seizure, muscle tetanization, effect protein synthesis and cell membranes, causing further death. The hyperexcitation of the nervous system also cause the masking of pheromones responsible for the mating process. The phytochemicals that acting by ingestion alter the physiological rhythm of the digestive system, preventing the contraction of the muscles of the intestine, causing his paralysis and hemolysis. There are components that act as repellents to block and inhibit the ability to search and locate food (antifeedant effect) reducing the amounts ingested and increased parasitism and predation by staying longer exposed to the environment and weak; repellency may be regarding the use of systems of chemical interaction between plant-insect chemical; the alomones, that plants synthesize when interacting with individuals of another species (insect pests, for example) induce them respond with physiological change or behavioral modifying which favors only the plant. The mechanism by which the repellent activity occurs could also be due to a mixed action for an unpleasant effect on the sensory endings as well as a chemical blocking of the perception that insect use for guidance.

The phytochemicals that cause lethal toxicity against insects larvae affect on any of the following target sites: midgut epithelium, gastric caeca, malpighian tubules, and in the nerve axon because disruption of channel sodium whose result in the insect is hyperactivity and seizure. The mechanism of action involves disruption of metabolism both through inhibiting the transport of electrons and uncoupling the ATP transport system, depolarization of the membrane potential, effect on calcium channel with sustained muscle contraction and inhibition of acetylcholinesterase (Shaalan et al., 2005; Weinzierl, 2000). Other phytocompounds asset, have a high effect of "knockdown", causing that the insect to stop feeding, become paralyzed and die of starvation soon after being in contact with the product or treated surfaces.

In experimental tests with sublethal concentrations of the extracts or active compounds of plants, there is often an extension of the period of biological development of the insects under study, making it possible to determine the characteristics effects of botanical extracts classified as regulator of growth, which contain phytoecdysones, phytojuvenoids and juvenile hormone causing prolongation of the stages of development, affecting the size, adult emergence, the physiology of reproduction by disrupting the reproductive system, fertility and hatching of larvae, resulting in effective control (Shaalan et al., 2005). The effect of phytochemicals that cause growth inhibition in various stages of development of insect pests act through inhibiting larval and pupal molt, longer duration of larval and pupal stage, morphological abnormalities and mortality during the molt among other effects (Shaalan et al., 2005).

Morphological abnormalities are observed in different development stage of insect, such as damage in the process of melanization in larvae and pupae, death in the intermediate stage of a larva and pupa (in this case can be observed organisms with the head of a pupa and the abdomen of a larva), death of adults with wings caught in the pupal exuviae and adult difficulties to fully emerge (Shaalan et al., 2005), these anomalies indicate an inhibitor effect on metamorphosis, probably due to disruption of hormonal control, and interference in the synthesis of chitin during the molting process (Pushpalatha & Muthukrishnan, 1999; Saxena & Sumithra, 1985). In the embryonic stage usually observe dehydration on eggs, bleeding, and death of embryo.

The biological effects of the phytocompound mentioned above are manifested individually or in combination depending of the chemical enrichment of plant species with potential pesticide and interactions that exists between the compounds. Many of the botanicals products that exhibit combined effects, such as the simultaneous damage in the larval development time and adult emergence, occasionally extend to the progeny of the larvae exposed to these treatments (Shaalan et al., 2005).

Boeke et al. (2004), validated the toxic and repellent effect of 33 plants used in Africa since the antique of empirical and traditional manner, for beetle *Callosobruchus maculatus* control.

The laboratory evaluation showed that the powders of *Nicotiana tabacum*, *Tephrosia vogelii*, and *Securidaca longepedunculata* significantly reduced the number of beetle progeny and the species *Clausena anisata*, *Dracaena arborea*, *T. vogelii*, *Momordica charantia* y *Blumea aurita* had repellent activity, as reported experimentally that the majority of species assessed, provided effective control against *C. maculatus*.

Certain compounds are well known for their mechanisms of action, as quassin, a triterpene isolated from the wood of *Quassia amara* (Simaroubaceae). The quassin is an insecticide that show effects on the mosquito larval *Culex quinquefasciatus* through the inhibition of tyrosinase enzyme activity and consequently alter the development of the cuticle (Evans & Raj, 1991). This compound has also been tested successfully in cereal crops to control aphids (Sengonca & Brüggen 1991) by the mechanism of inhibition of enzymes of the insect.

Species of the family Meliaceae are source of azadarachtin, a limonoid marketed and appreciated by their biological activities pesticides, such as the antifeedant effect, the regulation of growth, as ovicidal and larvicidal, among others. The main effect of azadirachtin is to inhibit development, especially affecting the molt, by inhibiting the hormone ecdysone. Scott et al. (1999), showed that azadirachtin caused inhibition of voltaje K^+ channel in cultured rat neurons, this compounds has also shows antimitotic affect on *Sf9* insect cell line, resulting in prolongation of repolarization (Salehzadeh et al., 2003). Microscopic studies have indicated that azadirachtin interfere with the formation of the mitotic spindles and in the assembly of microtubules in the axoneme during microgametogenesis of *Plasmodium berghei* (Billker et al., 2002).

The family Piperaceae has been used as sources of pesticides to contain piperamides, several lignans, and derivates of benzoic acid. The piperamides, are molecules with dual biological activity, the amide group is neurotoxic and secondly the group methylenedioxyphenyl (MPD) is an inhibitor of cytochrome P450 in the insect pest, which participates in the metabolism of fatty acids and steroids (Scott et al., 2003).

Commercial botanical insecticide, rhodojaponin-III, islated from *Rhododendron molle* effect on more than 40 species of insect pests being antifeedant, oviposition, ovicidal, inhibitor of growth and change and toxic by ingestion and through contact. Previous studies indicate that this compound inhibits proliferation of *Sf9* insect cell (isolated from pupal ovariantissue of *Spodoptera frugiperda*) dose-dependent effect. Besides interfering with cell division, the concentration of [Ca^{2+}], and intracelular pH (Cheng et al., 2011).

4. Pesticide compounds

Plant extracts and their derivatives are a source of many chemical compounds with potential insecticide or insectistatic and processed forms of botanical insecticides are isolated and purified compounds through extractions and distillation. For instance, nicotine and limonoid are distilled from plant extracts (Weinzierl, 2000).

Plants produce a vast and diverse reserve of secondary metabolites actives on different animals and plants of other species, allowing them to maintain relations of cohabitation (attractants) or defense (toxic or repellent substances) (Kutchan & Dixon, 2005). These secondary metabolites are not essential for growth and development of plants, but they are required for interaction with the environment and to respond to pressures such as scarcity of water and nutrients, extreme temperatures, to deter to the herbivores microorganisms and viruses; also serve as signals to communicate with other organisms (Felton et al., 2008; Wink & Schimmer, 1999).

The demand dynamic of biotic and abiotic environment gives the natural plasticity to the secondary metabolism and encourages the evolution of genetic diversification of the plant and thus generating a abundant group of natural products with variety of chemical structures (Kutchan & Dixon, 2005) many case bioactive (Macías et al., 2007).

The biosynthesis of secondary metabolites and storage of these compounds is regulated in space and time, so the growing tissues are more vulnerable and more protected than the old or senescent tissues. For instance, is usually observed in seeds, latent and period of germination, flower buds and young tissues retain a certain amount of specific compounds or are actively synthesized. The organs that are important for the survival and multiplication, such as flowers, fruits and seeds, are almost always a rich source of chemical defenses (Wink, 1999). In addition, the metabolic profile usually varies between parts of a plant, including developmental stages, sometime during the day, the geographic location of the plant species and between plant species (Wink, 1999).

Many secondary metabolites have biological activities such as insecticides, fungicides, and phytotoxic properties that can be employed in agriculture (Wink, 1999) either alone or in combination with other chemical and biological (Trysyono & Whalon, 1999; Weinzierl, 2000). Particularly during the past 20 years, phytocompounds such as terpenes, alkaloids, rotenone and pyrethrum have gained commercial importance for the development of botanical insecticides (Isman, 2006).

Macías et al. (2007), mention that it was until the twentieth century when the study of plant compounds and their mechanism of action is made relevant. The development of spectroscopic technique allowed the isolation and identification of pure active compounds such as (5E)-ocimenone from *Tagetes minuta* (1978), rotenone from *Derris elliptica* (1983), azadirachtin from *Azadirachta indica* (1981), capillin from *Artemisia nilagirica* (1990), quassin from *Quassia amara* (1991), neolignans from *Piper decurrens* (1996), arborine, a new bioactive compound related to quinazolone alkaloid, from *Glycosmis pentaphylla* (1999) and goniothalamin From *Bryonopsis laciniosa* (2003) (Shaalan et al., 2005).

Kathuria and Kaushik (2005), determinedthe antifeedant effect of etanol extracts of leaves from *Eucaliptus camaldulensis* y *Tylophora indica* en *Helicoverpa armigera* (Hûbner) and found that the alkaloids identified in *T. indica* are responsible for this activity. In another study, extracts were evalued red maple (*Arce rubrum*) resulting assets over *Malacosama disstria* larvae, causing antifeedant affect. Gallates derivatives (1-O-galatoil-L-ramnosa) present in the plant were compounds responsible for this activity (Zaid & Nozzolillo, 2000).

5. Mexican medicinal plants

According to estimates published up to now, Mexico is the third country worldwide with a diversity of vascular plants. Of the 250 000 species located around the world, in the Mexico there are 22 411 (10%), not including nearly a thousand species (Villaseñor & Magaña, 2002; Vovides et al., 2010). Diversification, is back to geological times and have been possible by the variety of soil conditions, climate and topography of the country, as well as plant genetics and anthropogenic activities of conservation, introduction, selection and plant breeding.

In general terms, the biological, ecological and cultural diversity of Mexico has led to the generation of empirical and scientific knowledge, the first has its origins in ancient times with the practices of observation to the nature and experimentation through trial and error, inheritance transmitted from generation to generation through texts or stories. Through the inventory made under the empirical system made were possible the first classifications of plants with data on their ecology, biological importance and usefulness (Gómez-Pompa, 2010). In Mexico the codices written by important pre-Hispanic groups are transcendental. With regard to the Azteca codex De la Cruz-Badiano is a record conceptual and illustrative of the medicinal plants used in New Spain of the Sixteenth Century, regarded worldwide as one of the best collections of Mexican folk medicine, this wealth of literature has fractured and disrupted on several occasions, however, has been rescued, preserved and expanded by the country's ethnic groups and has now increased interest to validate through experimental science (Bye & Linares, 1999). Scientists from Mexico and other countries have used the codices, herbal, picked and general ethnobotanical practices for various purposes, among these, botanists have been interested in reviewing corroborated and enrich the etnoflora catalogs, describing the location, uses regional and popular names of plants and the phytochemical have used ethnobotanical studies as a reference for the location of plants with biological significance and the search for new phytocompounds useful in protecting, and preserving food un pre- and post-harvest either as pesticides and botanical repellents, as well as raw materials for pharmaceutical, cosmetic, chemical, beverage, food and bioprocesses. A current record, provides that Mexico has about 7 000 species of vascular plants with some use for various purposes (Caballero & Cortés, 2001).

Importantly, there are still many regions of Mexico to explore thoroughly, to have an updated inventory of plants, a situation that reflects the potential in the many uses of these resources. In these sense, diversity and identification of endemic, native, and introduced strengthen several areas of research, local and foreign plant extracts or their derivatives. Of the plants with some kind of use, 3 300 species have medicinal use (Pérez, 2001); in addition to its therapeutic properties, many of these plants have the potential to be used in the management of pests and phytopathogens of agricultural and livestock importance, ancient practice that originated with the beginning of agricultural activities. The global ecological problem that exists in modern times, mankind has created demand for residue-free agricultural products and alternatives to reduce agrochemicals use, so that the development of conservation and sustainable agriculture was necessary and this favors the development and commercialization of these botanical pesticides.

6. Ethnobotanical study of Mexican medicinal plants with insecticide potential

Traditionally, the plants located in each geographic region of Mexico, are used for different purposes. Many have multiple applications and properties, the literature quotes are cite both for its medicinal properties as insecticides and antiparasitic properties. It is estimated that in Mexico there are about 7 000 useful plant species, representing 31% of vascular plants located in the country (Caballero & Cortés, 2001).

Ethnobotany is considered as a source for research of phytopesticides of interest to the agricultural and livestock with production sustainable and alternative.

This paper conducted a literature search and review of the publications on ethnobotanical studies in the country, plants that farmers and people in general routinely used to protect crops, stored grain, and ornamentals (Table 1). To confirm the medicinal use of plants

PLANT	Common name	Other use	Municipality or Community/ Reference	Plant part used	Preparation	Application forms	Species/location of control
ASTERACEAE							
Senecio salignus	Chilca	Remedy (foliage) andornamental	Tzental Region, Chiapas/Miranda, 1952				Corn and bean weevil (*Acanthoscelides obtectus* y *Zabrotes subfasciatus*)/store
Artemicia ludoviciana	Mugwort wormwood	Medicinal and pesticide (CONABIO, 2009)	Ixtapan de la sal/Rodríguez, 2008	Whole plant	Drying	Among the sacks of corn	Weevil/store
CAPRIFOLIACEAE							
Sambucus mexicana	Elder	Ceremonial, medicinal	Santos Reyes Nopala, Oaxaca	Fresh or dried leaves	Pulverized leaves	Arrange altérnate layers of leaves, then corn	Pest of stored maize and beans
FABACEAE							
Eritryna americana	Zompantle	Insect repellent, living fence, medicinal, ceremonial	/Hasting, 1990; Rodríguez, 2008	Seed	Combustion	Use of smoke	Corn and bean weevil /store

Table 1. Plants with potential pesticide used in different regions of Mexico

PLANT	Common name	Other use	Municipality or Community/ Reference	Plant part used	Preparation	Application forms	Species/location of control
MELIACEAE							
Cedrela spp.		Timber Medicinal	Cuetzálan, Puebla y Chicontepec, Veracruz/ Rodríguez, 2008	Leaves and seed	Dust	Mix with the beans stored	Corn and bean weevil /store
Melia azedarach	Tree of Paradise	Medicinal	Martínez de la torre, Veracruz/ Rodríguez 2008	Dried leaves	Dust	Mixed with corn	Corn and bean weevil /store
Trichilia havanensis	Xopiltetl		Tuzamapan de Galeana, Puebla/Rodríguez, 2008; López-Olguín, 1997	Leaves and fruit	Dust	Muxed with corn and beans	Corn and bean weevil /store
PIPERACEAE							
Piper auritum Kunth	Mumo, yerba santa	Medicinal	Chatino territory, Oaxaca/ Miranda, 1952	Whole plant	Dried and ground		Maize weevil/Storage
			Tepetate, Veracruz/ Ortega & Rodríguez, 1991	Whole plant	Powdery		Significant effect on the control of *S. frugiperda*, after four applications for a week/ Field

Table 1. Plants with potential pesticide used in different regions of Mexico

PLANT	Common name	Other use	Municipality or Community/ Reference	Plant part used	Preparation	Application forms	Species/location of control
Piper sanctum	homeoquelite	Medicinal	Cuetzálan, Santiago Yancuitlalpan y San Miguel Zinecapan, Puebla/ Rodríguez, 2008	Leaves	Dried	Cover the soil with a thin layer of partially dehydrated leaves, then a layer of corn and so on to accommodate the entire crop	
POLYPODIACEAE							
Pteridium aquilinum		Medicinal	Los Altos de Chiapas, México/ Ramírez *et al.*, 2006	Whole plant	Aqueous extracts by infusion 5%	Infusion applied to cabbage plants infested with larvae	Larvae of the second stage of *Leptophobia aripa* Elodia. Cause 27% mortality
RUTACEAE							
Zanthoxyllum liemmanianum	Colopahtle (tongue grass)	Remed for amoebiases and helminthic	Valle de Tehuacán, Puebla				Wood

Table 1. Plants with potential pesticide used in different regions of Mexico

PLANT	Common name	Other use	Municipality or Community/ Reference	Plant part used	Preparation	Application forms	Species/location of control
SAPINDACEAE							
Dondonaea viscosa			/ Lagunes *et al.*, 1984				Cause 40% mortality and reduces weight more than 50% in larvae of *S. frugiperda*//Labor atory tests
SMILACEAE							
Smilax aristolochiaefolia	*Sarsaparrilla*	Medicinal	/ Martinez, 1983				Control of neonates larvae of *S. frugiperda*//Labor atory tests
			/ Lagunes *et al.*, 1984	Whole plant	Maceration		Cause 40% mortality and reduces weight more than 50% in larvae of *S. frugiperda*//Labor atory tests
S. morarense	*sarsaparrilla*	Medicinal	/ Martinez, 1983				Control of neonates larvae of *S. frugiperda*

Table 1. Plants with potential pesticide used in different regions of Mexico

PLANT	Common name	Other use	Municipality or Community/ Reference	Plant part used	Preparation	Application forms	Species/location of control
S. morarense	*sarsaparrilla*	Medicinal	/ Lagunes *et al.*, 1984	Whole plant	Maceration		Cause 40% mortality and reduces weight more than 50% in larvae of *S. frugiperda*
SOLANACEAE							
Capsicum spp.	Chile	Insect repellent, dye, medicinal, cosmetic	Oaxaca/ Rodríguez H. C. 2008	Dried fruit	The fruit is roasted	The smoke is passed through the corn stored, locally know as "mats" to repel insects	Weevil /store
Cestrum anagyris	Huele de noche	Medicinal	/Ortega & Rodríguez, 1982	plant, leave, flower and the mix of leaf-flower	Infusion and maceration		Mortality of fourth instar larvae of *Culex quinquefasceatus*// Laboratory tests
			Lake Texcoco (laboratory and field test) / Rodríguez & Lagunes, 1987	Leave	Maceration	Bioassay and application of macerated in trays distributed later in southeast shore of lake	Field: mortality of fourth instar larvae of *Culex quinquefasceatus* (75%)

Table 1. Plants with potential pesticide used in different regions of Mexico

PLANT	Common name	Other use	Municipality or Community/ Reference	Plant part used	Preparation	Application forms	Species/location of control
Cestrum roseum		Medicinal	Lake Texcoco (laboratory and field test) / Rodríguez & Lagunes, 1987	Leave	Maceration	Bioassay and application of macerated in trays distributed later in southeast shore of lake	Field: mortality of fourth instar larvae of *Culex quinquefasceatus* (52%)
Cestrum thyrsoideum		Medicinal	Lake Texcoco (laboratory and field test) / Rodríguez & Lagunes, 1987	Leave	Maceration	Bioassay and application of macerated in trays distributed later in southeast shore of lake	Field: mortality of fourth instar larvae of *Culex quinquefasceatus* (41%)
Datura stramonium	Toloache	Medicinal	/Rodríguez, 2011	Whole plant		Intercalated species in cultivation of *Nicotiana tabacum*	Whitefly/field
Solanum cervantesii			/ Lagunes *et al.*, 1984		Maceration		Cause 40% mortality and reduces weigh more than 50% in larvae of *S. frugiperda* /Laboratory tests

Table 1. Plants with potential pesticide used in different regions of Mexico

PLANT	Common name	Other use	Municipality or Community/ Reference	Plant part used	Preparation	Application forms	Species/location of control
STERCULIACEAE							
Guazuma tomentosa	Cuahulote	Medicinal, craft, cosmetics, fuel, fodder, fiber, ceremonia, flavoring, and sugar industry	Laboratory tests/ Lagunes *et al.*, 1984	Whole plant	Macerated		Cause 40% mortality and reduces weight more than 50% in larvae of fall armyworm (*S. fugiperda)*
TROPAEOLACEAE							
Tropaeolum majus	*Capuchina* Mastuerzo	medicinal	Tarahumara of México Region/ Rodríguez, 2011	Fresh plant	Macerated aqueous 10% with paste soap 0.1%		Whitefly control in vegetables
TURNERACEA							
Turnera diffusa			Field trials/Jiménez &Villar, 1990		Infusions	Tests with one and three applications per week	Significant *S. fugiperda* control, compared to grain yield

Table 1. Plants with potential pesticide used in different regions of Mexico

concerned are consulted databased of Plant Atlas of Traditional Mexican digital library of Mexican Traditional medicine of the National Autonomous University of Mexico with access at www.medicinatradicionalmexicana.unam.mx, as well as the book "The scientific investigation of the Mexican medicinal herbs" (Aguilar et al., 1993) and publications with information ethnobotany.

7. Studies of insect pests of agricultural importance

In Mexico and many parts of the world, people field for various decades have been consistently observed in their environment, and empirically they have selected plants that are not attacked by diseases and pests, many of which can be used as repellents and pesticides. Among the more promising botanical insecticides from the standpoint of its regulation, marketing and use, are products derived from plants that have already been validated by their pharmacological activity and insecticide, as the powdered of leaves and seed from neem (Grain Protector®) and garlic extract (Biocrack®) (Silva et al., 2002).

According to Dev and Koul (1997) worldwide about 2 000 plant species have insecticidal active compounds with significant, mainly distributed in 61 families, of which we have identified for Mexico around 14 families of vascular plants by the number times cited in total publications consulted in this review, they are Asteraceae, Meliaceae, Convolvulaceae, Flacourtiaceae, Liliaceae, Solanaceae, Euphorbiaceae, Fabaceae, Lamiaceae, Rutaceae, Myrtaceae, Verbenaceae Burceraceae, Caricaceae (Table 2), despite diversity of resources with propierties worldwide, only a few of these species have commercial value in the market phytoinsecticides. Some authors like Isman (2006) mention that in modern times should restructure the search for new species with insecticidal or insectistatic activity and concentrate on the validation, regulation and marketing of phytoinsecticides already known for their potential. In developing countries like Mexico, is possible that the search of species with potential for pest control play an important role in food production (agricultural and livestock) and public health and livestock, because of empirical and traditional in several regions have been using some native species with this potential, either in the form of hedges, crude extracts, combustion products, powders, resins, latex, sap, poison baits or live plants interspersed throughout the orchards.

Although Mexico exist isolated investigations on the search for plants with insecticidal activity (in some case having as antecedent pharmacological activity),there are well established research groups from different institutions of the country, for several years, have established this area as its research. A clear example is found in the Postgraduate College (Montecillo, Texcoco, State of Mexico) where Dr. Cesáreo Rodríguez Hernández, Dr. Laura D. Ortega Arenas and the group of contributors, since 1981 have worked consistently for the validation of plans that have traditionally been used since ancient times in rural communities across the country. About 30 rears, Dr. Rodríguez has collected and documented information from various parts of the country about the type local vegetation, plants with properties, uses, controlling pest species and forms of preparation. Generally, the information is recorded as prescription practices used among rural workers, agricultural technicians and promoters of organic farming, which details the use of local flora for the preparation of powders, baits or extracts, using materials available in the field. These research ranging from the intensive search for potential plant species present in a community insecticide and conducting toxicity tests on one or more species of insect pests of worldwide importance such as *Spodoptera frugiperda* and the complex of while fly, or a local impact, such as *Leptophobia aripa elodea* (Table 3). The evaluations have been conducted in species of insect pests warehouse, public health and agricultural, using different parts of the candidate plants for preparations carrying out tests in laboratory and field level in several states. The information that Dr. Rodríguez and other working groups with whom he has worked, is recorded in different memories of the event "national and international symposium on plant and mineral substance in pest control" performed periodically in Mexico and is also published in scientific journals.

In this sense, Villavicencio-Nieto and colleagues (2010), have determined that the State of Hidalgo there is much dependence on farmers for the local flora, the Autonomous University of Hidalgo State investigated the traditional use of 124 species of plants in the region, specifically for the pest control, only 97 of them being medicinal and 11 are used as insecticides. This research found that these plants have different uses in other regions of Mexico, including pharmacologic, as is the case *Galphimia glauca,* which have been used all its parts in different products (extracts, powders, essencial oils and resins) used in the management of pests of livestock agriculture, and health, such as human lice. Plant species most used in the communities of Hidalgo were *Trichilia havanensis, Psidium guajava, Nicotiana tabacum, Tagetes erecta, Mentha rotundifolia, Ipomoea stans, Tagetes lucida, Parthenium hysterophorus,* and *Schinus molle.* As a result of surveys conducted in this investigation, Villavicencio-Nieto and colleagues found that the plants with insecticide potential under study, are used to control 29 different pest species such as lice, fleas, weevils, ants, mosquitoes, cockroaches, among others, and are toxic to vertebrates such as dogs, squirrels, rats, snakes, and raccoons. This marks the importance of promoting the proper use of botanicals among communities.

At the Center of Development of Biotic Products (CEPROBI) National Polytechnic Institute, Dr. Camino Lavín, developed his research on finding alternatives to the use of synthetic pesticides and in 1985 founded the department of plant-insect interactions, which among other line, encourages the development of phytoinsecticides. Currently, this line of research continues the group of collaborators and has evaluated *Ficus goldmanii, Ficus petiolaris* (Moraceae), *Cochlospermun vitifolium* (Bixaceae), *Croton ciliatoglanduliferus* (Euphorbiaceae), *Crescentia alata* (Bignoniaceae), *Phitecellobium dulce,* species of the genus *Tagetes* (Asteraceae) and also species in the Sierra Huautla, at the State of Morelos, as *Prosopis laevigata* (Fabaceae) and species of the genus *Bursera* (Burseraceae) *and Lupinus* (Fabaceae), which is known that several species have compounds with insecticidal and medicinal activity. They have also evaluated the biological activity of seeds of different varieties of *Carica papaya* (Caricaceae), which present effect insecticide e insectistatic against *Spodoptera frugiperda* (Franco et al., 2006).

In the Autonomous University of San Luis Potosi, have been assessed by laboratory tests, powdered of leaves and flowers from 81 plant species belonging to the Asteraceae family, the selection was made considering that this family includes many species with insecticidal activity or deterrent and also because they have pharmacological activities, the evaluations were conducted on *Sitophilus zeamais.* Of the 169 powder tested 50 were promising, highlighting the powder of leaves from *Zinnia acerosa* and *Z. peruviana,* in terms of insectistatic activity highlighted *Bahia absintifolia, Stevia pilosa* and *Jefea brevifolia* (Juárez-Flores et al., 2010).

Trichilia havanensis (Meliaceae) is a species found from southern Tamaulipas to Tabasco and Chiapas, in considered native to Mexico and given its relationship with *Azadirachta indica* and *Melia azaderach* belonging to the same family, has been studied for over 15 years in the Benemerita Autonomous University of Puebla. The assessments are aimed at finding alternatives to control *Ceratitis capitata,* fruit pest species with cosmopolitan distribution and quarantine regulations in several countries, his control is restricted to the use of insecticidal organophosphates and pyrethroids. Other insects that have been used for the evaluations are *Spodoptera exigua,* especies del género *Phyllophaga, Leptinotarsa decemlineata, Thrips tabaci, Helicoverpa armígera, Spodoptera litorali* and *Hypotenemus hampei.* Actually, after years of experimentation and validation is likely to be patented and marketed a bioinsecticide obtained from the fruit species (López-Olguin et al., 1997; López-Olguin et al., 1998; López-Olguin et al., 2002).

The National Autonomous University of Mexico there is also consolidated groups of researchers in this area. The Department of Naural Products Chemistry Institute have among their line of validation of natural products with antifeedant and insecticidal activity, particularly plant species of the Labiatae, Burseraceae and Verbenaceae family. Have evaluated the activity of the purified active compounds are present in species such as *Vitex hemsleyi.* The tests were done in neonate larvae of *S. frugiperda* (Villegas *et al.,* 2009). In the Faculty of Sciences, is studying the antifeedant activity of plant extracts from *Acacia cornigera, Bursera* species and some species of Solanaceae, the evaluations are performed on neonate larvae of *S. frugiperda,* and is also looking for alternatives to control *Boophilus microplus.*

Northern Sierra of Oaxaca, community groups have received government support for production to tomatoes and other vegetables, have been advised by engineers and technician from the Institute of Technology in the Oaxaca Valley, the presence of whiteflies in the crop has been controlled with the use of extracts and infusions of garlic, onions, marigolds, basil, pepper, rue, chamomile, and others, the advantages are clear as reduces the investment cost and the food product developed under the organic system can be sold at higher prices.

In the highlands of Chiapas cultivation of cabbage (*Brassica oleracea*) is of economic importance are usually affected mainly by the cabbage worm *Leptophobia aripa elodia* to control in these communities have used synthetic pesticides, to reduce costs, health problems and pollutation, El Colegio de la Frontera Sur has sought alternative biological control. This region has recorded around 1650 medicinal plant species, however, there are no studies on the effect of extracts of these species at different developmental stage of *L. aripa elodia,* a situation that prompted the selection of 15 wild species of insecticidal activity history ethnobotanical and medicinal use. The results showed no significant activity on *L. aripa elodia* although some of the species tested showed activity against *Locussta migratoria* and *Trichoplusia ni,* therefore should continue investigating the potential of these species in pest management (Ramírez-Moreno, et al., 2001). There has also been collecting traditional knowledge of indigenous Tzeltal farmers of Chiapas highlands, on the management of agricultural pests (ants, *Phyllophaga* spp., *S. frugiperda, Doru taeniatum, Diphaulaca wagnerii* y *L. Aripa elodia*) four of the most common crops in the region, this led to the evaluation of the sensitivity of these pest species and 64 medicinal wild plants belonging to the basic list of useful plants from this ethnic group, the idea to promote local and regional control ecological these pests (Trujillo-Vázquez & García-Barrios, 2001).

In the Biological Control Laboratory, Biotechnology Research Center, of the Autonomous University of Morelos State (UAEM), for 15 years under the initial coordination of Dr. Eduardo Aranda Escobar+, we have developed the research of plant extracts with biological activity on insect pests. Most plants have been collected in the State of Morelos, many of which have pharmacological properties (Table 4). Among the species tested include the genus *Ipomoea* (Convolvulaceae) bioassays have been done on *S. frugiperda* y *Bemisia tabaci* at different stages and we have observed different biological activities of the extracts, some *Ipomoeas* cause lethal toxicity against larvae and nymphs between 2-100% mortality (*I. carnea, I. pauciflora, I. intrapilosa, I. cuernavacensis, I. murucoides*), others cause decrease in weight of the larvae of *S. frugiperda* between 90-15% reduction (*I. murucoides, I. carnea* e *I. pauciflora*) and others affect the life cycle (*I. carnea*: cause malformation of pupae and adult difficulty to emerge, *I. pauciflora*: prolonged pupal development time). We also conducted tests on the establishment *in vitro* of Ipomoeas with potential, as an option to develop biotechnological technique for various purposes; one is to optimize the use of phytocompounds responsible for biological activity on insect pests (Toledo, 2001; Aguirre, 2008; Gaona, 2009; Vera et al., 2009; Guzmán-Pantoja et al., 2010).

Although they are abundant records of plants with insecticidal potential, before recommending its use should be tested for biosafety and formulation, it is important to the safety of these products in non-target species and the health of domestic animals and humans. Although most species with a history of drug use in communities has an apparent safety backup, remember the legacy of Paracelsus (1567) "the dose makes the poison". Another factor to consider is the stock of plants because it could jeopardize the survival of these species in the ecological environment, in this regards is necessary to implement strategies for the compounds responsible for biological activity according to the phenological stage of the plant and seasonality is needed to establish the dates of collection and, if possible, establish community gardens for intensive planting of these plants with potential insecticide would have continuous availability of phytoinsecticides.

8. References

Aguilar C.A., Martínez A.M.A. (1993). Los herbarios medicinales de México. En: La investigación científica de la herbolaria medicinal mexicana. Secretaría de Salud (Ed.), México, pp. 89-102.

Aguirre, M.A. (2008). Actividad insecticida de tejidos callogénicos de *Ipomoea murucoides* (Roem. Et Schult) (Convolvulaceae), sobre *Spodoptera frugiperda* (Lepidoptera: Noctuidae). Tesis de maestría. Centro de Investigación en Biotecnología. Universidad Autónoma del Estado de Morelos. Cuernavaca, Morelos, México, 60 p.

Aldana, L.L., Hernández, R.M. & Gutiérrez, O.M. (2007). Evaluación en vivero de extractos de tres especies de *Lupinus* sobre gusano cogollero *Spodoptera frugiperda* (Lepidoptera: Noctuidae). *Procceding of* X Congreso Internacional de Ciencias Agrícolas. Mexicali B. C., México.

Aldana, L.L., Hernández, R. M. & Gutiérrez, O.M. (2008). Efecto de polvos y extractos vegetales sobre *Scyphophorus acupunctatus* plaga del nardo y agave, *Procceding of XI Congreso Internacional de Ciencias Agrícolas Mexicali*, Baja California, México, 2008.

Aldana, L.L., Hernández, R.M. & Gutiérrez, O.M. (2008). Efecto de *Prosopis laevigata* sobre *Spodoptera frugiperda* plaga del maíz. 2008. *Procceding of* VII Congreso Internacional, XIII Congreso nacional de Ciencias Ambientales. Cd. Obregón, Sonora, México, 2008.

Aldana, L.L., Salinas, S.D., Valdés, E.M., Gutiérrez, O. M. & Valladares, C.M. (2010). Evaluación bioinsecticida de extractos de *Bursera copallifera* (D.C.) Bullock y *Bursera grandifolia* (Schltdl) Engl. en gusano cogollero *Spodoptera frugiperda* J.E. Smith (LEPIDOPTERA:NOCTUIDAE). *Polibotánica*, 29:149-158.

Ayala, O.J. (1985). Evaluación de sustancias vegetales contra el gusano cogollero del maíz *Spodoptera frugiperda* (J. E. Smith) (Lepidoptera: Noctuidae). *Tesis de Maestría en Ciencias*. Colegio de Posgraduados. *Chapingo*. México.

Billker, O., Shaw, M. K., Jones, I. W., Ley, S. V., Mordue A. J. & Sinden R.E. (2002) Azadirachtin disrupts formation of organised microtubule arrays during microgametogenesis of *Plasmodium berghei*. *Journal Eukaryotic Microbiology*, 49 (6): 489-497.

Boeke, S., Baumgart, I., van Loon, A.J., van Huis, M., Dicke & Kossou, D. (2004). Toxicity and repellence of African plants traditionally used for the protection of stored cowpea against Callosobruchus maculatus. *Journal of Stored Products Research*, 40(4):423-438.

Bye, R. & Linares, E. (1999). Plantas medicinales del México prehispánico. *In*: *Arqueología mexicana*, Vol. VII, Núm. 39. México. pp. 4-13.

Caballero, J. & Cortés, L. (2001). Percepción, uso y manejo tradicional de los vegetales en México. *In*: Rendón-Aguilar, B., Rebollar-Domínguez, S., Caballero-Nieto, J. y Martínez-Alfaro, M. A. (eds), *Plantas, cultura y sociedad estudio sobre la relación entre seres humanos y plantas en los albores del siglo XXI*, pp. 79-100. Universidad Autónoma Metropolitana-Iztapalapa y Secretaría del Medio Ambiente, Recursos Naturales y Pesca, pp. 315, ISBN: 970-654-782-7, México, D. F.

Camarillo, G., Ortega L., Serrato, M. & Rodríguez, C. (2009). Actividad biológica de Tagetes filifolia (Asteraceae) en Trialeurodes vaporariorum (Hemiptera:Aleyrodidae). *Revista Colombiana de Entomología* 35(2):177-184

Carballo, M. & Quiroga, R. (1986). Evaluación de extractos vegetales para el combate del gusano cogollero *Spodoptera frugiperda* (J. E. Smith) en villaflores, Chiapas. *XXI Congreso Nacional de Entomología*. Monterrey, Nuevo León, México, p. 134.

Céspedes, C., Calderón, J., Lina, L. & Aranda, E. (2000). Growth inhibitory effects on fall armyworm *Spodoptera frugeperda* of some limonoids isolated from *Cedrela* spp. (Meliaceae). *Journal Agricola Food Chemistry*, 48:1903-1908.

Céspedes, C., Rodrigo, Salazar J., Martínez, M. & Aranda, E. (2005). Insect growth regulatory effects of some extracts and sterols from Myrtillocactus geometrizans (Cactaceae) against Spodoptera frugiperda and Tenebrio molitor. *Phytochemistry*, 66:2481-2493.

CONABIO. (2009). *Malezas de México*. Heike, V. (ed.), retrieved from http://www.conabio.gob.mx.

Dayane, F.E., Cantrell, C.L. & Duke, S.O. (2009). Natural products in crop protection. *Bioorganic and Medicinal Chemistry*, 17: 4022-4034.

De la Torre, A. (2008). Agricultura sustentable en comunidades de la Sierra Norte de Oaxaca. Hernández M. (ed), *In: Manual de capacitación para la participación comunitaria*, pp. 31, México.

Dev, S. & Koul, O. 1997. *Insecticides of Natural Origin*. Harwood Academic Publishers The Netherlands. pp. 365

Evans D.A., Raj R.K. (1991). Larvicidal efficacy of quassin against Culex quinquefasciatus. Indian Journal Medical Research, 93: 324–327.

Felton, G.W. & Tumlinson, J.H. (2008). Plant–insect dialogs: complex interactions at the plant–insect interface. *Current Opinion in Plant Biology*, 11:457–463.

Franco, A.S., Jiménez, P.A., Luna, L.C. & Figueroa, B.R. (2006). Efecto tóxico de semillas de cuatro variedades de *Carica papaya* (Caricaceae) en *Spodoptera frugiperda* (Lepidoptera:Noctuidae). *Folia Entomológica Mexicana*, 45(2): 171-177.

Gaona, H.M. (2009). Actividad biológicas de extractos de *Ipomoea carnea* (Jacq.) sobre *Spodoptera frugiperda* Smith (Lepidóptero: Nuctuidae). Tesis de Licenciatura en Biología. Facultad de Ciencias Biológicas. Universidad Autónoma del Estado de Morelos, México, pp. 140

García, A. J., Verde, S. M. & Heredia, N. (2001). Traditional uses and scientific knowledge of medicinal plants from Mexico and Central America. *Journal of herbs, Spices & Medicinal Plants*, 8:37-89

García, M. R., Pérez, P. R., Rodríguez, H. C. & Soto, H. M. (2004). Toxicidad de alcaloides de *Erythrina americana* en larvas de mosquito *Culex quinquefasciatus*. *Revista Fitotecnia Mexicana*, 27(4):297-303

Gaugler, R. (1997). Alternative paradigms for comercializing biopesticides *Phytoparasitica* 25(3):179-182.

Gómez-Pompa, A. 2010. Las raíces de la etnobotánica. *Acta Biologica Panamensis*, 1: 87-100.

Gómez, M.A. (2004). La agricultura en México y en el mundo. CONABIO. *Biodiversitas*, 55: 13-15.

Gómez, C.M, Rindermann, R.S., Gómez, T.L., Arce, C.I., Morán, V.Y. & Quiterio, M.M. (2001). *Agricultura orgánica de México. Datos básicos*. Centro de Estadística Agropecuaria de la Secretaría de Agricultura, Ganadería, Desarrollo Rural, Pesca y Alimentación (SAGARPA), Centro de Investigaciones Económicas, Sociales y Tecnológicas de la Agroindustria y la Agricultura Mundial (CIESTAAM) de la Universidad Autónoma Chapingo (UACH). 2da. edición. México, D.F. 45 p.

Golob, P., Moss, C., Dales, M., Fidgen, A., Evans J. & Gudrups, I. (1999). The use of spices and medicinals as bioactive protectants for grains. *Food and Agriculture Organization of the United Nations Rome BULLETIN No.* 137, pp. 158, FAO, Viale delle Terme di Caracalla, 00100, ISBN 92-5-104294-2, Rome, Italy.

González, G.O. 1986. Evaluación de métodos tecnificados y no tecnificados para el combate del gusano cogollero del maíz *Spodoptera frugiperda* (J. E. Smith) y del gorgojo del maíz (*Sitophilus zeamais* (Motsch) en la Chontalpa, Tabasco, México. *Tesis de Maestría en Ciencias*. Colegio Superior de Agricultura Tropical, Cárdenas, Tabasco.

Grainge, M. & Ahmed, S. (1988). *Handbook of plants with pest control*. John Wiley. & Sons, New York, N.Y. 469.

Grainge, M., Ahmed, S., Mitchell, W.C. & Hylin, J.W. (1985). Plant species reportedly possessing pest-control properties-An. EWC/UH Database, pp. 1-249, *Resource Systems Institute*. ISBN: 0866380647, Honolulu and University of Hawaii, USA.

Guzmán-Pantoja L.E., Guevara-Fefer P., Villarreal O.M., León R. I., Aranda E.E., Martínez, P.R., Hernández, V.V. 2010. Biological activity of *Ipomoea pauciflora* Martens and Galeotti (Convolvulaceae) extracts and fractions on larvae of *Spodoptera frugiperda* J. E. Smith (Lepidoptera: Noctuidae). *African Journal of Biotechnology,* 9(24): 3659-3665, (June, 2010), ISSN 1684–5315.

Hasting, R.B. (1990). Medicinal legumes of México: Fabaceae, Papilionoideae, Part one. Econ. Bot, 44: 336-348.

Isman, BM. (1997). Neem and other botanical insecticides: barriers to comercialization. *Phytoparasitica,* 25(4):339-344.

Isman, BM. (1999). Neem and related natural products. Hall, F. & Menn,J.J. (eds), *In: Methods in Biotechnology,* Vol. 5: Biopesticides: Use and Delivery. Humana Press, Totowa . N.J. USA. p. 139-153.

Isman, M. B. (2006). Botanical insecticides, deterrents, and repellents in modern agriculture and an increasingly regulated world. *Annual Review of Entomology,* 51: 45–66.

Isman, M.B. (2008). Perspective botanical insecticide: for riche, for poorer. Pest Management Science, 64: 8-11.

Jackson, M.D. & Peterson, J.K. (2000). Sublethal effects of Resin Glycosides from the periderm of sweetpotato storage roots on *Plutella xylostella* (Lepidoptera: Plutellidae). *Journal of Economic Entomology,* 93 (2): 388-393.

Jiménez, C.M. & Rodríguez, H. C. (1990). Acción tóxica del piquerol A (terpeno) y sus derivados sobre larvas de *Culex quinquefasciatus, Aedes aegypti* y *Spodoptera frugiperda.* Resúmenes del II Simposio Nacional sobre sustancias vegetales y minerales en el combate de plagas. *Sociedad Mexicana de Entomología,* Oaxaca, México, p. 11.

Jiménez, C.F. & Villar, M.C. (1990). Utilización de dos especies de plantas con propiedades tóxicas, para el combate del gusano cogollero del maíz *Spodoptera frugiperda* (J. E. Smith) en el C.A.E.E.A., ciclo primavera-verano.1988. Resúmenes del II Simposio Nacional sobre sustancias vegetales y minerales en el combate de plagas. *Sociedad Mexicana de Entomología,* Oaxaca, México, p. 16.

Juárez-Flores B.I., Jasso-Pineda Y., Aguirre-Rivera J-R. & Jasso-Pineda I. (2010). Efecto de polvos de Asteráceas sobre el gorgojo del maíz (*Sitophilus zeamais* Motsch). *Polibotánica,* 30:123-135

Kumul, D. E. (1983). Búsqueda de plantas silvestres del Estado de Veracruz, con propiedades tóxicas contra gusano cogollero del maíz *Spodoptera frugiperda* J. E. Smith y mosquito casero (*Culex quinquefasciatus* Say). *Tesis profesional.* Departamento de Parasitología Agrícola. UACH, México, 76 p.

Kutchan, T. & Dixon, R.A. (2005). Physiology and metabolism Secondary metabolism: nature's chemical reservoir under deconvolution. *Current Opinion in Plant Biology,* 8: 227–229.

Lagunes, T. A, Domínguez, R. R. & Bermudes, V. L. (1982). Búsqueda de plantas nativas del Estado de México con propiedades tóxicas contra gusano cogollero, *Spodoptera frugiperda* J. E. Smith y mosquito casero, *Culex quinquefasciatus* Say. *Chapingo,* 7 (37):35-39.

Lagunes, T., Arenas, A., Arenas, L. & Rodríguez, H. C. (1984). Extractos acuosos y polvos vegetales con propiedades insecticidas. CONACyT-CO-UACH-INIA-DGSV. Centro de Entomología y Acarología, Colegio de Posgraduados, Chapingo, México.

Lagunes, T.A. & Rodríguez, H.C. (1989). Búsqueda de tecnología apropiada para el combate de plagas de maíz almacenado en condiciones rústicas. *Informe del proyecto CONACYT PTV/AI/NAL/85/3149. CONACYT-CP*, 150 P.

Llorente-Bousquets, J. & Osegueda, S. (2008). Estado del conocimiento de la biota en Capital natural de México. Vol I: *Conocimiento actual de la biodiversidad.* CONABIO, México, pp. 283-322.

López-Olguín, J., Budia, F., Castañera, P. & Viñuela, E. (1997). Actividad de *Trichilia havanensis* Jacq. (Meliazeae) sobre larvas de Spodoptera littoralis (Boisduval) (Lepidoptera: Noctuidae). *Boletín de Sanidad Vegetal Plagas,* 23: 3-10.

López, P, E. & Rodríguez, H. C. (1999). Actividad de la chilca *Senecio salignus* (Asteraceae) en el combate del gorgojo mexicano del frijol *Zabrotes subfasciatus* (Coleoptera: Bruchidae). Rodríguez, H. C. (ed.), *Procceding of* Memorias del Simposio Nacional sobre substancias vegetales y minerales en el combate de plagas. (5, 1999, Aguascalientes, México). p. 93-99.

López-Olguín, J., Adán, A., Ould-Abdallahi, E., Budia, F., Del Estal, P. & Viñuela, E. (2002). Actividad de *Trichilia havanensis* Jacq. (Meliazeae) en la mosca mediterranea de la fruta *Ceratitis capitata* (Diptera:Tephritidae). *Boletín de Sanidad Vegetal Plagas,* 28:299-306.

López, P, E. & Rodríguez, H. C. (2006). Actividad biológica de la raíz de *Senecio salignus* contra *Zabrotes subfasciatus* en frijol almacenado. *Agrociencia,* 41:95-102.

Machado, C.H. & Rodríguez, H.C. (1991). Toxicidad de *Hippocratea* spp (Hippocrateaceae) en larvas de *Culex quinquefasciatus, Aedes aegypti* (Diptera:Culicidae) y *S. frugiperda* (Lepidoptera: Noctuidae) en el laboratorio. Resúmenes del III Simposio Nacional sobre sustancias vegetales y minerales en el combate de plagas. *Sociedad Mexicana de Entomología,* Veracruz, México, p. 40.

Macías, F.A., Galindo, J.L. & Galindo, J.C. (2007). Evolution and current status of ecological phytochemistry. Phytochemistry, 68: 2917–2936.

Magaña, P. & Villaseñor, J. L. (2002). La flora de México, ¿se podrá conocer completamente?. *Ciencia,* 66: 24-26.

Martínez, P. S. (1983). Búsqueda de plantas medicinales con propiedades insecticidas contra el gusano cogollero *Spodoptera frugiperda* (J. E. Smith) (Lepidoptera: Noctuidae). *Tesis de licenciatura.* Depto. de parasitología agrícola. UACH, Chapingo, México, 83 p.

Martínez-Tomás, S., Pérez-Pacheco, R., Rodríguez Hernández, C., Ramírez-Valverde, G. & Ruíz-Vega, J. (2009). Effects of an aqueous extract of Azadirachta indica on the growth of larvae and development of pupae of Culex quinquefasciatus. *African Journal of Biotechnology,* 8(17): 4245-4250.

Miranda, F. 1952. *La Vegetación de Chiapas.* Ediciones del Gobierno del estado de Chiapas, pp.319, Tuxtla Gutiérrez, Chiapas, México.

Navarrete, A., Reyes, B., Sixto,C., Rodríguez, C. & Estrada E. (1991). Alfa-Sanshool principio activo larvicida de la corteza de *Zanthoxyllum liebmannianum* (ENGL.) P. Wilson. *Procceding of* Memorias del III Simposio Nacional sobre sustancias vegetales y minerales en el combate de plagas, p. 41, Veracruz, México.

Ortega, A. L. & Hernández, R. C. (1991). Evaluación en campo de polvos vegetales contra el gusano cogollero del maíz (Spodoptera frugiperda (J.E. Smith) (Lepidoptera: Noctuidae) en Tepetates, Veracrúz. *Procceding of* Memorias del tercer Simposium

Nacional sobre sustancias Vegetales y Minerales en el Combate de Plagas, Veracrúz, México. p. 1-5.

Ortega, A.L. & Rodríguez, H.C. (1991). Utilización de gordolobo *Gnaphalium inortatum* (Asteraceae) para la protección de maíz almacenado en condiciones rústicas. Resúmenes del III Simposio Nacional sobre sustancias vegetales y minerales en el combate de plagas. *Sociedad Mexicana de Entomología,* Veracruz, México, pp. 15-19.

Ortega, A.L., Rodríguez, H.C. & Tamayo, M.F. (1998). Extractos acuosos de Nim *Azadirachta indica* como alternativa de manejo de la mosquita blanca en el cultivo de tomate. Resumen del I Simposio Internacional y IV Nacional sobre sustancias vegetales y minerales en el combate de plagas. *Sociedad Mexicana de Entomología,* Acapulco, Gro., México, pp. 39-48.

Osuna, L.E. (2005). Uso del Neem para la elaboración artesanal de plaguicidas. *Folleto Técnico No. 10.* Ed. Instituto Nacional de Investigaciones Forestales, Agrícolas y Pecuarias, Centro de Investigación Regional del Noroeste, Campo Experimental Todos Santos, La Paz, B.C.S., México. pp. 32.

Pacheco, S. C., Villa, A. P., Rodríguez, H. C., Zamilpa, Á. A, Hernández, G. H. & Jiménez, P. A. (2009). Respuesta del picudo del agave *Scyphophorus acupunctatus* Gyll. hacia extractos hidroalcohólicos de higuerilla *Ricinus communis* L. *Procceding of* Quinto Congreso Estatal: La Investigación en el Posgrado. Universidad Autónoma de Aguascalientes. Aguascalientes, Ags. México.

Paéz, L.A. (1987). El uso de polvos vegetales e inertes minerales como una alternativa para el combate del gorgojo del maíz *Sitophilus zeamais* Mots. (Coleotera: Curculionidae) en maíz almacenado. *Tesis de Maestría.* Colegio de Postgraduados, Chapingo, México, 102 p.

Pedraza, F.J.J. & Albarrán, M.M. (1986). Utilización de sustancias acuosas vegetales para el combate del gusano cogollero del maíz *Spodoptera frugiperda* J.E. Smith (Lepidoptera: Noctuidae) en San Antonio del Rosario. Tlatlaya Estado de México. *Tesis de Licenciatura.* UAEM. Facultad de Ciencias Agrícolas, Cerillo, México.

Pereda-Miranda, R. & Bah, M. (2003). Biodynamic constituents in the Mexican morning glories: purgative remedies transcending boundaries. *Current Topics in Medicinal Chemistry,* 3: 111-131.

Pérez, H. M. A. (2001). Prólogo. *In:* Rendón, A. B., Rebollar, D. S., Caballero, N. J. y Martínez, A. M. (eds.), Plantas, cultura y sociedad estudio sobre la relación entre seres humanos y plantas en los albores del siglo XXI, pp. 7-11, Universidad Autónoma Metropolitana-Iztapalapa y Secretaría del Medio Ambiente, Recursos Naturales y Pesca, pp. 315, ISBN: 970-654-782-7, México, D. F.

Philogène, B. J., Regnault-Roger, C. & Vincent. C. (2003). Productos fitosanitarios insecticidas de origen vegetal: promesas de ayer y de hoy. *In:* C. Regnault-Roger, B. J. Philogène, C. Vincent (eds.), Biopesticidas de origen vegetal., Mundi Prensa. pp. 1-18, México.

Prakash, A. & Rao, J. (1997). *Botanical pesticides in agriculture.* Ed. Lewis Publishers, New York, USA, 461p.

Pushpalatha, E. & Muthukrishnan, J. Efficacy of two tropical plants extracts for the control of mosquitoes. *Journal of Applied Entomology,* 1999; 123: 369–73.

Ramírez-Moreno, L., García-Barrios, L., Rodríguez, C., Morales, H. & Castro, R. A. (2001). Evaluación del efecto insecticida de extractos de plantas sobre *Leptophobia aripa elodia*. *Manejo Integrado de Plagas*, 60:50-56.

Ramos, L. M., Pérez, G. S., Rodríguez, H. C., Guevara, F. P. & Zavala, S. M. (2010). Activity of *Ricinus communis* (Euphorbiaceae) against *Spodoptera frugiperda* (Lepidoptera:Noctuidae). *African Journal of Biotechnology*, 9(9): 1359-1365.

Rodríguez, H, C., Lagunes, T. A., Domínguez, R. R. & Bermúdez, V. L. (1982). Búsqueda de plantas nativas del Estado de México con propiedades tóxicas contra el gusano cogollero, Spodoptera exigua J.E. Smith, y mosquito casero, Culex quinquefasciatus Say. *Chapingo*, 37-38:35-39

Rodríguez, H.C. (1990). Actividad insecticida de cancerina (*Hippcratea excelsa*: Hippocrateaceae) en siete especies de insectos de importancia económica. Resúmenes del II Simposio Nacional sobre sustancias vegetales y minerales en el combate de plagas. *Sociedad Mexicana de Entomología*, Oaxaca, México, p. 10.

Rodríguez, H. C. (1990). Perspectivas del uso de plantas con propiedades insecticidas. *Procceding of* Memorias del Simposio Nacional sobre sustancias vegetales y minerales en el combate de plagas, (11, 1990, Oaxaca, México). p. 176-187.

Rodríguez, H.C. (1991). Evaluación en campo de polvos vegetales y minerales contra el gusano cogollero del maíz (*Spodoptera frugiperda* (J. E. Smith) (Lepidoptera: Noctuidae)) en Tepetates, Veracruz. Resúmenes del III Simposio Nacional sobre sustancias vegetales y minerales en el combate de plagas. *Sociedad Mexicana de Entomología*, Veracruz, México, p. 1.

Rodríguez, H. C. & Lagunes, T. A. (1992). Plantas con propiedades insecticidas; resultados de pruebas experimentales en laboratorio, campo y granos almacenados. *Agroproductividad* (México), 1:17-25.

Rodríguez, H. C. (1993). Fitoinsecticidas en el combate de insectos: Bases prácticas de la agroecología en el desarrollo centroamericano. *In:* Manejo de plagas en el sistema de producción orgánica. Guatemala, ALTERTEC/HELVETAS/ CLADES. p. 112-125, México.

Rodríguez, H. C. (1996). Recetas para el control de insectos. *In:* Control alternativo de insectos plaga. Rodríguez H, C. (ed), Colegio de Postgraduados and Fundación Mexicana para la educación ambiental, A.C. p. 46-51, Tepoztlán, Edo. de México, México.

Rodríguez, H. C. (1997). Insecticidas vegetales y agricultura orgánica. *In*: Evento de aprobación en certificación de agricultura orgánica. Colegio de Postgraduados. p. 162-179, Montecillo, México.

Rodríguez, H.C. (1999). El paraíso *Melia azedarach* (Meliaceae) como alternativa de manejo de plagas. *Avances en la investigación 1999*, Colegio de Postgraduados, Instituto de Fitosanidad, México, pp. 1-3.

Rodríguez, H. C. (2000). La higuerilla: una alternativa contra plagas. *Boletin de RAPAM*, 28: 7-11.

Rodríguez H, C., Lagunes, T,A., Domínguez, R. & Bermúdez, V.L. (1982). Búsqueda de plantas nativas del Estado de México con propiedades tóxicas contra el gusano cogollero, *Spodoptera exigua* J.E. Smith, y mosquito casero, *Culex quinquefasciatus* Say. *Revista Chapingo* 7 (37-38):35-39.

Rodríguez, H. C. & López, P. E. (2001). Actividad insecticida e insectistática de la chilca (*Senecio salignus*) sobre *Zabrotes subfasciatus*. *Manejo Integrado de Plagas*, 59:19-26.
Rodríguez, H. C. (2006). Plantas Contra Plagas 1. Potencial Práctico de Ajo, Anona, Nim, Chile y Tabaco. Ed. 30 Colegio de Post Graduados Red de Acción sobre plaguicidas y Alternativas en México (RAPAM) y Red de Acción en Plaguicidas y sus Alternativas para América Latina (RAP-AL). Texcoco, Edo. de México, México.
Rodríguez-López, V., Figueroa-Suárez M., Rodríguez T. & Aranda E. (2007). Insecticidal activity of *Vitex mollis*. *Fitoterapia*, 78:37-39.
Rodríguez, H, C. (2008). Alternativas para el manejo integrado de gorgojos en graneros rústicos. LEISA *revista de agroecología*, Marzo: 32-35.
Rodríguez, H.C. (2008). Opciones biorracionales para el manejo de plagas. In: *Manejo integrado de plagas*. Toledo J. & Infante F. (Eds). Ed Trillas. pp. 183-191.
Rodríguez, H. C. (2011). Curso básico para inspectores en agricultura orgánica. Celaya, Guanajuato, México. pp. 24.
Romo, O.J., Rodríguez, H.C. (1988). Combate d la conchuela del frijol *Epilachna varivestis* Muls. (Coccinellidae: Coleoptera) con extractos acuosos vegetales en Chango, Edo. de México. Resúmenes del *XXIII Congreso Nacional Entomología*. Morelia, Michoacán, México. p. 282.
Salehzadeh, A., Akhkha, A., Cushley, W., Adams, R.L.P., Kusel, J.R. & Strang, R.H.C. (2003). The antimitotic effect of the neem terpenoid azadirachtin on cultured insect cells. *Insect Biochemistry and Molecular Biology*, 33: 681–689.
Saxena, S.C. & Sumithra, L. (1985). Laboratory evaluation of leaf extract of a new plant to suppress the population of malaria vector Anopheles stephensi Liston (Diptera: Culicidae). *Current Science*, 54:201- 2.
Sengonca, C. & Brüggen, K.U. 1991. Untersuchungenüber die Wirkung wäßriger Extrakte aus Quassia amara (L.) auf Getreideblattlä use. *Jorunal of Applied Entomology*, 112, 211–215.
Scott, R.H., O'Brien, K., Roberts, L., Mordue, W. & Mordue, L. J. (1999). Extracellular and intracellular actions of azadirachtin on the electrophysiological properties of cultured rat DRG neurones. *Comp. Biochem. Physiol. C Pharmacol Toxicol Endocrin*, 123, 85–93.
Scott, I.M., Jensen, H., Scot, J.G., Isman, M.B., Arnason, J.T. & Philogèine, B. J. (2003). Botanical insecticides for controlling agricultural pests: Piperamines and the Colorado Potato Betle *Leptinotarsa decemlineata* Say (Coleoptera: Chysmelidae). *Archives of insect Biochemistry Physiology*, 54: 212-225.
SEMARNAT. (2011). URL: http://app2.semarnat.gob.mx/tramites/Doctos/DGGIMAR/Guia/07-015AD/riesgos.pdf.
Sengonca, C., Bru, S. A., Akhkha, A., Cushley, W., Adams, R.L., Kusel, J.R. & Strang, R.H. (2003). The antimitotic effect of the neem terpenoid azadirachtin on cultured insect cells. *Insect Biochemistry Moleculra Biology*, 33, 681–689.
Shaalan, E., Canyon, D., Faried, M.W., Abdel-Wahab, H. & Mansour, A. H. (2005). A review of botanical phytochemicals with mosquitocidal potential. *Environment International*, 31: 1149-1166.

Silva, A. G., Lagunes, T. A., Rodríguez, M. C. & Rodríguez, L. D. (2002). Insecticidas vegetales: una vieja y nueva alternativa para el manejo de plagas. *Manejo Integrado de Plagas y Agroecología*, (Costa Rica), 66: 4-1 2.

Singh, R.N. & Saratchandra, B. (2005). The development of botanical products with special reference to seri-ecosystem. *Caspian Journal of Environmental Sciences*, 3 (1): 1-8.

Siqueira, H., Alvaro, A., Guedes, Raul, N.C. & PicanÇo, M.C. (2000). Insecticide resistance in population of *Tuta absoluta* (Lepidoptera: Geleiidae). *Agricultural and Forest Entomology*, 2: 147-153.

Toledo, T.E. (2001). Propiedades insecticidas de algunas especies de *Ipomoea* (Convolvulaceae) del Estado de Morelos. Tesis de Licenciatura. Facultad de Estudios Superiores Iztacala. Universidad Nacional Autónoma de México. Edo. de México, México, pp. 51.

Trujillo, V. R., & García-Barrios, L. (2001). Conocimiento indígena del efecto de plantas medicinales locales sobre las plagas agrícolas de los altos de Chiapas, México. *Agrociencia*, 35(6):685-692.

Trysyono, A. & Whalon, M. (1999). Toxicity of neem applied alone and in combinations with *Bacillus thuringiensis* to Colorado potato beetle (Coleoptera: Chysomelidae). *Journal of Economic Entomology*, 92: 1281-1288.

Vera, C.L., Hernández, V.V., León, R.I., Guevara, F.P. & Aranda, E.E. (2009). Biological activity of methanol extracts of *Ipomoea murucoides* Roem et Schult on *Spodoptera frugiperda* J. E. Smith. *Journal of Entomology*, 6(29): 109-116.

Villavicencio-Nieto, M. A., Pérez- Escandón, B. E. & Gordillo-Martínez, A. J. (2010). Plantas tradicionalmente usadas como plaguicidas en el Estado de Hidalgo, México. *Polibotánica*, 30:193-238.

Villegas, E.S. (1989). Incorporación de *Hippocratea excelsa* (Hippocrateaceae) y cuatro polvos minerales en maíz encostalado para evitar el daño de insectos en Lerma, Estado de México. *Tesis de Licenciatura de Ingeniero Agrónomo*, Especialidad en Parasitología Agrícola. Universidad Autónoma Chapingo, Departamento de Parasitología Agrícola, México, 76 p.

Villegas, C., Martínez, V. M. & Baldomero, E. (2009). Antifeedant activity of anticopalic acid isolated from *Vitex hemsleyi*. *Journal of Biosciences*, 64:502-508.

Villanueva, J.J.A. (1988). Actividad biológicas de extractos acuosos de frutos vegetales sobre larvas de primer instar del gusano cogollero del maíz *Spodoptera frugiperda* (J. E. Smith) (Lepidoptera: Noctuidae), bajo condiciones de laboratorio. *Tesis profesional*. Departamento de Parasitología Agrícola-UACI I, Chapingo, México, 77 p.

Vyvyan, J.R. (2002). Allelochemicals as leads for news herbicides and agrochemicals. *Tetrahedron*,58: 1631-1646.

Vovides, A. P., Linares, E. & Bye, R. (2010). *Jardines botánicos de méxico: historia y perspectivas*. Ed. Secretaría de Educación de Veracruz del Gobierno del Estado de Veracruz de Ignacio de la Llave, pp. 232. ISBN: 978-607-7579-18-2, Veracruz, México.

Xing-An, C., Jian-Jun, Xie, Mei-Ying, Hu, Yan-Bo, Z. & Jing-Fei, H. (2011). Induction of Intracellular Ca2+ and pH Changes in Sf9 Insect Cells by Rhodojaponin-III, A Natural Botanic Insecticide Isolated from *Rhododendron molle*. *Molecule*, *16*: 3179-3196.

Wink, M. & Schimmer, O. (1999). Modes of action of defensive secondary metabolites. *In*: Michael Wink (ed.), Functions of plant secondary metabolites and their exploitation in biotechnology. *Annual Plant Reviews*, Vol. 3., Sheffield Academic Press LTD. p. 16-130, USA-Canada.

Weinzierl, R.A. (2000). Botanicals insecticides, soaps, and oils. *In*: Rechcigl J.E., Rechcigl, N.A. (ed.), Biological and Biotechnological Control of Insect Pests. CRC Press LLC. Boca Raton, Florida, p. 101–121, EE. UU.

Zaid, M. & Nozzolillo, C. (2000). 1-o- galloyl-L-rhamnose from A*cer rubrum*. *Phytochemistry*, 52: 1629-1361.

Part 2

Phytochemicals and Bioactive Compounds

4

Standardization of Herbal Drugs Derivatives with Special Reference to Brazilian Regulations

Wagner Luiz Ramos Barbosa[1] et al.*
[1]*Universidade Federal do Pará,*
Brazil

1. Introduction

The development of herbal medicine requires a careful selection and unambiguous identification of plant species that will be the exclusive active principle, either as extract or as fraction, embedded in the product. An isolated substance, even if obtained from natural sources, does not give rise to a phytomedicine.

The technical standardization of an intermediary of a phytomedicine is a decisive step for the quality standard that the product will show. After the validation of the alleged use, popular form of use, posology and agronomic certification of the plant material, for which phytochemical and pharmacognostic pattern will be developed to monitor the physical, chemical and physico-chemical characteristics of the plant, ensuring homogeneity of samples and the similarity to specimens tested in experimental stage. The plant material is then extracted and the obtained extract is used in the development of the formulation. This extract must be in accordance to the Brazilian Pharmacopoeia, respecting as far as possible the characteristics of the popular form of use. Before the next step, the pharmacotechnical handling, the extract will be phytochemically analysed, in order to determine the metabolic substance classes present in the sample. Then it must be pharmacologically investigated to assure that its activity, is similar to that originally alleged and experimentally tested; its physical and physico-chemical characteristics will be determined, and, subsequently, the extract undergoes chemical and chromatographic analysis to have identified substances that could characterize the plant and serve as chemical and, preferably, pharmacological quality markers. Substances which are chemically stable, responsible for the activity to be presented by the phytomedicine and able to be detectable and quantifiable by usual analytical methods, such as chromatography and ultraviolet spectroscopy or mass spectrometry, are potential candidates to be used as markers.

To compose a pharmacopoeial monography of a medicinal plant it is recommended to describe the characteristics concerning the anatomy of organelle or tissues of the plant organ to be notified or from which a medicine will be developed. These structures of the herbal

* Lucianna do Nascimento Pinto[1], Luiz Cláudio Silva Malheiros[1], Patricia Miriam Sayuri Sato Barros[1], Christian Barbosa de Freitas[1], Jose Otavio Carrera Silva Junior[1], Sandra Gallori[2] and Franco Francesco Vincieri[2]
[1]*Universidade Federal do Pará, Brazil*
[2]*Università degli Studi di Firenze, Italy*

drug can be observed in microscopic anatomical analysis and can be depicted as a micrography which is the document to be added to the monography.

2. Microscopic anatomical description of leaves of *Echinodorus macrophyllus*

The information produced from these analyses helps to standardize the raw material utilized in the production of a phytomedicine, this is illustrated by the anatomical description of leaves of *Echinodorus macrophyllus* which is used to produce several phytotherapeutical products in Brazil. To obtain the anatomical slices the dried plant material was rehydrated for 24h in distilled water and sectioned with stainless steel blade in different regions of the leaf and midrib. The sections were clarified in 20% NaClO and stained with Astra blue and basic fuchsin (MACHADO et al., 1988).

Fractographs were obtained in light microscope Axiolab model ZEISS coupled to a Canon Power Shot model A640 digital camera for registration of anatomical characters. The electron micrographs of the material were prepared using the process of critical point and metallization with gold dust deposition and suitably organized in circular metal holders (stubs), the images were captured in the scanning electron microscope model LEO 1450 VP (KRAUS & ARDUIN, 1997).

The following figures show the photographs of the cuts obtained by optical microscopy at the referred enlargement (10X or 40X). The leaf shows discrete epicuticular wax deposition of granulation aspect. In frontal view, the epidermal cells on both sides, adaxial and abaxial, are irregularly shaped, ranging from square and rectangular, with tiny and slightly sinuous walls. In transverse section the epidermis of both surfaces are uniseriate, with rectangular cells with flat anticlinal and periclinal walls; they are heterodimensional (Figure 1).

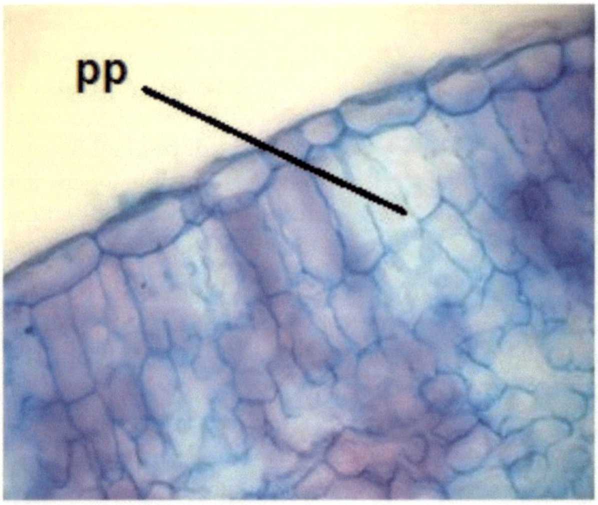

Fig. 1. Transverse section of leaf showing the upper epidermis and palisade parenchyma (pp) in frontal view (40X).

The parenchyma is dorsiventral, consisting generally of two strata of homogeneous cells, slightly Sinuous anticlinal and smooth periclinal walls the first layer being more organized, with cells elongated, juxtaposed and perpendicular to the epidermis; the second layer palisade tissue consists of cells of the same format, but different in size, apparently less than the first. The cells of spongy parenchyma present thin walls, are heterodimensional showing different formats, in addition to well-developed intercellular spaces (Figure 2).

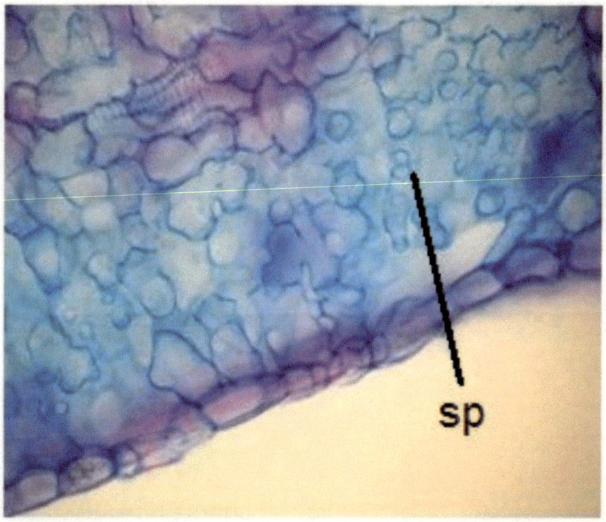

Fig. 2. Transverse section of the leaf showing the lower epidermis with sinuous anticlinal walls and spongy parenchyma (sp) (40X).

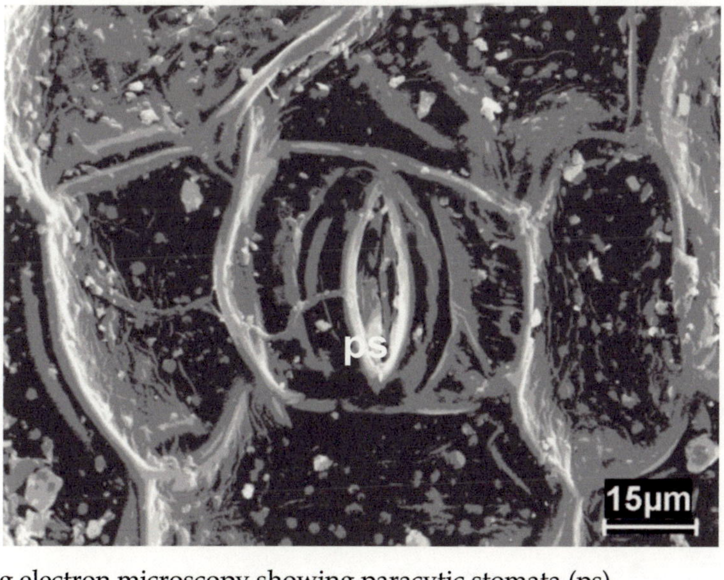

Fig. 3. Scanning electron microscopy showing paracytic stomata (ps).

In the parenchyma paracytic stomata can be observed, where stomatal complex is formed by a pair of lateral subsidiary cells connected to the guard cells, corroborating the description made by Tomlinson (1982). Picture obtained by electronic microscopy (Figure 3).

The vascular bundles have xylem at the upper face and phloem occurring at the opposite side, in polar regions cells of sclerenchyma can be seen. This set appears enclosed in a sheath of parenchyma.

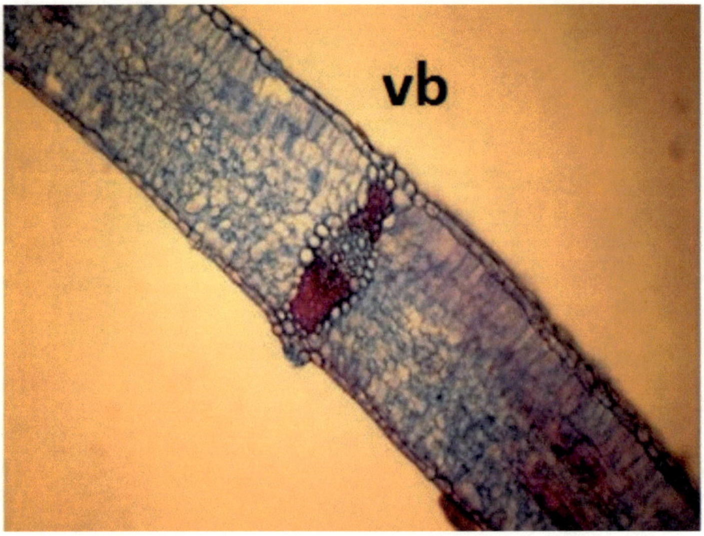

Fig. 4. Transverse section of leaf showing vascular bundle (vb) (10X).

The next figures show the transverse section of a petiole, which exhibits triangular to hexagonal shape, anatomically resembling the petiole of *Sagittaria lancitolia,* also an Alismataceae (TOMLINSON, 1982) (Figure 5).

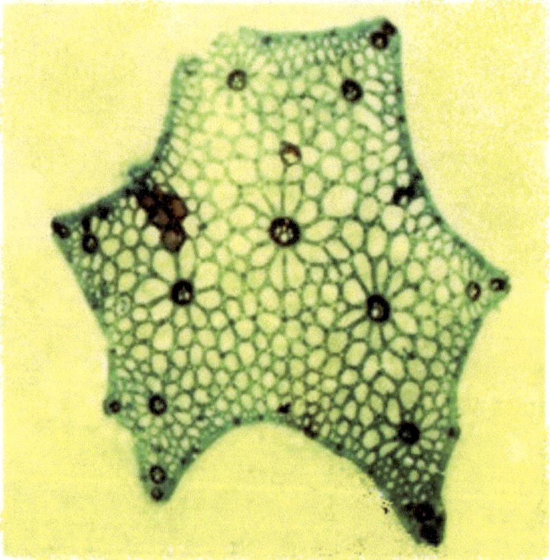

Fig. 5. Transverse section of petiole showing the hexagonal shape (10X).

Figure 6 displays a thin cuticle, showing a uniseriate epidermis, with polygonal shaped cells, and smooth walls. Reference to this format of petiole in this species has already been made by Matias (2007).

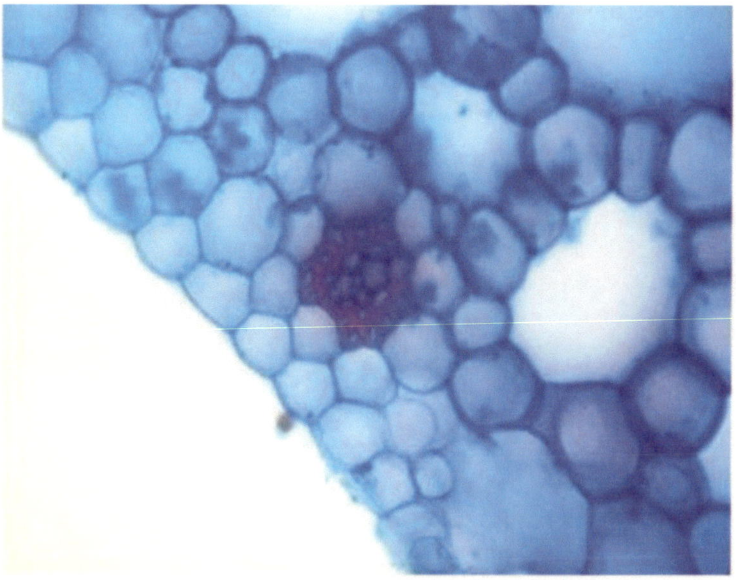

Fig. 6. Transverse section of petiole showing the epidermis (40X).

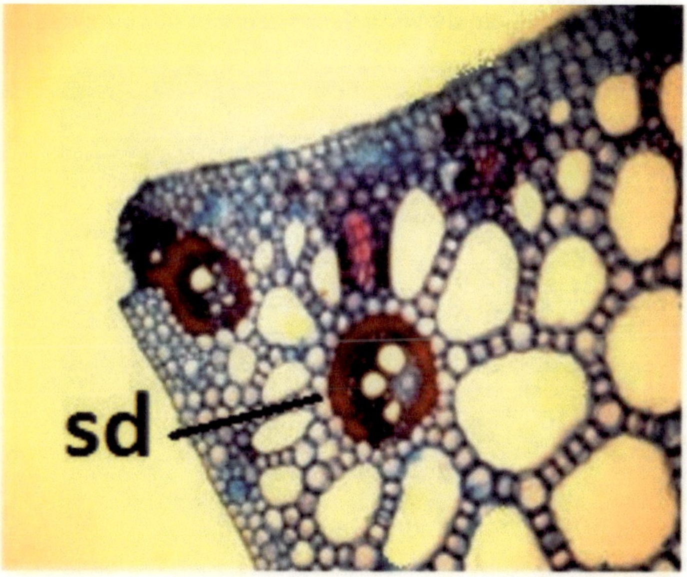

Fig. 7. Transverse section of the petiole highlighting the presence of secretory ducts (sd) (10X).

The figure 7 shows that the petiole has two to three layers of compact parenchyma cells, in which secretory ducts are to see as well vascular bundles that have smaller diameter than the ones observed in the leaf's parenchyma. This plant organ presents a great amount of parenchyma formed by a layer of isodiametric parenchyma cells, where bundles of different sizes are distributed, as seen in the figure.

In the parenchyma of the petiole diaphragms can be observed (Figures 8 and 9). These structures are septate braciform cells that interrupt the existing intercellular spaces, preventing the collapse of the organ if there is an injury in the submerged part of the plant. Leite (2007) describes in less detail this structure.

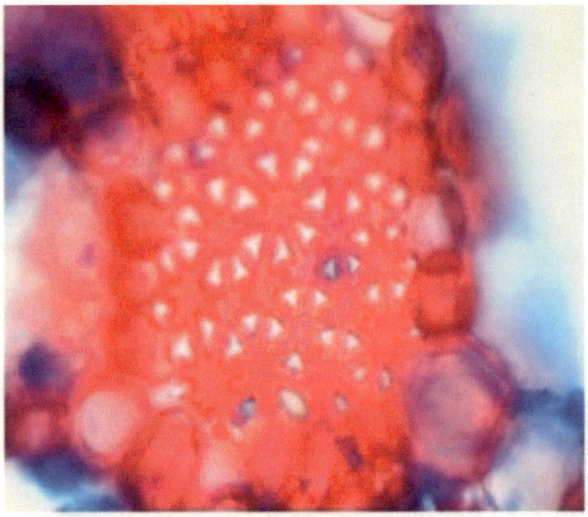

Fig. 8. Transverse section of petiole showing the presence of diaphragms. 40X.

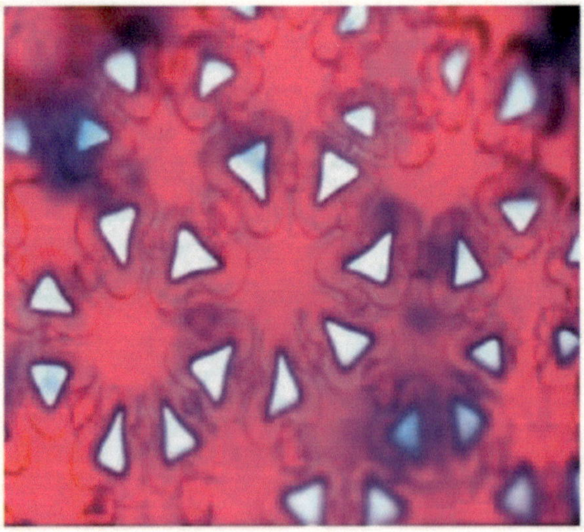

Fig. 9. Details of diaphragms in a higher enlargement (100X).

The presence, in the analysed sample, of petioles with different sizes and shapes could also be observed. Figure 10 illustrates this observation since the shape of the organ differs from that showed in figure 5. The characteristic of the petiole here presented, according to Matias

(2007), seems closely similar to that from *E. subalatus* and *E. palaefolius*, indicating a possible introduction of parts of one of these species in the commercial sample, object of this study.

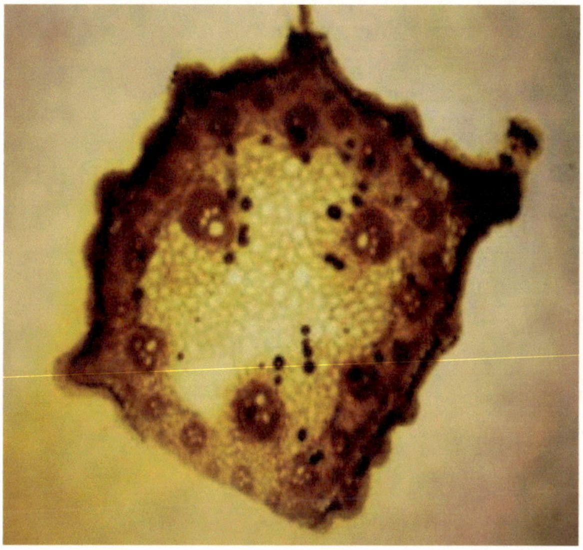

Fig. 10. Transverse section of a petiole showing a shape different from that already described (10X).

As a conclusion about the results here presented it could be assumed that the raw material to be used in the production of a phytomedicine must be analysed by microscopic anatomical techniques to ensure the identity of the species here in question. More specifically, although most of the fragments analysed can be attributed to *Echinodorus macrophyllus*, there is the possibility that fragments of petiole from *E. subalutus* and *E. palaefolius* were introduced in the material supplied for the work reported in this section. Anyway, it is important to note that for the production of herbal medicines based on *E. macrophyllus*, the part used is the leaf, where the chemical markers and the possible active principles are present, which this feature can threaten the credibility of the medicines prepared having a medicinal plant as active pharmaceutical matter.

Once the raw material is anatomically characterized, in case of the development of a phytomedicine, a set of procedures is followed, which includes processing of plant material providing the herbal drug, that is used to obtain an extract, both drug and extract, are physically and physico-chemically analysed. Afterwards, or simultaneously, this extract undergoes the next steps in developing the proposed medicine, where chemical markers, or rather, pharmacological active markers, must be detected, characterized and quantified in the herbal drug derivative - a tincture, for instance.

3. Characterization of potential markers for an *Eleutherine* species using TLC, LC-DAD e NMR

The following case illustrates the characterisation of pro-oxidizing components found in an *Eleutherine* species (Iridaceae) that presents an excellent anti-protozoan activity in its extract. The substances belong to a class of metabolites which is easily detectable and quantifiable by hyphenated techniques like LC-DAD. A tincture prepared from this medicinal plant was phytochemically investigated and provided two components which have been characterized by LC-DAD and by NMR. As the substances have this biochemical characteristic, induce oxidative stress, which allows combating microorganisms and protozoa, and can support the use of the plant as antiprotozoal agent, they can be used as markers for derivatives and products derived from this species.

In attention to Brazilian regulation the marketing of herbal drugs for use in the form of tea, the phytochemical approach of an extract obtained from the medicinal plant in question and its chloroform fraction was performed and shows the presence of naphthoquinones.

Metabolic class	Crude extract	Chloroform
Steroids & Triterpenoids	+	+
Azulen	+	+
Reducer Sugars	+	-
Anthraquinones	+	+
Naphthoquinones	+	+

Table 1. Metabolic classes detected by phytochemical analysis.

The lyophilized chloroform fraction prepared from the tincture, was used in a sequence of chromatographic experiments performed using normal phase silica gel column chromatography and preparative Thin Layer Chromatography - TLC, with chloroform and acetone as mobile phase and with an 10% ethanolic solution of KOH for TLC monitoring of the separation and isolation of the naphthoquinones. The characterisation of the substances was achieved by comparison of the ^{1}H e ^{13}C NMR spectra of them with the spectra of substances already isolated from other species of Eleutherine

Still in compliance with the Brazilian standards for herbal drugs (BRASIL, 2010), TLC analyses were conducted aiming to establish the chromatographic profile of the crude extract (EE), Hexan Fraction (HF) and the Chloroform Fraction (CF), and thus contribute to the quality control of drugs and their derivatives. Figure 10, observed under visible light, shows two zones of yellow color at Rfs 0.31 and 0.25, and pink areas at 0.44 pink Rf 0.62, both in EE and CF.

When the chromatogram is observed under ultraviolet light at 254 nm, three absorption zones in EE and CF can be observed with the following retention factor (Rf) 0.25 and 0.31 0.44, respectively. The chromatograms, after treatment with a 10% KOH methanolic solution, which is the spray reagent to detect quinones in the sample, show brownish coloured zones at Rf 0.25, 0.31 and 0.44 when observed under day light, this feature indicates the presence of naphthoquinones (WAGNER; BLAT .2001) in EE and CF.

Naftoquinones are chemical compounds that present biological activities such as bactericide, fungicide, giardicide and amebicide and in recent years have aroused interest in the medicinal chemistry because they can induce oxidative stress, causing apoptosis (cell death) via topoisomerase inhibition (ANAZETTI; MELO, 2007). The isolated naftoquinones had their antioxidant capacity evaluated through the reaction with 2.2-diphenyl-1-picrilhidrazil (DPPH. +) a stable free radical. The reaction was monitored by colour change and the

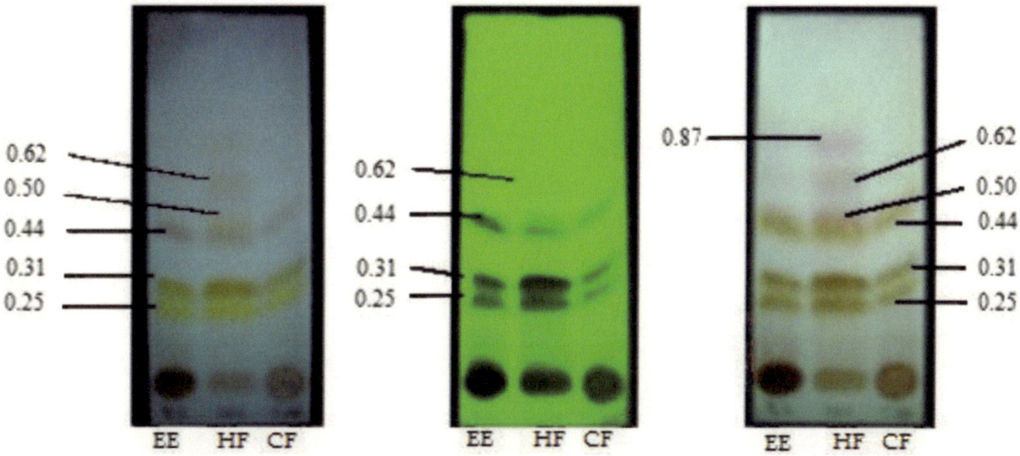

Fig. 11. Chromatograms obtained on normal sílica gel using as eluent Chloroform/Aceton 99:1. From left: observed under visible light; b) ultraviolet light by 254 nm, and c) after treatment with 10% metanolic KOH.

activity was measured by absorbance decrease of the sample measured at 517nm in relation to the corresponding blank (BLOIS, 1958).

In order to verify the suitability of the substances to function as quality markers, the chromatographic profile of chloroform fraction and ethanolic extract was determined by High Performance Liquid Chromatography. To accomplish this task a Merck Hitachi® LaChrom7000 chromatographic system equipped with a diode array detector (DAD) was employed. The analysis were performed on a Agilent LiChrospher100 (250mmx 4.6 mm) column using ultra purified water (A) and acetonitrile (B) as mobile phase, which was pumped at 1.0mL/min., in gradient, starting with 15% of B during 10 minutes, followed by periods of 10 minutes by 30%, 50% and 80%. The detection range was set between 200nm and 400 nm, using the method developed by Paramapojn et al (2008), adapted to our sample conditions.

The chromatogram of EE registered at 250nm presented two peaks (Ep1 and Ep2) of high intensity with Rt=18.93min. and 20.83min., areas of 45854675 and 60180902 and purity of 99.97% and 99.72% (fig. 12).

The chromatogram of the chloroform fraction presents as more intense peaks those with Rt of 19.12min. (Ep2) and 21.18min. (Ep1), areas of 1900571 and 7813739 and purity of 98.29% and 99.75, respectively, (Fig. 13).

Substances Ep1 and Ep2 were analysed by HPLC under the same conditions as EE and CF, and showed peaks at Rt of 18.13min. and 21.71 min., areas of 3641711 and 24727851 and purity around 99.14% and 99.92% respectively. Using the reversed search function where recorded data are compared to others stored in the equipment library, it could be observed that peaks 01 in EE (fig. 12) and CF (fig. 13) present a similarity correlation of 97.40% and 99.89%, respectively, to substance Ep2. The peaks 02 in EE (fig. 12) and CF (fig. 13) showed correlation of 99.84% and 99.98% to substance Ep1.

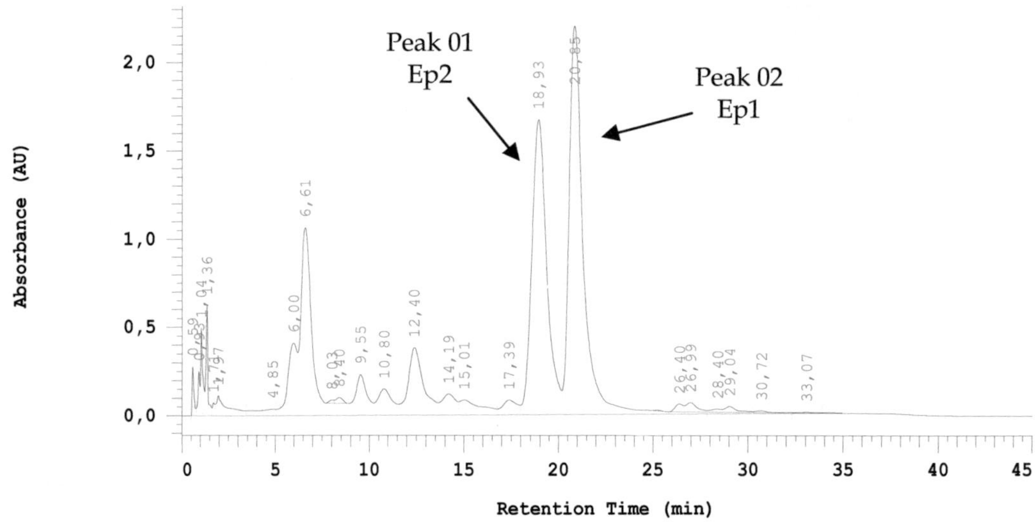

Fig. 12. CLAE - Chromatogram registered at 250nm from EE.

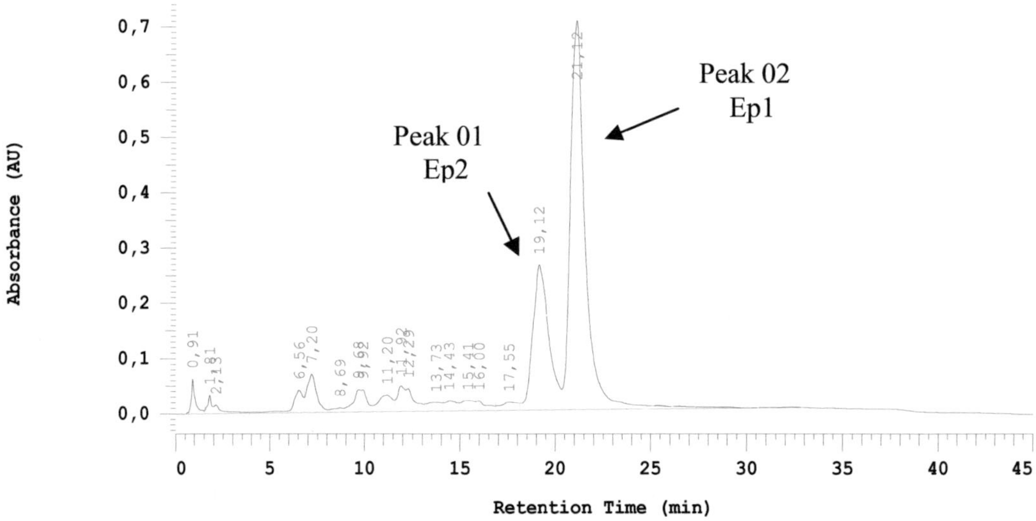

Fig. 13. HPLC - Chromatogram obtained from the Chloroform Fraction, registered at 250nm.

The detection of these substances by LC-DAD is based on diode arrangement and generates a diagram showing retention time, wavelength and absorbance as the three dimensions considered in the picture, which evidence the resolution of the chromatogram in the region where the two naphthoquinones are eluted (Figure 14).

3.1 Characterization of substance Ep1 as isoeleutherol

The Hydrogen Nuclear Magnetic Resonance spectrum obtained from Ep1 shows at δ= 1.74ppm a duplet, due to a coupling with H-1, corresponding to three equivalents Hydrogen atoms from the Methyl group at C-1 in the furan ring. H-1 (δ 5.72ppm) couples with the

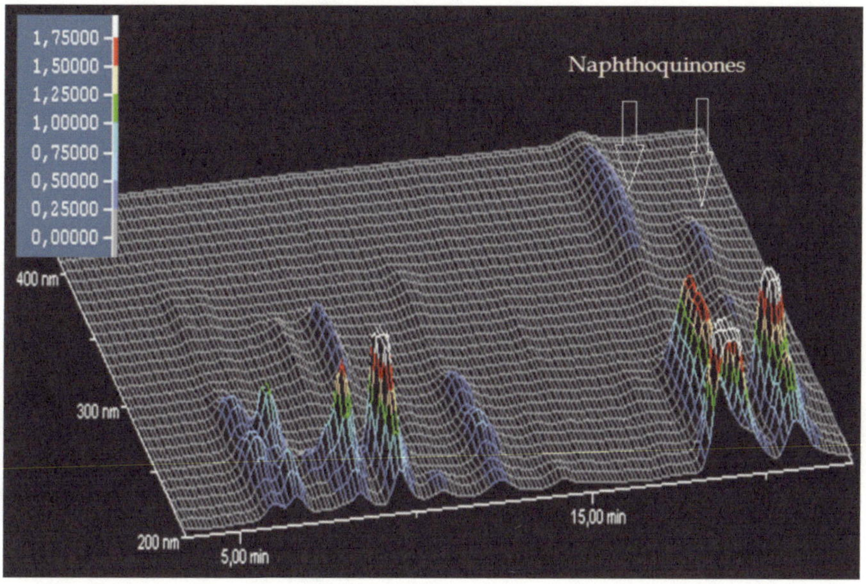

Fig. 14. Chromatographic diagram showing the chemical constituents of EE. In detail the two isolated naphthoquinones and the absorbance scale.

three Methyl Hydrogen atoms and produces a quadruplet. Furthermore four non equivalent aromatic Hydrogen atoms, *e. g.* H-4, H-6, H-7 and H-8 (Fig. 15) can also be observed. H-4 appears as a singlet by δ= 7.86ppm, H-5 (δ= 6.93ppm) couples with H-6 (δ= 7.40ppm) giving rise to a duplet, H-6 besides the coupling with H-5 also couples with H-7 (δ= 7.54ppm) originating a signal like a superposed double duplet or false triplet, H-7 couples with H-6 and produces a duplet. The Hydrogen atoms from the Methoxyl group at C-8 (δ= 4.11ppm) appears as a singlet. Finally a phenolic Hydrogen atom generates a singlet at δ= 9.64.

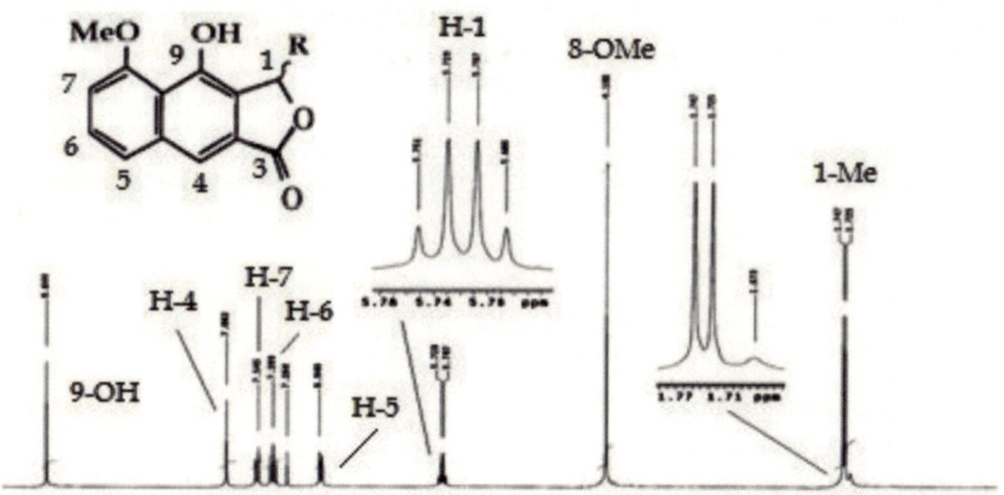

Fig. 15. ^{1}HNMR spectrum of Isoeleutherol.

The ^{1}HNMR data registered for Isoeleutherol isolated from *Eleutherine americana* MERR. et HEYNE by Hara et al (1997), agrees with that obtained from the substance here described as Ep1, in consequence we can affirm that Ep1 is Isoeleutherol and this is the first report of the occurrence of this substance in the *E. plicata* Herb

Hydrogen Atom	Ep1 δ(ppm)	Isoeleutherol δ(ppm)	Multiplicity	J (Hz)
1-Me	1.74	1.73	d	6.5
8-OMe	4.11	4.11	s	
H-1	5.72	5.70	dd	6.5
H-5	6.93	6.93	d	7.7
H-6	7.40	7.39	dd	7.7
H-7	7.54	7.54	dd	7.7
H-4	7.86	7.84	s	
9-OH	9.64	9.63	s	

From: Hara et al, 1997.

Table 2. ^{1}HNMR data Ep1, in comparison to Isoeleutherol.

Because Isoeleutherol can show an adequate stability and seems to be one of the major chemical constituent of the tincture prepared from the bulbs of *Eleutherine plicata* EE, this substance can be used as a marker for the standardization of the herbal drug and its derivatives, probably linked to the antimoebian activity alleged to the plant.

3.2 Structural characterization of Ep2 as isoeleutherine

The substance Ep2 was analysed by ^{1}HRMN, and the characterization of its structure was made by comparison of the obtained spectral data with that found in the literature. In table 3 it can be seen that the Hydrogen atoms H-6, H-7 and H-8 in the aromatic ring, appear at δ=7.73, δ=7.64 and δ=7.27 respectively, with identical coupling constant $J_{6H\text{-}8H}$= 6.7. The signal attributed to 6-H appears in the form of a duplet coupling with H-7, which in turn appears in the form of triplet due to the coupling with 6-H and h-8. The Hydrogen atoms of the Methyl group attached to C-1 and 1-H appear as duplet with δ= 1.33 and δ= 1.54, respectively and the Hydrogen atoms of Methyl group at C-3 appear as a duplet by δ= 1.34.

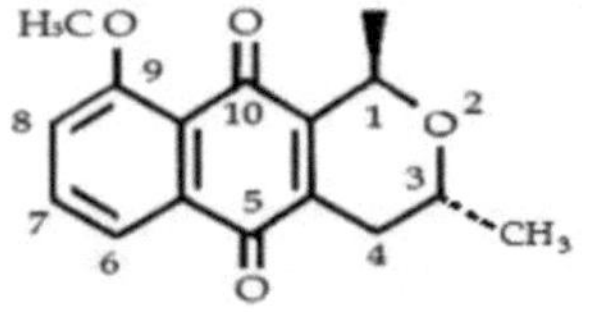

Fig. 16. Chemical structure of isoeleutherine

The bulbs of *Eleutherine plicata* Herb., vernacular "marupazinho", are widely used in inland areas of the State of Pará, as a tea to treat diarrhoea possibly caused by *Giardia* and/or *Entamoeba*. The isolation of isoeleutherine from the Chloroform fraction of the tincture, suggests that the antiamoebian and antigiardian activity alleged by the population may be due to this chemical constituent, also found in the aqueous extract. Besides isoeleutherol,

Hydrogen Atom	Ep2 δ(ppm)	Isoeleutherine δ(ppm)	Multiplicity	J (Hz)
3-ME	1.33	1.34	d	6.1
1-ME	1.53	1.53	d	6.7
4-βH	2.23	2.23	dd	11.0-19.0
4-αH	2.69	2.68	dd	3.5-19.0
3-H	3.95	3.96	m	- - -
9-OME	4.0	4.0	s	- - -
1-H	5.0	5.01	q	6.7
8-H	7.27	7.27	d	6.7
7-H	7.64	7.64	t	6.7
6-H	7.73	7.74	d	6.7

Based on Hara et al, 1997.

Table 3. ^{1}HNMR data from Ep2 in comparison to isoeleutherine.

already known to inhibit HIV replication in H9 lymphocytes, these chemical constituents can be used as chemical markers for the quality control of the herbal drug and its derivatives.

4. Characterization of Flavonoid glycosides as potential markers for a Vitaceae using LC-MS

Another plant species widely recognized in Brazil, the *Cissus* species (Vitaceae) used in treating stroke sequels and to control diabetes, had its tincture analysed by LC-MS and is under evaluation for developing a phytomedicine. The tincture was obtained from dried leaves according to the methods described in the Brazilian Pharmacopoeia 5th edition (200g dried plant material macerated in 1 L ethanol 98°GL) (FARMACOPEIA BRASILEIRA, 2010). The analyses were performed in a HPLC system equipped with a diode-array detector. The compounds were separated on a RP-18 column using a mobile phase in linear gradient prepared with Acetonitrile, Methanol and Water (Table 4) containing HCOOH (pH 3.2); the flow rate was 0.8 mL min-1.

Time (min)	H20+ %	MeOH%	CH_3CN%	Flow (mL/min.)
0.1	100	0	0	0.8
5	85	0	15	0.8
25	75	0	25	0.8
40	75	0	25	0.8
42	0	100	0	0.8
47	0	100	0	0.8

Table 4. Mobile phase composition and flow

The tincture of *C. verticillata* was filtered on a PTFE membrane filter before analysis. The UV-Vis spectra were recorded at the range of 190-450nm, and chromatograms were acquired at 230, 254, 280, 330 and 350 nm. Typical chromatograms at 350 nm of *Cissus* (I) and Passionflower (II-reference) samples are reported in Figure 17.

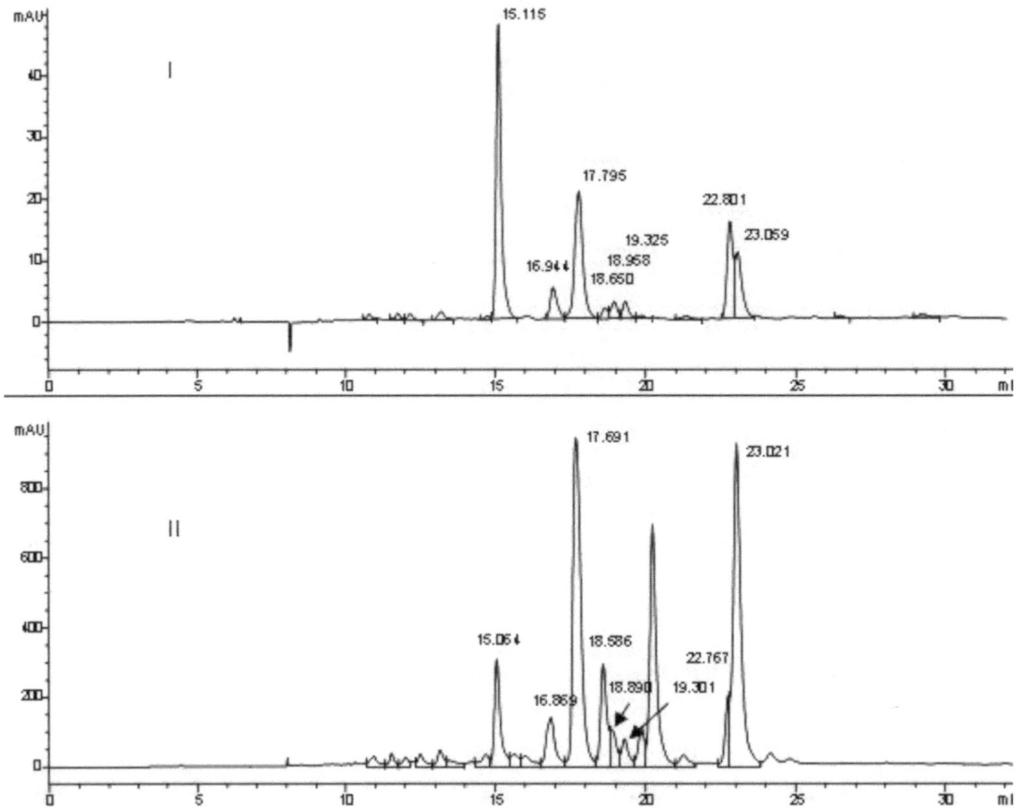

Fig. 17. Chromatograms at 350 nm of *Cissus* (I) and Passionflower (II) (reference) tincture.

The HPLC system described above was interfaced with atmospheric pressure chemical ionization (APCI)-electrospray mass-selective detector (MSD). The interface geometry with orthogonal positioning of the nebulizer relative to the capillary inlet, enabled the use of analytical conditions similar to those used for HPLC-DAD analysis. The conditions used for mass spectrometry (gas temperature 350°C at a flow rate of 10Lmin-1, nebulizer pressure 30psi, quadrupole temperature of 30°C and capillary voltage 3500 V) were optimized to achieve the maximum sensitivity of ESI values. The column, time period, and flow rate used were the same as those described above, without appreciable variation of the chromatographic profile. Full scan spectra from m/z 100 to 800 were obtained in positive-ion mode; the scan time was 1s. The volume of sample solution injected was 10μL.

Identification of all constituents was performed by HPLC-MS analysis and/or by comparison of the retention times of peaks in the extracts with those of the authentic reference samples. Peak purity was checked by examination of the mass spectra and/or by use of HPLC with diode-array detection (UV spectra of the peaks were compared with those of authentic reference samples).

Table 5 shows the comparison of LC-MS data obtained from *Cissus verticillata* tincture to those from *Passiflora incarnata* which allows the characterization of the compounds listed therein (BILIA et al, 2002). Peaks A, B, C, D, G and H show very similar retention time in both chromatograms (Figure 17).

Cissus verticillata				Passiflora incarnata		
	[M+H]+	Rt	Substance		Rt	Substance
A	595	15.11	Vicenin-2 (apigenin 6,8-di-C-glucoside)	A′	15.06	Apigenin 6,8 di-C-glycoside (probably vicenin-2)
B	565	16.94	Isoschaftoside (apigenin 6-C-arabino-8-C glucoside)	B′	16.87	Isoschaftoside
C	565	17.79	Schaftoside (apigenin 6-C-glucosyl-8-C arabinoside)	C′	17.69	Schaftoside
D	-	18.65	Homoorientin (luteolin 8-C-glucoside)	D′	18.64	Homoorientin
E	565	18.96	structural isomer of isoschaftoside	E′	18.97	Not reported
F	565	19.32	structural isomer of schaftoside	F′	19.30	Not reported
G	433	22.80	Vitexin (apigenin 8-C-glucoside)	G′	22.72	Vitexin
H	433	23.06	Isovitexin (apigenin 6-C-glucoside)	H′	23.02	Isovitexin

Table 5. LC-MS data of *C. verticillata* compared to *P. Incarnata*

Comparing mass spectra of these substances to those obtained from *P. incarnata* and using the information available in the literature the flavonosides of *C. verticillata* could be characterized. The peaks A and A′ presented analogous mass spectra exhibiting [M+H]+ and [M+Na]+ ions at m/z 595 and 617. These data suggest the presence of an apigenin nucleus bounded to two glucose moieties, and thus it could be characterized as vicenin-2. Peaks B/B′ and C/C′ exhibited [M+H]+ and [M+Na]+ ions at m/z 565 and 587. These data suggest the presence of an apigenin nucleus plus a pentose and glucose. However, the absence for both peaks spectra of the fragment ions [M+H-162]+, [M+H-132]+ or [M+H-(162+132)]+ at m/z 403, 433 and 271 (corresponding to the aglycone apigenin) suggest that peaks B, B′, C and C′ are 6,8-C-glycosides of apigenin. These suggestions were confirmed by the typical fragment ions [M+ H-H2O]+ and [M+H-2H2O]+ that were evidenced at m/z 547 and 529.

Another characteristic fragment ions [M+H- 2H2O-CH2O]+, [M+H-5H2O-CH2O]+ and [M+H- 6H2O-CH2O]+ were also evidenced at m/z 499, 445 and 427. From these data, peak B was identified as 6-C-arabinosyl-8-C-glucosylapigenin (isoschaftoside) and the peak C was identified as 6-C-glucosyl-8-C-arabinosylapigenin (schaftoside). Peaks D (minor constituent) and D′ were identified as homoorientin, by comparison of chromatographic and spectroscopic data with authentic samples.

Peaks E (minor constituent) and F (minor constituent) exhibited [M+H]+ and [M+Na]+ ions at m/z 565 and 587. These data suggested the presence of an apigenin nucleus plus a pentose and glucose. However, the absence for both peaks spectra of the fragment ions [M+H-162]+, [M+H-132]+ or [M+H-(162+132)]+ at m/z 403, 433 and 271 (corresponding to the aglycone apigenin) suggested that peaks E and E′ were 6,8-C-glycosides of apigenin. These suggestions were confirmed by the typical fragment ions [M+ H-H2O]+ and [M+H-2H2O]+ that were evidenced at m/z 547 and 529.

The fragment ions [M+H- 2H2O-CH2O]+ and [M+H-5H2O-CH2O]+ were also evidenced at m/z 499 and 445. No differentiation was found between mass spectra of isoschaftoside and compound E and between mass spectra of schaftoside and compound F. From these data, the minor constituents, peaks E and F, were identified as apigenin-6,8-di-C-glycoside (probably structural isomers of isoschaftoside and schaftoside respectively).

The peaks at 23,06min and 22,80 min in the LC-DAD chromatograms of *Cissus*, suggest the presence of isomers vitexin and isovitexin when compared with the respective standards, therefore the mass spectra shows the fragmentation pattern. These mass spectra show important fragmentations that help to differentiate the position of the pyranose unit in the ring of flavone apigenin characterizing the detection of vitexin and isovitexin in the analyzed samples.

The signal registered at 22.8 min in the *Cissus* chromatogram was characterized by comparison to that observed for commercial *Passiflora incarnata*. The mass spectra showed the same fragmentation pattern. Base peak coincided with molecular ion (433 [M+H]), the spectra also showed fragmentation of the pyranose ([M+H-120]+) and the loss of two molecules of water ([M+H-18]+, [M+H-36]+), characterizing the structure of the vitexin. Similarly, the signal at 23,06 min, corresponds to a mass spectrum which shows the loss of 120 amu ([M+H-120]+), that can be attributed to the fragmentation of part of the glucose molecule; the spectrum also showed three typical peaks of losses of three molecules of water from the glucose unit ([M+H-18]+, [M+H-36]+ e [M+H-54]+, indicating to be due to isovitexin.

Peaks G and G' exhibit [M+H]+ and [M+Na]+ ions at m/z 433 and 455. Peak G and H were identified as vitexin and isovitexin respectively also by comparing their chromatographic and spectroscopic data with that provided by authentic samples.

On basis of these results it can be stated that the ethanol tincture at 98ºGL of *Cissus verticillata* (L) Nicolson & C. E. Jarvis) contains at least eight flavonoid glycosides which can be used as markers to monitor the quality of plant material, its derivatives and products. The detection and characterization of these substances in pharmacopoeial preparations, using LC-DAD and LC-MS, can be very useful in developing phytomedicines, once the isolation and characterization of these substances by chromatographic and spectrometric usual methods are expensive and demand more time.

5. Characterization of a metabolic class as potential marker by UV-spectroscopy: Validation of a new quantification method according to Brazilian regulation

The standardization of plant extracts, which contain chemical substances without the necessary chemical characteristics to be used as quality markers, can be accomplished using chemical groups, or metabolic classes, found in the intermediary as active pharmaceutical constituent. This is the case, for example, of an Apocynaceae that composes a phytomedicine widely used in Brazil and has as its active principle, alkaloids. The complexity of the alkaloid fraction present in the intermediate and the instability of the substances when isolated indicated that the development of a method based on the alkaloid fraction, using ultraviolet spectroscopy to standardize this extract would be the best solution.

A species from the genus *Himatanthus*, popularly known as "agoniada", has its bark commonly used in the form of decoction to produce a phytomedicine indicated to treat uterine congestion; irregular, difficult and painful periods and uterine cramps, besides other associated symptoms (CRUZ, 1985).

The aqueous extract prepared with the barks of the plant, after concentration and drying, was treated with 1% aqueous HCl and filtered, then the solution was made alkaline with concentrated ammonium hydroxide to pH 10. The alkalinised solution was partitioned with chloroform. The chloroform fraction filtered through anhydrous sodium sulphate and concentrated without heating under reduced pressure, was used to prepare a methanol solution at 30 mg/mL which was used to quantify the total alkaloids fraction.

The observation of an absorption maximum at 281nm by the UV analysis of the alkaloid fraction allowed to choose Yohimbine as external standard for the quantification process, because of its absorption maxima at 281nm (OLIVEIRA, 1994). In addition the substance is an indole alkaloid, which is also present in Apocynacee species (SOUZA, 2008), and is able to be acquired in the market as chemical reference substance (CRS). This substance was also utilized to produce a series of dilutions in methanol, which could be utilized to determine linearity of the method and to compose the calibration curve.

5.1 Brazilian guidelines to define validation procedures

Despite of the technique used to characterize markers, and the fact that they are isolated or in the form of a chemical group - metabolic class, the method developed for their quantification must be validated in order to ensure that this analytical method generates reliable information about the analysed sample (RIBANI, et al. 2004). Analytical method validation is the confirmation by examination and provision of objective evidence that the specific requirements for an intended specific use are met (NBR ISO/IEC/17025, 2001). Validation is intended to demonstrate that the method is appropriate for qualitative, semi-quantitative and/or quantitative determination of drugs and other substances in pharmaceuticals (BRASIL, 2003).

All regulatory agencies in Brazil and in other countries require the validation of the analytical methodology for the registration of new products (RIBANI, et al. 2004). In Brazil, there are two certification agencies, ANVISA (National Agency for Sanitary Surveillance) and INMETRO (National Institute of Metrology, Standardization and Industrial Quality) which verify the competence of analytical laboratories. These bureau provide guidelines to define the validation procedures of new analytical methods, respectively, the resolution No. 899, from 5/29/2003 (BRASIL, 2003) and the document INMETRO DOQ-CGCRE-008, June 2007, which aims at guiding the validation of analytical methods.

Here we adopted the criteria described by the resolution No. 899 of ANVISA, as the basis for the development of a quality control method for the aqueous extract prepared from *Himatanthus* sp. According to this resolution there are four set of tests for validation of a new method, as follows:

1. Quantitative assays for the determination of an active ingredient in pharmaceuticals or raw materials;
2. Quantitative tests or limit test for the determination of impurities and degradation products in pharmaceuticals and raw materials;

3. Performance tests (e.g. dissolution, active substance release);
4. Identification tests

A method that aims at the quantification of a marker in a phytomedicine fits category I and can be considered validated when the following parameters: selectivity/specificity, linearity, interval, precision, limit of detection (sensitivity), accuracy, robustness are determined and verified.

5.1.1 Selectivity/specificity

A segment of the UV spectrum obtained from the alkaloid fraction of *Himatanthus* sp aqueous extract (30 µg/mL), the Yohimbine hydrochloride (22 µg/mL) and methanol solvent in the range between 200nm and 400nm is shown in Figure 18 and discloses the absorption maximum at 281nm just to Yohimbine and the alkaloid fraction. Herewith, it could be confirmed that at this wavelength it is selectively possible to quantify the reference substance and the alkaloid fraction even in the presence of other components.

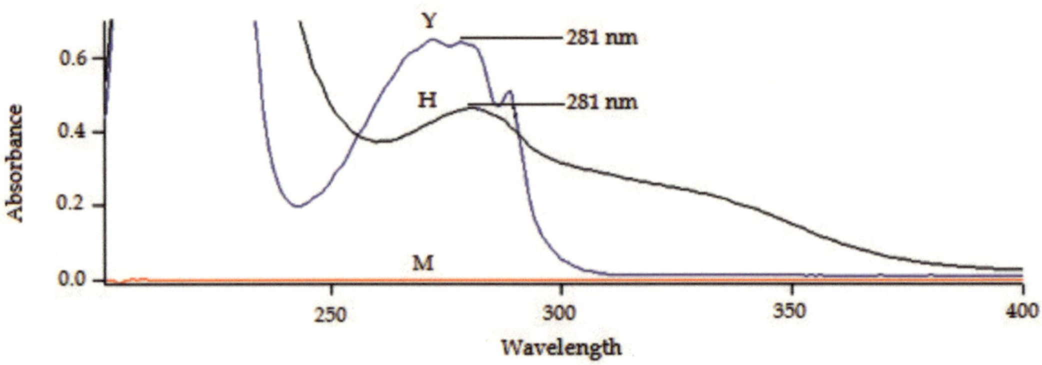

Fig. 18. Segment of UV spectra of Yohimbine (Y) and the alkaloid fraction of the aqueous extract of *Himatanthus sp.* (H), in comparison to the methanol solvent (M) showing the selectivity of the developed method.

5.1.2 Linearity

The spectrophotometric method presented linearity at 281nm for the concentrations tested. The linearity of the method, the coefficient of determination (R2) and correlation (r) to Yohimbine are expressed in Figure 19.

The value of the correlation coefficient itself is not sufficient to ensure the adequacy of the linear adjustment to the calibration curve, because calibration models with high residue in the analytic signal, or unevenly distributed points along the calibration range can nevertheless offer a good correlation coefficient (RIBEIRO, et al., 2008). For that reason the analysis of residue of the data used for the determination of the method linearity was performed and could demonstrate a uniform data distribution, constant variance (homocedastity), average zero and absence of atypical samples (Figure 20) observed in homogeneous distribution of points along the axis of the chart indicating that the curve is well adjusted.

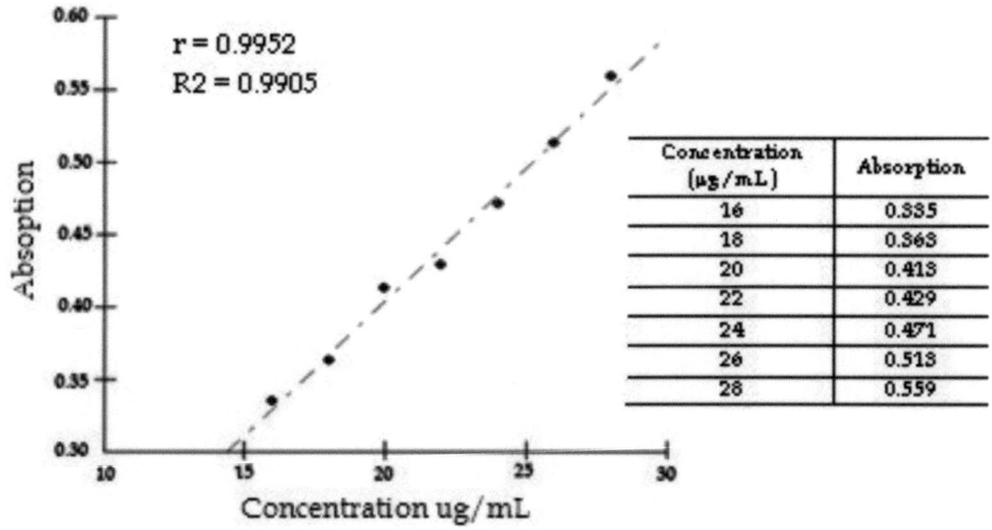

Concentration (µg/mL)	Absorption
16	0.335
18	0.363
20	0.413
22	0.429
24	0.471
26	0.513
28	0.559

Fig. 19. Graphical representation of the linearity method for the series dilution of Yohimbine in methanol at 281nm, in detail, the used concentrations and their absorbance.

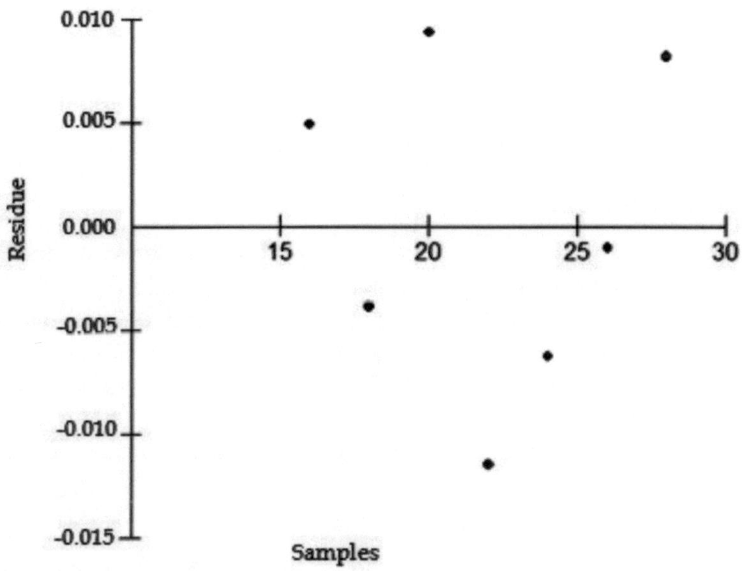

Fig. 20. Graphical representation of the residues of method's linearity data using the dilution series of Yohimbine.

5.1.3 Interval

Interval means the range between the maximal and minimal limits of quantification of an analytical method. Typically, it is derived from the study of linearity and depends on the intended application of the method (BRASIL, 2003). Thus, the range employed for the standardization of the aqueous extract of *Himatanthus sp* (16 to 28 µg/mL) was established in accordance with the average of absorptions found for Yohimbine (range of 80% to 120%).

5.1.4 Calibration curve

The analytical curve, with the respective line equation and Pearson correlation coefficient (r) for Yohimbine is demonstrated in Figure 21.

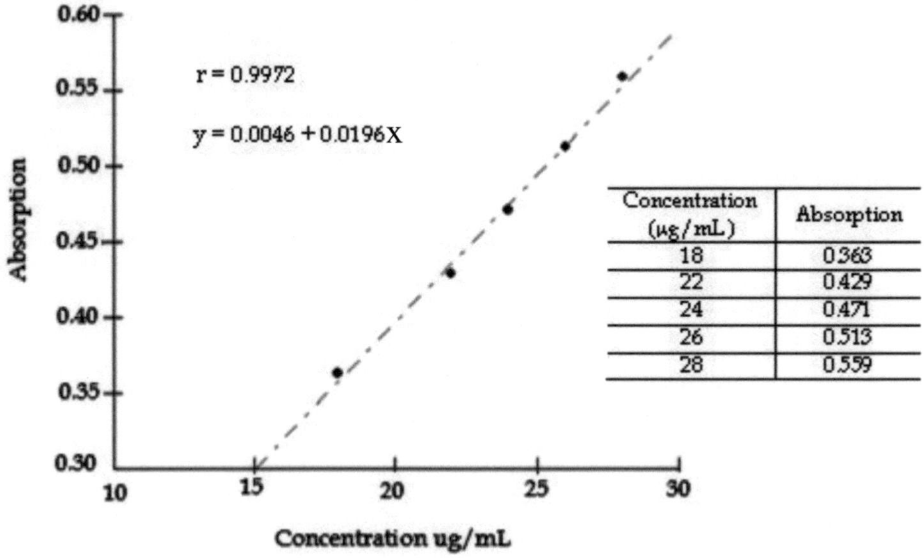

Fig. 21. Graphical representation of the calibration curve obtained using the dilution series with Yohimbine.

5.1.5 Precision and accuracy

Data of repeatability (intra-run), intermediate precision (inter-run) and accuracy are demonstrated in Table 6 where it can be seen that the relative standard deviation values found vary from 0.19% to 2.09% and that the accuracy values found oscillate between 98% and 102.90%. ANVISA establishes that the precision variation may not exceed 5% and that the accuracy should not be less than 95% (BRASIL, 2003). These data confirm that the proposed method for the quantification of total alkaloids of aqueous extract of *Himatanthus sp.* by UV spectrophotometry is in accordance with current legislation and provides reliable results.

5.1.6 Detection limit

It is the lowest amount of analyte present in a sample which can be detected, but not necessarily quantified, under the established experimental conditions. In the case of instrumental methods the estimation of the detection limit can be determined by the equation:

$$DL = \frac{SDa \times 3}{IC}$$

Where: SDa is the standard deviation of the y-intercept of at least 3 calibration curves built containing concentrations of the drug near the supposed limits of quantification and IC is the inclination of the calibration curve. The value of the detection limit estimated by the equation for the here proposed method is 4.59 μg/mL.

$$DL = \frac{0.03 \times 3}{0.0196} = 4.59\,\mu g / mL$$

Test	Calculated Concentration. (µg/ml)	N	C (µg/ml)	DP	DPR (%)	Accuracy (%)
Repeatability	16	3	15.698	0.030	0.19	98.00
	20	3	19.864	0.181	0.90	99.32
	28	3	27.724	0.392	1.41	99.01
Intermediate precision Day 1	16	3	16.448	0.205	1.25	102.80
	20	3	20.580	0.257	1.25	102.90
	28	3	28.373	0.245	0.86	101.33
Intermediate precision Day 2	16	3	16.213	0.339	2.09	101.33
	20	3	20.345	0.054	0.27	101.72
	28	3	28.391	0.271	0.96	101.39

(C) average concentration of (N) determinations; (SD) standard deviation; (RSD %) Relative Standard Deviation.

Table 6. Results of repeatability, intermediate precision and accuracy of the developed UV-Spectrophotometric method to determine the total alkaloids fraction contained in the aqueous extract of *Himatanthus* sp.

5.1.7 Quantification limit

It is the lowest amount of analyte in a sample, which can be determined with acceptable accuracy and precision under the established experimental conditions and can be expressed by the equation:

$$QL = \frac{SDa \times 10}{IC}$$

Where: SDa is the standard deviation of the y-intercept of at least 3 calibration curves built containing concentrations of the drug near the supposed limits of quantification and IC is the inclination of the calibration curve. The quantification limit of the reported method is 15.31µg/mL.

5.1.8 Robustness

The robustness of the proposed method was evaluated by changing the supplier of the solvent used to prepare the sample (Table 7). Three determinations were made in low (16 µg/mL), middle (20 µg/mL) and high (28 µg/mL) concentrations, with three replicates each. The absorption maxima at 281nm obtained for these Yohimbine solutions prepared with solvents from two different suppliers were compared and no variation in the obtained spectra could be observed. The data are shown in table 7 and were submitted to a statistical variance analysis, which provided a p value of 0.5694, evidencing no significant statistical difference, because $p > 0.05$, thus demonstrating a robust method.

Solvent supplier	Calculated Concentration (μg/mL)	N	Determined Concentration (μg/ml)	Absorption
1	16	3	16.448	0.293
	20	3	20.580	0.373
	28	3	28.373	0.523
2	16	3	16.217	0.261
	20	3	19.651	0.315
	28	3	28.141	0.449

(C) average concentration of (N) determinations

Table 7. Results of the evaluation of robustness of the developed UV-Spectrophotometric method for the determination of total alkaloids contained in the aqueous extract of *Himatanthus* sp.

5.2 Quantification of total alkaloids fraction present in the aqueous extract of a *Himatanthus* sp.

The analysis of a methanolic solution at 30μg/mL of an alkaloid fraction obtained from the aqueous extract of a *Himatanthus* species barks; performed in triplicate, in a spectrophotometer, at 281nm, provided an average absorption of 0.462. Using the equation deduced from the calibration curve ($y = 0.0046 + 0.0196x$), it is possible to calculate the amount of total alkaloids present in the sample; the results are condensed in Table 8.

Material	Herbal Drug	Dry aq. extract	Alkaloid Fraction	Total Alkaloid
Weight	25000mg	9549mg	26.74mg	20.80mg
I	100%	....		0.0832% (832ppm)
II		100%		0.218%
III			100%	77.79%

Table 8. Amount of total alkaloids on the powdered bark of *Himatanthus* sp employed for the preparation of dried herbal drug (I), in relation to dried aqueous extract (II) and in relation to total alkaloid fraction obtained (III).

The proposed quantification method could be validated, since it shows selectivity at 281nm for the alkaloid fraction from the *Himatanthus* species aqueous extract, giving reliability to the quantification of total alkaloids fraction in the plant material. In addition it is a robust method, according to the parameters established by the legislation in use in Brazil. The correlation between absorbance and concentration, according to the equation obtained, is linear, at a given wavelength; the quantification method is also exact and precise, as well as accessible and easy to be applied.

In Brazil, the National Health Surveillance Agency - ANVISA - responsible for regulating the use of medicinal plants and their derivatives, protects and promotes the health of the population, ensuring the safety of health products and services. This control seeks to deconstruct the idea that herbal medicines are products of less quality or without toxic potential risk, because it evaluates various parameters as quality, safety and efficacy, demanding requirements similar to those required for synthetic medicines. The Collegiate

Direction Resolution (RDC) No. 14/2010 from ANVISA regulates the registration of phytomedicines in Brazil and defines how to achieve standardization of intermediates used in the galenic development of herbaceous medicines. The developed methods, in this process, shall be validated according to the rules described in the Special Resolution (RE) No. 899/2003, also from ANVISA, which indicates as validation parameters for herbal extracts: selectivity of the method to detect the marker, calibration curve and linearity by the quantification of the marker, precision by the calculation of the content of the marker, limits of detection and quantification of the marker in the sample, and robustness of the method regarding modifications in its routine.

6. Quantification of isolated substances using HPLC

The method for the quantification of marker compounds isolated from active pharmaceutical ingredients (APhI) that will give rise to phytomedicines must have the same validation criteria presented in section 5.1. These substances should be ideally associated to the alleged activity of the medicinal plant although for the registration of the product, according to the Brazilian legislation, this fact is not decisive.

The presence of the marker shall be characterized in the matrix (extract from which the phytomedicne will be developed) as demonstrated in section 3, by thin-layer chromatography (TLC) and high performance liquid chromatography (HPLC) data. The structure of the substance must be elucidated or characterized by spectroscopic techniques such as UV, infrared and nuclear magnetic resonance (NMR) as in 3.1 and 3.2 and by mass spectrometry as described in section 4, where the technique was applied hyphenated to HPLC. Once the structural characteristics of the candidate substance to be used as a marker are described and the analytical conditions by HPLC defined, a calibration curve using this technique and a dilution series containing the potential marker can be drawn, by correlating the peak area of the substance registered on the chromatogram, to the concentration of the solution employed to register it. Once the area of the substance in the chromatogram of the APhI is registered, this value shall be applied to the straight line equation defined by the calibration curve (as in section 5.1.4).

The validation of a quantification method based on isolated markers demands the same criteria previously described and exemplified in section 5.1. HPLC methods for the standardization of herbal extracts used to develop phytomedicine produces more accurate results, since the most common source of error, in this technique, is the preparation of samples and components of the eluent, steps prepared by human operators. These possible deviations can be minimized by obtaining data in replicate.

7. References

Machado RD, Costa CG, Fontenelle GB 1988. Foliar anatomy of *Eugenia sulcata* Spring ex Mart. (Myrtaceae). Acta Bot Rev 1: 275-285.

Kraus JE; Arduin M. 1997. Manual básico de métodos em morfologia vegetal. Rio de Janeiro: EDUR. 25p.

Tomlinson PB 1982. Anatomy of the Monocotyledons. VII. Helobiae (Alismatidae). Clarendon Press: Oxford.

Matias LQ 2007. The genus Echinodorus (Alismataceae) from caatinga of Brazil. Rodriguésia 58: 743-774.

Leite JVP, Pepper DS, Gomes RSDL, Barros AMD 2007. Contribution to the pharmacobotanical study of *Echinodorus macrophyhllus* (Kunt) Micheli (hat-in-leather) - Alismataceae. Farmacogn Rev 17: 242-248.

Brasil, 2010. Ministério da Saúde, Agencia Nacional de Vigilância Sanitária, Resolução da Direção Colegiada n° 10/2010. Brasília, Brasil.

Wagner, H; Bladt, S. Plant drug analysis: A thin layer chromatography atlas. 2ª ed. Springer, p.275-279, 2001.

Anazetti MC; Melo PS. 2007. Morte celular por apoptose: uma visão bioquímica e molecular. Metrocamp pesquisa, 1, 1, 37-58.

Blois, S. 1955. A note on free radical formation in biologically occurring quinones. Biochimica et Biophysica Acta, 18, , Page 165, ISSN 0006-3002, (http://www.sciencedirect.com/science/article/pii/000630025590038X).

Paramaponj, S. et al. Analysis of naphthoquinone derivatives in the Asian medicinal plant Eleutherine americana by RP-HPLC and LC-MS. Journal of Pharmaceutical and Biomedical Analysis, v. 47, p. 990-993, 2008. access: www.elsevier.com/locate/jpba accessed em: 15 ago 2008.

Hara, H. et al. Elecanacin, a novel new naphthoquinone from the bulb of Eleutherine americana Merr. Et Heyne. Chemical Pharmaceutical Bulletin, v. 45, nº. 10, p. 1774-1776, 1997.

Farmacopeia Brasileira, 2010. Ministério da Saúde, Agência Nacional de Vigilância Sanitária, Farmacopeia Brasileira, Brasilia.

Bilia AR, Bergonzi MC, Gallori S, Mazzi G, Vincieri FF, 2002. Stability of the constituents of Calendula, Milk-thistle and Passionflower tinctures by LC-DAD and LC-MS, Journal of Pharmaceutical and Biomedical Analysis 30, 613–624 www.elsevier.com/locate/jpba.

Cruz, GL Dicionário das Plantas Úteis do Brasil. 3ª ed. Rio de Janeiro: Editora Civilização Brasileira S. A., 1985.

Oliveira, AJB. 1994. Estudo de quatro espécies do gênero Aspidosperma por cromatografia gasosa de alta resolução acoplada à espectrometria de massas. MSc Dissertation. Universidade Estadual de Campinas, São Paulo. http://biq.iqm.unicamp.br/arquivos/teses/ficha21388.htm. Access 22/02/2009.

Souza, WM. 2008. Estudo químico e das atividades biológicas dos Alcalóides indólicos de *Himatanthus lancifolius* (Muell. Arg.) Woodson, Apocynaceae - (agoniada). 173f. Doctoral Thesis. Universidade Federal do Paraná, Curitiba.

Ribani, M. 2004. Validação em métodos cromatográficos e eletroforéticos. Quim. Nova, 27, 5, 771-780.

NBR ISSO/IEC 17025. 2001. Requisitos Gerais para a Competência de Laboratórios de Calibração e de Ensaios. Rio de Janeiro.

Brasil. 2003. Ministério da Saúde. Agência Nacional de Vigilância Sanitária. Resolução Especial n° 899/2003. Dispose on the Guidelines for validation of analytical and bioanalytical methods. http://e-legis.anvisa.gov.br.

Ribeiro, FAL et al. 2008. Planilha de validação: uma nova ferramenta para estimar figuras de mérito na validação de métodos analíticos univariados. Química Nova, 31, 1, 164-171.

5

The Phytochemical and *In Vitro* Pharmacological Testing of Maltese Medicinal Plants

Everaldo Attard[1] and Pierpaolo Pacioni[2]
[1]*University of Malta, Institute of Earth Systems, Division of Rural Sciences and Food Systems,*
[2]*Universita' degli Studi di Perugia, Facoltà di Agraria,*
[1]*Malta*
[2]*Italy*

1. Introduction

1.1 General background

The Maltese archipelago is composed of a small number of islands with a total surface area of approximately 457 km^2. Albeit this small size the Maltese islands host a vast number of plant and animal species. Plant biodiversity, with its 1264 vascular species, is mainly attributed to the strategic position of Malta within the Mediterranean, in which throughout the years several conquerors and civilisations sought to possess Malta particularly for military purposes. In part, the plant diversity of Malta is attributed to introductions brought about by various military forces, as an aid during injury and sickness. Naturally, the phytodiversity has an inclination towards the Mediterranean type of flora with an approximately 66% of the Maltese flora pertaining to this region (E. Attard, 2004). Typical Mediterranean medicinal plants include conifers (*Pinus halepensis* and *Cupressus sempervirens*), broad-leaved trees (*Laurus nobilis, Morus nigra* and *Tamarix gallica*), fruit trees (*Ceratonia siliqua, Citrus* trees, *Nerium oleander, Olea europaea* and *Punica granatum*), and others (*Allium sativum, Aloe ferox, Capparis spinosa, Opuntia ficus-indica, Origanum vulgare, Papaver somniferum, Phytolacca decandra* and *Pistacia lentiscus*). The other portion (34%) is attributed to plants originating from the warm North African (*Cynomorium coccineum, Ficus carica* and *Myrtus communis*) and the colder South Europaean regions (*Crataegus monogyna, Populus alba* and *Salix species*).

There are approximately 458 medicinal taxa, used in the past to treat one or more ailments (Lanfranco 1993; Lanfranco 1975). Most popular treatments were for the gastrointestinal system, nervous system, cardiovascular system and dermatological conditions. The most predominating plant family within this group is the Asteraceae family, followed by the Lamiaceae and Fabaceae families (Attard, 2004). In spite of their use, these medicinal plants were administered on a trial and error basis. Today, with the advent of modern scientific techniques, the ethnobotanical attributes of a medicinal plant can be challenged by phytochemical and pharmacological testing.

1.2 Scientific evaluation of local medicinal and aromatic plants in relation to pharmacology

Locally, only 8 % out of the 458 taxa have been studied scientifically. However, the studies conducted were rather fragmented and covering one or two extracts from a specific plant. Plants include *Ecballium elaterium* (E. Attard et al., 2005; E. Attard & H. Attard, 2008), *Crataegus monogyna* (E. Attard & H. Attard, 2006), *Olea eurpoaea* (Mangion Randon & E. Attard, 2007), *Ephedra fragilis* (E. Attard & Vella, 2009) *Urtica dubia* (Rossi & E. Attard, 2011), *Tetraclinis articulata* (Buhagiar et al., 1999) and *Ricinus communis* (Darmanin, 2003) amongst others.

1.3 Technical approaches

The evaluation of plant species using different solvent systems has been widely exploited in previous studies (Rodriguez-Lopez et al., 2003; Kumarasamy et al., 2002; Calderon et al., 2003; Konning et al., 2004). A wide spectrum of solvents may be employed when a small number of plants (1-15) are investigated, but when investigating larger numbers or a new group of plants for the first time, the solvents used in ethno-medicine are preferentially selected (Punjani and Kumar, 2003; Guarrera, 2003).

Phytochemical analysis for major classes of metabolites is an important first step in pharmacological evaluation of plant extracts. Some journals require that pharmacological studies be accompanied by a comprehensive phytochemical analysis. Details of such analysis are found in several text books (Harborne, 1984; Evans, 2009). The main secondary metabolite classes include flavonoids, terpenoids and alkaloids, which have been widely tested by the acidified vanillin test, the Salkowski test and the Dragendorff's test, respectively.

Bench top bioassays have been devised to facilitate screening of a large number of samples (Meyer et al., 1982; Carballo et al., 2002). They are based on the principle that pharmacology is simply toxicology at low doses, while toxicology is pharmacology at high doses. Several researchers have used these bioassays for primary pharmacological screening of medicinal plants (Franssen et al., 1997; Kanegusuku et al., 2001; Javidnia et al., 2003). The brine shrimp lethality test (BST), which involves the exposure of brine shrimps to different extract concentrations, is considered as a useful tool for preliminary assessment of cytotoxicity (Jaki et al., 1999). It is a rapid (24 hours), inexpensive and simple technique. A positive correlation has been found between the brine shrimp test and cytotoxicity of the 9KB human nasopharyngeal carcinoma, and other cell lines (Meyer et al., 1982; Kim et al., 2000).

The DNA methyl green bioassay is a simple and comprehensive technique with a high throughput. Methyl green, binds quantitatively to DNA forming a DNA-methyl green complex, hence identifying agents with a high affinity for the DNA. This affinity determines the displacement of methyl green, hence leading to a colourless carbinol (N. Kurnick, 1950; B. Kurnick and Foster, 1950; Krey and Hahn, 1975).

1.4 Aims of study

We believe that Maltese medicinal and aromatic plants have a great pharmacological potential. This is based on the concept that, in the past, these plants had important medicinal uses. Therefore, we aimed our study at ethnobotanical research by:

1. Identifying plants cited in ethnobotanical research as active medicinal plants
2. Preparing five extracts using different solvents from each medicinal plant, and the subsequent determination of the classes of metabolites present in the different extracts.
3. Determining whether or not, the extracts obtained eventually possess pharmacological activity employing a primary screening programme.
4. Identifying plant extracts that possess DNA binding.

2. Materials and methods

2.1 Plant materials

Fifty-five authenticated plant specimens were collected locally during different seasons of the year. The plants were selected on their relative abundance, and collected during their flowering period. The plants were further identified at the Rural Sciences and Food Systems Division, Institute of Earth Systems. Voucher specimens are stored within the Institute. The botanical and ethnobotanical details of the medicinal plants and their voucher specimen code numbers are listed in Table 1.

2.2 Preparation of plant extracts

Fresh plants were cut and oven-dried for 48 hours at 35-40°C in a hot air convection oven. Five 300g samples of the dried plants were ground in a heavy duty blender for 20 minutes. 500 ml of solvent (distilled water, distilled water and ethanol (1:1) mixture, ethanol or chloroform or petroleum ether) were added to the respective sample, shaken for 48 hours at 210 rpm, and filtered through a Buchner funnel. Each filtered extract was concentrated at 38 °C under reduced pressure, and finally dried in an oven at 38 °C.

2.3 Phytochemical analysis: quantitative colorimetric assays

Although most phytochemical analysis carried out may have a qualitative importance, the methods were modified according to other authors to read aborbance values at a wavelength of 405 nm rather than visual examination. The MTP reader gave more concrete results, in the form of absorbance values. Therefore semi-quantification is possible through this process.

Four colorimetric tests were quantitatively used to determine the presence or absence of metabolites:

1. The Salkowski test for terpenoids. After the addition of chloroform and concentrated sulphuric acid, a reddish brown colouration at the interface forms, hence showing a positive result for the presence of terpenoids (Edeoga et al., 2005);
2. The Dragendorff's test for alkaloids (Steinberg et al., 1997) gives a brown coloration;
3. The Acidified Vanillin test for flavonoids. Under acidic conditions, vanillaldehyde condenses to flavan-3,4-diols, flavan-3-ol monomers and proanthocyanidins to give a cherry-red product (Deshpande et al., 1986);
4. The ninhydrin test was used for proteins (Delhaye & Landry, 1992). The α-amino acids typically give a blue-purple product.

Voucher specimen number	Botanical Name, family	Maltese, (English) Names	Part/s used, preparation and Maltese Traditional uses
IOA-AMP-002	*Acanthus mollis* L., Acanthaceae	Ħannewija (Common bear's breeches)	Herb/Emollient as skin softener (Borg, 1927)
IOA-AMP-015	*Aloe vera* L., Liliaceae	Sabbara (Yellow aloe)	Leaf Juice in child weaning, laxative, increases menstruation (Penza, 1969; Cassar Pullicino, 1947; Cassar, 1964)
IOA-AMP-026	*Anagallis arvensis* L., Primulaceae	Ħarira ħamra or Ħarira kaħla (Scarlet pimpernel or Blue pimpernel)	Herb and seeds as sudorific and in rabies (Penza, 1969; Gulia, 1855)
IOA-AMP-037	*Antirrhinum siculum*, Mil., Scrophulariaceae	Papoċċi bojod (Sicilian snapdragon)	Leaves as astringent, diuretic and in chest problems (Penza, 1969; Borg, 1927)
IOA-AMP-036	*Antirrhinum tortuosum* L., Scrophulariaceae	Papoċċi ħomor (Red snapdragon)	Leaves as astringent, diuretic and in chest problems (Penza, 1969; Borg, 1927)
IOA-AMP-049	*Asparagus aphyllus* L., Liliaceae	Spraġ selvaġġ (Wild asparagus)	Herb as diuretic (Penza, 1969)
IOA-AMP-453	*Aster squamatus* (Sprengel) Hieron, Asteraceae	Settembrina selvaġġa (Narrow leaved aster)	A very abundant plant, said to be introduced to the Maltese Islands sometime around the 1930s
IOA-AMP-068	*Calendula arvensis* L., Asteraceae	Suffejra Selvaġġa (Wild or woody marigold)	Herb in coughs and colds, chiblains, sudorific, warts and calluses, jaundice (Lanfranco, 1993; Penza, 1969)
IOA-AMP-071	*Calendula suffruticosa* L., Asteraceae	Suffejra Selvaġġa (Wild or woody marigold)	Herb in jaundice (Penza, 1969)
IOA-AMP-081	*Carlina gummifera* (L.) Les., Asteraceae	Xewk tal-miskta (Stemless atractylis)	Herb is poisonous (Lanfranco, 1993)
IOA-AMP-091	*Ceratonia siliqua* L., Mimosaceae	Ħarruba (Carob)	Decoction of unripe pods as astringent for the gums and in cough (Penza, 1969; Lanfranco, 1980)
IOA-AMP-145	*Cynoglossum creticum* Miller, Boraginaceae	Ilsien il-kelb (Southern hound's tongue)	Root decoction and leaf poultice for joint pain and burn relief (Penza, 1969)
IOA-AMP-153	*Diplotaxis erucoides* (L.) DC., Brassicaceae	Ġarġir (White rocket)	Herb as a stimulant (Penza, 1969)
IOA-AMP-463	*Diplotaxis tenuifolia*, Brassicaceae	Ġarġir (perennial wall rocket)	Herb as a stimulant (Penza, 1969)
IOA-AMP-223	*Dittrichia viscosa* (L.) Greut., Asteraceae	Tulliera Komuni (Sticky Fleabane)	Leaf decoction, liquid preparation and oil as haemeostatic, wound healing, itching, improve eye sight; pain, depurative and venereal diseases (Penza, 1969; Lanfranco, 1980; Gulia, 1855; Cassar Pullicino, 1947)
IOA-AMP-460	*Eucalyptus globulus*, Myrtaceae	Ewkaliptus (Tasmanian Blue	Oil as astringent and expectorant (Lanfranco, 1993)

Voucher specimen number	Botanical Name, family	Maltese, (English) Names	Part/s used, preparation and Maltese Traditional uses
		Gum)	
IOA-AMP-459	*Ferula communis*, Apiaceae	Ferla (Giant fennel)	Herb (Penza, 1969)
IOA-AMP-185	*Foeniculum vulgare* Miller, Apiaceae	Busbies (fennel)	Seeds and herb as flavouring agent in liquid preparations and treatment of colic pain (Penza, 1969)
IOA-AMP-191	*Fumaria capreolata*, Fumariaceae	Daħnet l-art (Fumitory)	Herb infusion as tonic, taenifuge, stomachic, kidney stones, in bath for sick children (Borg, 1927; Penza, 1969; Gulia, 1855)
IOA-AMP-190	*Fumaria officinalis* L., Fumariaceae	Daħnet l-art (Fumitory)	Herb infusion as tonic, taenifuge, stomachic, kidney stones, in bath for sick children (Borg, 1927; Penza, 1969; Gulia, 1855)
IOA-AMP-454	*Galactites tomentosa* Moench, Asteraceae	Xewka bajda (Boar thistle)	Herb consumed as a monofloral boar thistle honey
IOA-AMP-197	*Gladiolus italicus* Gaud., Iridaceae	Gladjoli salvaġġ (Common cornflag)	Leaves and bulb as galactogogue, aphrodisiac and emmenagogue (Penza, 1969; Borg, 1927)
IOA-AMP-101	*Glebionis coronaria* Tzvelev, Asteraceae	Lellux or Żigland (Crown daisy)	Herb (Lanfranco, 1993)
IOA-AMP-202	*Hedera helix* L., Araliaceae	Liedna (Ivy)	Gum and leaves in wound healing and as astringent (Penza, 1969)
IOA-AMP-461	*Holoschoenus vulgaris, Cyperaceae*	Simar tal-boċċi (*roundhead bulrush*)	A common plant in halophytic environments
IOA-AMP-213	*Hyoscyamus albus* L., Solanaceae	Mammażejża (White henbane)	Leaf poultice and ointment as sedative, in haemorrhoids and wound healing (Penza, 1969)
IOA-AMP-217	*Hypericum aegyptiacum* L., Guttiferae	Fexfiex il-baħar (Egyptian St. John's wort)	Herb Juice in wound healing, urinary tract infections and increases menstrual flow (Penza, 1969)
IOA-AMP-450	*Inula crithmoides* L., Asteraceae	Xorbett (Golden samphire)	Herb (Gulia, 1855)
IOA-AMP-462	*Lactuca sativa*, Asteraceae	Ħassa salvaġġa (Wild lettuce)	Leaf poultice as sedative (Penza, 1969)
IOA-AMP-236	*Lactuca virosa*, Asteraceae	Ħassa salvaġġa (Wild lettuce)	White latex as sedative (Penza, 1969)
IOA-AMP-234	*Laurus nobilis* L., Lauracea	Rand (Laurel)	Seed oil and leaf decoction in rheumatic pain and neuralgia; stomachic; diaphoretic, depurative (Penza, 1969; Cassar Pullicino, 1947; Lanfranco, 1980; Cremona, 1971)
IOA-AMP-238	*Leontodon tuberosus*, Asteraceae	Żigland (Tuberous hawkbit)	Herb as diuretic and tonic (Lanfranco, 1993)
IOA-AMP-254	*Malva sylvestris* L., Malvaceae	Ħubbejża (Common mallow)	Leaf/flower poultices and root decoction in vaginitis, intestinal problems, depurative, skin and throat inflammation (Penza, 1969; Lanfranco, 1980)
IOA-AMP-268	*Mercurialis annua* L., Euphorbiaceae	Burikba (Annual mercury)	Juice as tonic and galactofuge (Penza, 1969; Lanfranco, 1975)

Voucher specimen number	Botanical Name, family	Maltese, (English) Names	Part/s used, preparation and Maltese Traditional uses
IOA-AMP-285	*Nerium oleander* L., Apocynaceae	Oljandru (Oleander)	Herb for skin itching (Cassar Pullicino, 1947)
IOA-AMP-290	*Olea europaea* L., Oleaceae	Żebbuġa (Olive)	Olive oil and leaves as laxative, wound healing, sunburn, antihypertensive, aching muscles (Penza 1969; Lanfranco, 1980)
IOA-AMP-286	*Opuntia ficus-indica* (L.) Mill., Cactaceae	Bgħajtar tax-xewk (Prickly pear)	Cladode/flower poultice in stomach pain, burnt skin, joint pain/headaches; astringent and antidiarrhoeal (Cassar Pullicino, 1947; Lanfranco, 1980; Lanfranco, 1975)
IOA-AMP-291	*Oxalis pes-caprae* L., Oxaliaceae	Ħaxixa ingliża, Cape sorrel	Herb juice as emetic and for acne (Lanfranco, 1975)
IOA-AMP-090	*Palaeocyanus crassifolius* (Bert.) Dost., Asteraceae	Widnet il-baħar (Maltese rock centaury)	National Plant of Malta
IOA-AMP-294	*Papaver somniferum* L. Papaveraceae	Xaħxieħ (Opium poppy)	Poppy heads and latex as sedative (Penza, 1969)
IOA-AMP-296	*Parietaria judaica*, Urticaceae	Xeħt ir-riħ (Pellitory of the wall)	Herb, decoction; herb boiled with garlic and chamomile in bronchitis, pharyngitis, pulmonitis and cough; catarrh; kidney stones; haemorrhoids (Borg, 1927; Penza, 1969; Cassar Pullicino, 1947)
IOA-AMP-304	*Phlomis fruticosa* L., Lamiaceae	Salvja tal-Madonna (Jerusalem sage)	Boiled leaves as cough remedy (Penza, 1969)
IOA-AMP-317	*Pinus halepensis* Miller, Pinaceae	Żnuber (Aleppo pine)	Inhalation and ointment for catarrh and as diuretic (Lanfranco, 1975)
IOA-AMP-319	*Pistacia lentiscus* L., Anacardiaceae	Deru (Mastic tree)	Mastic resin for filling of teeth (Gulia, 1855)
IOA-AMP-318	*Plantago lagopus* L., Plantaginaceae	Beżbula komuni (Hare's foot plantain)	Boiled leaves for wound healing, eye diseases and increases urination (Penza, 1969; Cassar Pullicino, 1947)
IOA-AMP-331	*Prasium majus* L., Lamiaceae	Te Sqalli (Mediterranean Prasium)	Infused leaves as diuretic (Penza, 1969; Gulia, 1855; Cremona, 1971)
IOA-AMP-345	*Psoralea bituminosa* L., Mimosaceae	Silla tal-blat (Bitumen pea)	Herb in rheumatic pain (Penza, 1969)
IOA-AMP-308	*Reicardia picroides*, Asteraceae	Kanċlita (Common reichardia)	Herb as diuretic and tonic (Lanfranco, 1993)
IOA-AMP-348	*Reseda alba* L., Resedaceae	Denb il-ħaruf (White mignonette)	Roots for painful gums (Borg, 1927; Penza, 1969)
IOA-AMP-360	*Ricinus communis* L., Euphorbiaceae	Riġnu (Castor oil tree)	Decoction of seeds, roots or leaves as laxative, rheumatism, neuralgic affections, ophthalmia; galactorrhoea (Penza, 1969)
IOA-AMP-374	*Schinus terebinthifolius*, Anacardiaceae	Bżar Falz (Drooping false pepper)	Ground fruit (Borg, 1927)
IOA-AMP-392	*Silybum marianum* (L.) Gaertn., Asteraceae	Xewk Bagħli (Milk thistle)	Herb as tonic, urinary tract, fever (Penza, 1969)

Voucher specimen number	Botanical Name, family	Maltese, (English) Names	Part/s used, preparation and Maltese Traditional uses
IOA-AMP-388	*Smyrnium olusatrum* L., Apiaceae	Karfus il-ħmir (Alexanders)	Herb as stimulant (Penza, 1969)
IOA-AMP-393	*Sonchus oleraceus* L., Asteraceae	Tfief (Sow thistle)	Herb as diuretic and purgative (Penza, 1969)
IOA-AMP-443	*Verbena officinalis* L., Verbenaceae	Buqexrem (Vervain)	Poultice/decoction for wound healing, astringent, diarrhoea, dysentery, diabetes (Penza, 1969)

Table 1. Botanical, ethnobotanical and voucher specimen code numbers for the fifty-five plants studied.

2.4 Brine Shrimp Test (BST)

In a set of 12-well plates, each well contained 10 nauplii, 1 ml sea water and 1 ml of extract diluted to final concentrations of 1%, 0.1%, 0.01%, 0.001% and 0.0001% respectively. The tests were set out in triplicate so that a total of fifteen wells per extract were used. numbers of living nauplii were counted after 24 hours. The LC_{50} values and 95 % confidence intervals were determined in µg/ml, using the Finney probit analysis computer program. A median lethal concentration (LC_{50}) smaller than 1000 µg/ml (Alkofahi et al., 1997) indicates pharmacological activity.

2.5 DNA-methyl green (intercalation) tests

DNA intercalation assay for DNA activity. Samples were incubated with 200 µl of DNA-methyl green in the dark at 25 °C for 24 h. The decrease in absorbance at 650 nm was calculated as a percentage of the untreated DNA-methyl green absorbance value. The median inhibitory concentration (IC_{50}) was calculated (Desmarchelier et al., 1996) through regression analysis. Cucurbitacin E and Dexamethasone were used as potent and moderate positive controls, respectively. Data was analyzed using Student's t-test.

3. Results and discussion

In this study, 55 plant species from 31 plant families were studied. The plant families ranked in the following order: Asteraceae (15 species), Apiaceae (3 species), Liliaceae, Scrophulariaceae, Mimosaceae, Brassicaceae, Fumariaceae, Euphorbiaceae, Lamiaceae and Anacardiaceae (2 species), Acanthaceae, Primulaceae, Boraginaceae, Iridaceae, Araliaceae, Solanaceae, Guttiferae, Lauracea, Malvaceae, Apocynaceae, Cactaceae, Oleaceae, Oxaliaceae, Papaveraceae, Urticaceae, Pinaceae, Plantaginaceae, Resedaceae, Verbenaceae, Myrtaceae and Cyperaceae (1 species). The distribution of plants within families was as broad as possible. However, the most abundant plant family of the Maltese flora (Attard, 2004) was given more importance than the other families.

3.1 Phytochemical analysis

The results for the four phytochemical classes are illustrated in table 2 and a generalised picture of the number of extracts, containing phytochemicals for each solvent system used, is illustrated in figure 1.

PLANT NAME	P. N°	Aqueous	Aqueous-ethanol	Ethanol	Chloroform	Petroleum ether
Acanthus mollis	002	TP	TP	TFP	TP	T
Aloe vera	015	-	-	TF	AF	-
Anagallis arvensis	028	P	P	P	FP	P
Antirrhinum siculum	037	P	TP	TP	TP	T
Antirrhinum tortuosum	036	TFP	TFP	TFP	T	TP
Arum italicum	046	TFP	TFP	TFP	T	T
Asparagus aphyllus	049	TFP	TFP	TFP	TFP	TAFP
Aster squamatus	453	FP	AFP	P	-	F
Calendula arvensis	068	TAP	TFP	AFP	-	F
Calendula suffruticosa	073	F	TFP	TFP	-	P
Carlina gummifera	081	TAFP	FP	A	-	TF
Ceratonia siliqua	091	AF	F	FP	TAF	AF
Cynoglossum creticum	145	FP	TFP	TFP	-	TP
Diplotaxis erucoides	153	P	P	T	-	-
Diplotaxis tenuifolia	463	TF	FP	FP	TF	T
Dittrichia viscosa	223	TFP	FP	TF	FP	AFP
Eucalyptus globulus	460	TFP	TFP	TFP	TFP	-
Ferula communis	459	TP	TP	TP	-	FP
Foeniculum vulgare	185	T	TP	TP	-	F
Fumaria capreolata	191	TP	TFP	TFP	TF	TP
Fumaria officinalis	190	TP	TP	TP	F	P
Galactites tomentosa	454	TFP	TFP	AP	-	TFP
Gladiolus italicus	197	-	-	TAF	-	TF
Glebionis coronaria	101	TFP	T	TAFP	-	TF
Hedera helix	202	-	TP	T	-	TF
Holoschoenus vulgaris	461	TFP	FP	F	F	T
Hyoscyamus albus	213	P	A	TP	-	TP
Hypericum aegyptiacum	217	FP	F	-	F	TP
Inula crithmoides	450	TFP	TFP	TFP	F	TF
Lactuca sativa	462	T	T	P	P	F
Lactuca virosa	236	-	P	-	TP	F
Laurus nobilis	234	F	T	T	-	TAF
Leontodon tuberosus	238	TFP	TFP	TF	F	F
Malva sylvestris	254	T	TP	T	-	-
Mercurialis annua	268	TF	TF	F	TFP	TF
Nerium oleander	285	TF	TFP	TFP	P	TF
Olea europaea	290	TFP	TFP	TF	TF	TFP
Opuntia ficus- indica	286	T	TP	TFP	P	TP
Oxalis pes-caprae	291	TF	TFP	TF	TF	A
Palaeocyanus crassifolius	90	TFP	TP	TP	TP	TFP
Papaver somniferum	294	FP	TP	TP	FP	TF

PLANT NAME	P. N°	Aqueous	Aqueous-ethanol	Ethanol	Chloroform	Petroleum ether
Parietaria judaica	296	F	FP	TFP	FP	AP
Phlomis fruticosa	304	TP	TFP	TFP	T	TFP
Pinus halepensis	317	P	-	TF	F	AF
Pistacia lentiscus	319	TFP	TF	P	-	-
Plantago lagopus	318	-	FP	AFP	TP	AP
Prasium majus	331	TFP	TFP	TFP	TP	P
Psoralea bituminosa	345	TP	TFP	T	T	P
Reichardia picroides	308	TFP	TFP	TP	F	TFP
Ricinus communis	360	TFP	TP	TFP	TF	-
Schinus terebinthifolius	374	TFP	TP	TP	P	TF
Smyrnium olusatrum	388	TFP	P	TFP	F	P
Sonchus oleraceus	393	TF	TF	TF	-	TF
Verbena officinalis	443	P	TP	TP	-	P

Table 2. The phytochemical analysis of the extracts under investigation for the main phytochemical classes: Flavonoids (F), Terpenoids (T), Alkaloids (A) and Proteins (P)

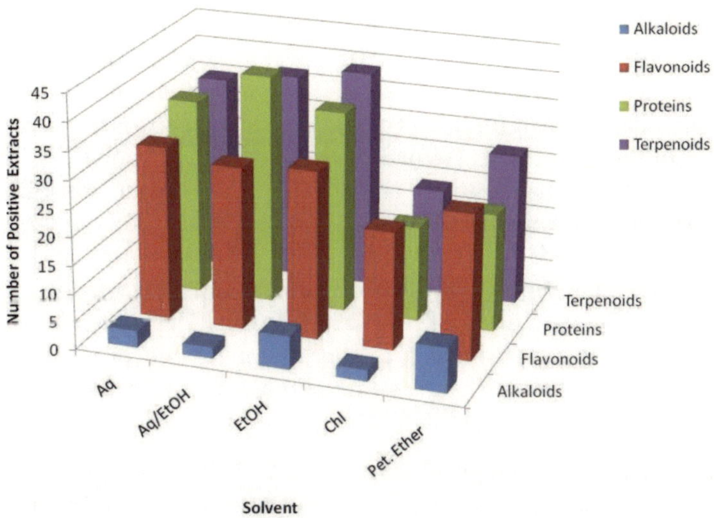

Fig. 1. A generalised profile of the number of extracts containing terpenoids, alkaloids, flavonoids and proteins for each solvent system used (n=280).

The predominating compound classes were terpenoids (56.07 %), followed by proteins (53.57 %) and flavonoids (48.93 %). Alkaloids were limited to a smaller number of extracts (7.50 %). The majority of the polar solvents, aqueous, aqueous-ethanol and ethanol contained terpenoids and proteins ($p<0.05$, n=4). The chloroform extract contained mainly flavonoids ($p<0.05$, n=4), while the petroleum ether extracts contained predominantly flavonoids and terpenoids.

The highest terpenoid contents were found in the ethanol and aqueous-ethanol extracts. In fact, it was observed that 70.70 % of the positive extracts were polar extracts, i.e. using water, water-ethanol and ethanol as extracting solvents. This is due to the fact that most terpenoids are present in the glycosidic form rather than the non-polar or low polarity terpene aglycone form. Some plants exhibited the presence of terpenes and related compounds in all solvent systems. Typical examples included *Acanthus mollis*, which mainly contains β-sitosterol as the triterpene-like compound (Loukis & Philianos, 1980), *Antirrhinum tortuosum*, with mono and sesquiterpene volatile derivatives (Nagegowda et al., 2008), *Arum italicum*, with the tetraterpene carotenoids (Bonora et al., 2000), *Asparagus aphyllus* with saponins and sapogenins (Shao et al., 1996), *Olea europaea* containing mainly triterpenoids (Caputo et al., 1974; Elamrani, 2011), *Palaeocyanus crassifolius* containing sesquiterpene lactones (Koukoulitsa et al., 2002) and *Phlomis fruticosa*, mainly containing mono- and sesquiterpenes (Amor et al., 2009). In the case of *Fumaria capreolata* the main constituents mentioned in previous studies were the alkaloids (Soušek et al., 1999; Maiza-Benabdesselam et al., 2007). In this present study, there was the strong presence of terpenoids.

The distribution of alkaloids in polar and non-polar solvents was almost equal (52.38 % and 47.62 %, respectively). Alkaloids may be present either as the non-polar organic form or as the polar ionised alkaloid salt. The highest content was recorded in the ethanol extract of *Gladiolus italicus* and in the chloroform extract of Aloe vera. For *Gladiolus*, this result goes in accordance with that obtained by Ameh and coworkers (2011) and for *Aloe*, a similar result was obtained by Waller and coworkers (1978). Other plants with an alkaloidal content include *Asparagus aphyllus* (Negi et al., 2010), *Calendula arvensis* (Shamsa et al., 2008), *Glactites tomentosa, Glebionis coronaria, Oxalis pes-caprae, Parietaria judaica, Carlina gummifera, Hyoscyamus albus* (Doerk-Schmitz et al., 1993), *Laurus nobilis* (Nayak et al., 2006), *Pinus halepensis* (Tawara et al., 1993) and *Plantago lagopus* (Hultin & Torssell, 1965). *Fumaria* species are known to contain alkaloids (Soušek et al., 1999; Maiza-Benabdesselam et al., 2007). However, no alkaloids were detected for *Fumaria officinalis* and *Fumaria capreolata* in this present study. Although *Ceratonia siliqua* is claimed to contain no alkaloids (El Hajaji et al., 2011), in this present study, alkaloids were detected in the aqueous, chloroform and petroleum ether extracts. It was also observed that for *Papaver somniferum* no alkaloids were detected in the leaves. This depends on several factors. Primarily, the wild variety might have a low potential for the production of morphinan alkaloids, and other plant parts such as the stem, roots and capsules, tend to accumulate more alkaloids than the leaves (Williams & Ellis, 1989).

For the flavonoid group, out of the positive responses, 65.69 % were polar extracts while the rest (34.41 %) were extracts derived from non-polar solvents. Typically, flavonoids are polyphenolic compounds that are highly soluble in aqueous and aqueous-alcohol solvents. However, flavonoids have been reported to be also extracted by chloroform and petroleum ether (Gudej & Czapski, 2009; Rajendran & Krishnakumar, 2010). Plants containing flavonoids in all extracts, consistent with other studies, include *Asparagus aphyllus* (Sun et al., 2007), *Ceratonia siliqua* (Papagiannopoulos et al., 2004; Vaya & Mahmood, 2006), *Dittrichia viscosa* (M.J. Martin et al., 1988), *Leontodon tuberosus* (Zidorn & Stuppner, 2001), *Mercurialis annua* (Aquino et al., 1987) and *Olea europaea* (Benavente-García et al., 2000). Almost all plant species exhibited the presence of flavonoids in one or more extracts, except for four plants, namely, *Antirrhinum siculum, Diplotaxis erucoides, Malva sylvestris* and *Verbena officinalis*. Other studies report the presence of flavonoids in *Diplotaxis erucoides* (Bennett et al., 2006), *Malva sylvestris* (Billeter et al., 1991) and *Verbena officinalis* (Rehecho et al., 2011).

The absence of flavonoids in these species for the current study may be due to several factors that include a different chemotype, different environmental conditions and the presence of these compounds below the detection limit, amongst others. *Antirrhinum siculum* is palely pigmented and this may contribute to the insignificant content of flavonoids (C. Martin et al., 2010).

Proteins prevail in many plants. Within the positive response group, 74.67 % were polar extracts while 25.33 % were non-polar extracts. This indicated that three-forths of the detected proteins were functional proteins including enzymes. *Anagallis arvensis, Asparagus aphyllus, Palaeocyanus crassifolius* and *Prasium majus* exhibited the presence of proteins in all their extracts. This goes in accordance with previous studies carried out on these plants (Alignier et al., 2008; King et al., 1990). Plants that were devoid of proteins in all their extracts include *Aloe vera, Gladiolus italicus, Laurus nobilis* and *Sonchus oleraceus*. In previous studies, *Aloe vera* revealed the presence of glutathione peroxidase (Sabeh et al., 1993), *Gladiolus italicus* contained arabinogalactan-protein (Gleeson & Clarke, 1979) and *Laurus nobilis* contained lipase (Isbilir et al., 2008). Although most plant material was collected at flowering time, the inclusion of seed protein in the extract would have been possible in cases where fruit were harvested alongside the flowers.

3.2 The Brine Shrimp Test

The results for the tested extracts are given in Table 3. Primary screening involves the use of bench-top bioassays. Extracts exhibiting LC_{50} values above 1000 µg/ml are generally regarded as ineffective extracts. In this study, 42.26 % of the extracts were therefore inactive (Table 4). The most inactive were the petroleum ether extracts, while the most active were the ethanolic extracts. Correlating the BST lethal concentrations to phytochemical classes, it was observed that inactive extracts contained several phytochemicals. The reason may be due to the low concentration or possible antagonistic activity between the phytochemicals from the different classes. 55.68 % of the extracts exhibited LC_{50} values below 1000 µg/ml. The most active were the ethanolic extracts (72.97 %), while the least active were the petroleum ether extracts (35.14 %). Four plants exhibited activity for all their five extracts. These were *Nerium oleander, Olea europaea, Opuntia ficus-indica* and *Pinus halepensis,* all exhibiting LC_{50} values below 0.01 µg/ml. These four plant species are amongst the most popular Maltese traditional medicinal plants. It was also observed that some extracts with non-detectable phytochemicals exhibited significant LC_{50} values. Typical examples include the aqueous extract of *Lactuca virosa,* the aqueous-ethanol extract of *Pinus halepensis,* the ethanolic extracts of *Hypericum aegypticum* and *Lactuca virosa,* and the chloroform extracts of *Ferula communis, Foeniculum vulgare* and *Pistacia lentiscus.* On the other hand, there were extracts that exhibited significant LC_{50} values as opposed to other studies. For example, for *Fumaria officinalis* aqueous-ethanol and ethanol extracts, in the present study, exhibited significant effects on brine shrimps as opposed to the ethanol extract reported in the study by Erdoğan (2009).

3.3 The DNA-methyl green assay

Table 5 shows the IC_{50} values obtained for the DNA-methyl green assay. Although low IC_{50} values have been reported for pure compounds (Burres et al., 1992) , such as rubiflavin and distamycin A (17 and 18 µg/ml, respectively), it is reasonable that in the case of extracts higher IC_{50} values are acceptable as for pyrido[2,3-d]pyrimidin-4(1H)-one and pyrido[2,3-d]triazolo[3,4-b]pyrimidine analogs (40 - 53 µg/ml) (Goda & Badria, 2005). Since plant extracts are complex matrices with several phytochemicals, IC_{50} values are expected to be higher than for pure compounds. Therefore, extracts with IC_{50} values below 70 µg/ml were considered as active (Figure 2). Only 15 % of the extracts displaced methyl green from the methyl green DNA complex. It is likely that these compounds act as intercalating agents at the DNA level. 86.67 % were active polar extracts with proteins predominating in these extracts. The other extracts either exhibited an IC_{50} value higher than 70 µg/ml or else a 50 % activity was never achieved. From the remaining 85 %, only one-third of the extracts exhibited values above 70 µg/ml. Alkaloids only featured in one active aqueous extract of *Ceratonia siliqua*. Terpenoids, flavonoids and proteins predominated mainly in aqueous and aqueous-ethanol extracts. For a few extracts, there was no correlation between the phytochemical class and DNA-methyl green activity. These include the aqueous-ethanol extract of *Gladiolus italicus*, the aqueous extract of *Hedera helix* and the ethanolic extract of *Hypericum aegyptiacum*. For example *H. aegyptiacum* contains hypericin that can inhibit DNA topoisomerase II (Peebles et al., 2001), but the naphthodianthrone was not detected by the phytochemical tests.

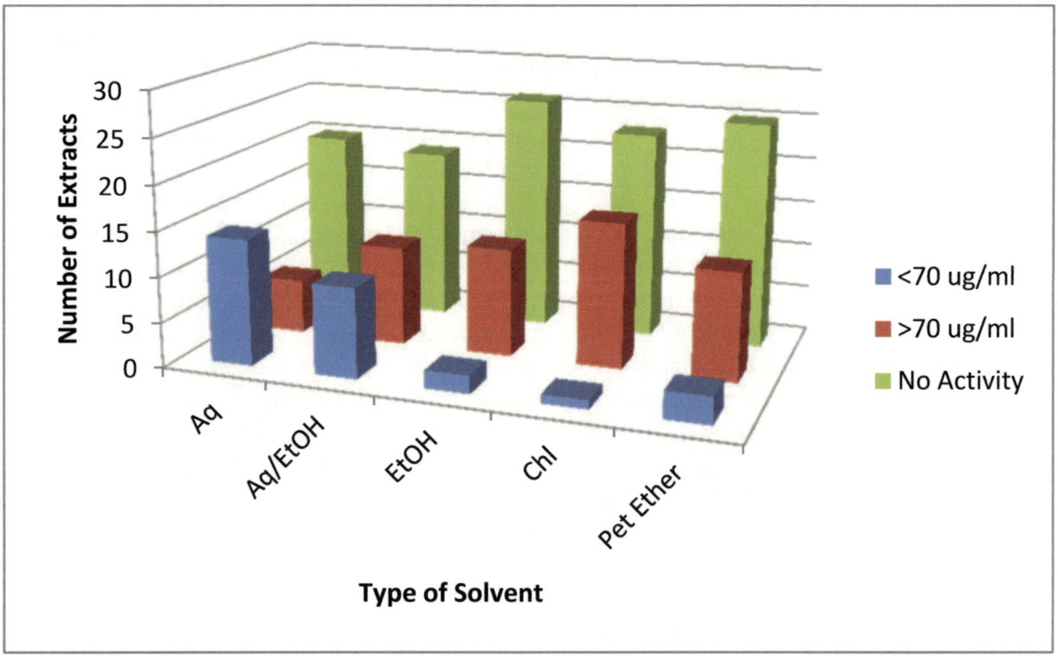

Fig. 2. The number of extracts classified as (a) below 70 µg/ml, (b) above 70 µg/ml range and (c) non-active extracts with the different solvent types for the DNA methyl green assay.

PLANT NAME	P. N°	Aqueous	Aqueous-ethanol	Ethanol	Chloroform	Petroleum ether
Acanthus mollis	002	<0.01	<0.01	<0.01	<0.01	>1000
Anagallis arvensis	028	460	<0.01	<0.01	>1000	>1000
Antirrhinum tortuosum	036	<0.01	>1000	<0.01	>1000	<0.01
Antirrhinum siculum	037	10	<0.01	<0.01	>1000	<0.01
Asparagus aphyllus	049	>1000	<0.01	<0.01	<0.01	>1000
Aster squamatus	453	>1000	>1000	>1000	>1000	>1000
Calendula arvensis	068	>1000	63	>1000	>1000	796
Carlina gummifera	081	>1000	>1000	>1000	>1000	>1000
Dittrichia viscosa	223	>1000	>1000	>1000	<0.01	>1000
Ferula communis	459	<0.01	<0.01	<0.01	<0.01	>1000
Foeniculum vulgare	185	>1000	<0.01	<0.01	<0.01	>1000
Fumaria officinalis	190	>1000	<0.01	<0.01	>1000	<0.01
Fumaria capreolata	191	>1000	>1000	<0.01	<0.01	>1000
Galactites tomentosa	454	>1000	>1000	>1000	>1000	>1000
Glebionis coronaria	101	>1000	>1000	93	131	>1000
Hyoscyamus albus	213	>1000	ND	<0.01	>1000	>1000
Hypericum aegyptiacum spreng	217	<0.01	<0.01	<0.01	>1000	>1000
Inula crithmoides	450	>1000	344	>1000	>1000	562
Lactuca sativa	462	<0.01	<0.01	<0.01	>1000	<0.01
Lactuca virosa	236	<0.01	<0.01	<0.01	>1000	>1000
Leontodon tuberosus	238	>1000	>1000	>1000	>1000	>1000
Nerium oleander	285	<0.01	<0.01	<0.01	<0.01	<0.01
Opuntia ficus- indica	286	<0.01	<0.01	<0.01	<0.01	<0.01
Olea europaea	290	<0.01	<0.01	<0.01	<0.01	<0.01
Oxalis pes-caprae	291	<0.01	<0.01	<0.01	<0.01	>1000
Palaeocyanus crassifolius	090	>1000	<0.01	<0.01	>1000	10
Papaver somniferum	294	<0.01	<0.01	<0.01	<0.01	>1000
Pinus halepensis	317	<0.01	<0.01	<0.01	<0.01	<0.01
Plantago lagopus	318	>1000	10	<0.01	>1000	0.07
Pistacia lentiscus	319	<0.01	<0.01	<0.01	<0.01	ND
Prasium majus	331	<0.01	<0.01	<0.01	<0.01	>1000
Psoralea bituminosa	345	<0.01	<0.01	<0.01	10	<0.01
Reichardia picroides	308	>1000	>1000	>1000	>1000	>1000
Reseda alba	348	>1000	<0.01	ND	10	>1000
Ricinus communis	360	>1000	<0.01	<0.01	<0.01	>1000
Schinus terebinthifolius	374	<0.01	<0.01	<0.01	<0.01	>1000
Sonchus oleraceus	393	>1000	>1000	>1000	>1000	>1000

Table 3. The result for the effect of extracts on the Brine Shrimp Test

	Percentage per extract type					Percentage of Total Extracts
BST result	Aqueous	Aqueous-ethanol	Ethanol	Chloroform	Petroleum ether	
>1000	51.35	27.03	24.32	48.65	59.46	42.16 %
0.01-1000	5.41	8.11	2.70	8.11	10.81	7.03 %
0.01	43.24	62.16	70.27	43.24	24.32	48.65 %
ND	0.00	2.70	2.70	0.00	5.41	2.16 %

Table 4. The percentage of results classified as (a) above 1000 μg/ml, (b) 0.01 – 1000 μg/ml range, (c) less than 0.01 μg/ml and (d) not determined (ND) with the different solvent types for the brine shrimp test.

PLANT NAME	P. N°	Aqueous	Aqueous-ethanol	Ethanol	Chloroform	Petroleum ether
Acanthus mollis	2	30.399	34.102	NA	131.005	34.354
Aloe vera	15	NA	278.589	270.983	NA	NA
Anagallis arvensis	28	28.658	43.534	NA	NA	NA
Antirrhinum tortuosum	36	63.354	156.171	314.838	38.065	354.278
Antirrhinum siculum	37	NA	NA	NA	NA	NA
Asparagus aphyllus	49	NA	52.985	NA	305.865	NA
Calendula suffruticosa	73	70.296	144.921	350.003	261.826	364.324
Ceratonia siliqua	91	23.230	NA	NA	134.563	NA
Cynoglossum creticum	145	45.941	50.063	NA	NA	NA
Eucalyptus globulus	460	NA	NA	NA	NA	NA
Ferula communis	459	NA	NA	NA	71.158	92.264
Foeniculum vulgare	185	NA	NA	NA	NA	NA
Fumaria capreolata	191	133.655	77.458	NA	596.272	NA
Fumaria officinalis	190	NA	346.108	NA	NA	79.496
Gladiolus italicus	197	NA	54.931	NA	143.109	251.228
Hedera helix	202	60.086	231.921	NA	NA	NA
Holoschoenus vulgaris	461	NA	91.229	NA	NA	NA
Hyoscyamus albus	213	NA	NA	195.094	NA	NA
Hypericum aegyptiacum	217	NA	NA	66.803	NA	443.799
Diplotaxis tenuifolia	463	NA	30.688	NA	NA	NA
Dittrichia viscosa	223	26.945	NA	108.418	171.989	NA
Laurus nobilis	234	50.835	NA	324.334	189.539	NA
Lactuca sativa	462	NA	166.722	326.359	NA	NA
Lactuca virosa	236	NA	NA	NA	NA	57.791
Malva sylvestris	254	NA	31.530	NA	NA	54.922
Mercurialis annua	268	NA	165.974	NA	NA	NA
Nerium oleander	285	NA	62.957	NA	105.401	163.761
Opuntia ficus- indica	286	41.899	85.339	NA	115.870	NA
Olea europaea	290	53.908	95.687	80.988	227.594	NA
Oxalis pes-caprae	291	NA	NA	64.089	223.200	171.288
Palaeocyanus crassifolius	90	122.931	NA	NA	NA	NA
Papaver somniferum	294	147.538	NA	NA	NA	131.727

Parietaria judaica	296	NA	NA	89.115	NA	NA
Phlomis fruticosa	304	137.404	NA	159.786	130.591	171.195
Pinus halepensis	317	NA	NA	NA	NA	NA
Plantago lagopus	318	NA	49.252	338.260	NA	NA
Pistacia lentiscus	319	NA	NA	NA	NA	NA
Prasium majus	331	48.142	103.372	273.826	92.489	279.194
Psoralea bituminosa	345	NA	59.332	NA	NA	177.895
Reseda alba	348	193.473	NA	NA	NA	NA
Ricinus communis	360	48.912	NA	NA	103.224	NA
Schinus terebinthifolius	374	NA	NA	NA	NA	181.849
Smyrnium olusatrum	388	104.605	NA	NA	NA	NA
Silybum marianum	392	NA	46.528	NA	NA	NA
Verbena officinalis	443	67.656	104.453	145.529	158.008	NA
Cucurbitacin E	-	19.12				
Dexamethasone	-	32.74				

Table 5. The median inhibitory concentration (IC_{50} in µg/ml) values obtained for the DNA-methyl green assay (NA no activity – 50% effect was never reached).

4. Conclusions

This study has confirmed the presence of useful phytochemicals and biological activities of several extracts from selected Mediterranean plants. It is expected that these results will serve as a stimulus for further investigations into the active phytochemicals.

5. Acknowledgment

This work was supported and funded by the Malta Council for Science and Technology, Malta (Project code: RTDI-2004-074).

6. References

Alignier, A., Meiss, H., Petit, S. & Reboud, X. (2008). Variation of post-dispersal weed seed predation according to weed species, space and time. Journal of Plant Diseases and Protection, Vol. 21, pp. 221-228, ISSN 1861-3829

Ameh, S.J., Obodozie, O.O., Olorunfemi, P.O., Okoliko, I.E. & Ochekpe, N.A. (2011). Potentials of *Gladiolus* corms as an antimicrobial agent in food processing and traditional medicine. *Journal of Microbiology and Antimicrobials,* Vol. 3, No. 1, pp. 8-12, ISSN 2141-2308

Amor, I.L.B., Boubakera, J., Sgaiera, M.B., Skandrania, I., Bhouria, W., Neffati, A., Kilani, S., Bouhlel, I., Ghedira, K. & Chekir-Ghedira, L. (2009). Phytochemistry and biological activities of *Phlomis* species. *Journal of Ethnopharmacology,* Vol. 125, No. 2, pp. 183-202, ISSN 0378-8741

Aquino, R., Behar, I., D'agostino, M., De Simone, F., Schettino, O. & Pizza, C. (1987). Phytochemical investigation on *Mercurialis annua. Biochemical Systematics and Ecology,* Vol. 15, No. 6, pp. 667-669, ISSN 0305-1978

Attard, E. & Attard, H. (2006). The Potential Angiotensin-Converting Enzyme Inhibitory Activity of Oleanolic Acid in the Hydroethanolic Extract of *Crataegus monogyna* Jacq. *Natural Product Communications,* Vol. 1, No. 5, pp. 381-386, ISSN 1934-578X

Attard, E. & Attard, H. (2008) Antitrypsin activity of extracts from *Ecballium elaterium* seeds. *Fitoterapia*, Vol. 79, No. 3, pp. 226-228, ISSN 0367-326X

Attard, E. & Vella, K. (2009). The Effects of Ephedrine and *Ephedra fragilis* Crude Extracts on Human Peripheral Lymphocytes. *Pharmacognosy Research,* Vol. 1, No. 2, pp. 38-42, ISSN 0974-8490

Attard, E., Brincat, M.P. & Cuschieri, A. (2005). Immunomodulatory activity of cucurbitacin E isolated from *Ecballium elaterium*. *Fitoterapia*, Vol. 76, pp. 439-441, ISSN 0367-326X

Attard, E. (2004). Status of Medicinal and Aromatic Plants in Malta, In: Baricevic, D., Bernath, J., Maggioni, L. and Lipman E. *Report of a Working Group on Medicinal and Aromatic Plants,* First Meeting, Gozd Martuljek, Slovenia, 12-14 September 2002, International Plant Genetic Resources Institute, Rome, Italy, pp. 85 – 87, ISBN 978-92-9043-812-0

Benavente-García, O., Castillo, J., Lorente, J., Ortuño, A. & Del Rio, J.A. (2000). Antioxidant activity of phenolics extracted from *Olea europaea* L. leaves. *Food Chemistry*, Vol. 68, No. 4, pp. 457-462. ISSN 0308-8146

Bennett, R.N., Rosa, E.A.S, Mellon, F.A. & Kroon, P.A. (2006). Ontogenic profiling of glucosinolates, flavonoids, and other secondary metabolites in *Eruca sativa* (salad rocket), *Diplotaxis erucoides* (wall rocket), *Diplotaxis tenuifolia* (wild rocket), and *Bunias orientalis* (Turkish rocket). *Journal of Agricultural and Food Chemistry*, Vol. 54, No. 11, pp. 4005-4015, ISSN 0021-8561

Billeter, M, Meier, B. & Sticher, O. (1991). 8-hydroxyflavonoid glucuronides from *Malva sylvestris*. *Phytochemistry*, Vol. 30, No. 3, pp. 987-990, ISSN 0031-9422

Bonora, A., Pancaldi, S., Gualandri, R. & Palmira Fasulo, M. (2000). Carotenoid and ultrastructure variations in plastids of *Arum italicum* Miller fruit during maturation and ripening. *Journal of Experimental Botany*, Vol. 51, No. 346, pp. 873-884, ISSN 0022-0957

Borg, J. (1927). *Descriptive Flora of the Maltese Islands,* Government Printing Office, Malta

Buhagiar, J.A., Podesta, M.T., Wilson, A.P., Micallef, M.J. & Ali, S. (1999). The induction of apoptosis in human melanoma, breast and ovarian cancer cell lines using an essential oil extract from the conifer *Tetraclinis articulata*. *Anticancer Research*, Vol. 19, No. 6B, pp. 5435-5443, ISSN 0250-7005

Burres, N.S., Frigo, A., Rasmussen, R.R. & McAlpine, J.B (1992). A colorimetric microassay for the detection of agents that interact with DNA. *Journal of Natural Products*, Vol. 55, No. 11, pp. 1582–1587, ISSN 0163-3864

Carballo, J.L., Hernandez-Inda, Z.L., Perez, P. & Garcia-Gravalos, M.D. (2002). A comparison between two brine shrimp assays to detect in vitro cytotoxicity in marine natural products. *BMC Biotechnology*, Vol. 2, pp. 17-25, ISSN 1472-6750

Cassar, P. (1964). *Medical History of Malta,* Wellcome Historical Medical Library, London

Cassar Pullicino, J. (1947). *An Introduction to the Maltese Folklore*, Malta

Calderon, A.I., Terreaux, C., Gupta, M.P. & Hostettmann, K. (2003). *In vitro* cytotoxicity of 11 Panamanian plants. *Fitoterapia*, Vol. 74, pp. 378 – 383, ISSN 0367-326X

Caputo, R., Mangoni, L., Monaco, P. & Previtera L. (1974). New triterpenes from the leaves of *Olea europaea*. *Phytochemistry*, Vol. 13, No. 12, pp. 2825-2827, ISSN 0031-9422

Cremona, A. (1971). *Ħxejjex ta' Mediċina Popolari fil-Gżejjer ta' Malta u Għawdex*, Leħen il-Malti, No. 16

Darmanin, S. (2003). Investigations of the Anti-Neoplastic Activity of a Bioactive Extract derived from *Ricinus communis*. University of Malta. Faculty of Medicine and Surgery. Department of Anatomy. (Unpublished)

Delhaye, S. & Landry, J. (1992). Determination of tryptophan in pure proteins and plant material by three methods. Analyst, Vol. 117, pp. 1875 - 1877, ISSN 0003-2654

Deshpande, S.S., Cheryan, M. & Salunkhe, D.K. (1986). Tannin analysis of food products. CRC Critical Reviews in Food Science & Nutrition, Vol. 24, pp. 401-449, ISSN 0099-0248

Doerk-Schmitz, K., Witte, L. & Alfermann, A.W. (1993). Tropane alkaloid patterns in plants and hairy roots of Hyoscyamus albus. Phytochemistry, Vol. 35, No. 1, pp. 107-110, ISSN 0031-9422

Edeoga, H.O., Okwu, D.E. & Mbaebie, B.O. (2005). Phytochemical constituents of some Nigerian medicinal Plants. *African Journal of Biotechnology*, Vol. 4, pp. 685-688, ISSN 1684-5315

El Hajaji, H., Lachkarb, N., Alaoui Cherrah, Y., Farah, A., Ennabili, A., El Bali, B. & Lachkar, M. (2011). Antioxidant activity, phytochemical screening, and total phenolic content of extracts from three genders of carob tree barks growing in Morocco. *Arabian Journal of Chemistry*, Vol. 4, No. 3, pp. 321-324, ISSN 1878-5352

Elamrani, A. (2011). The Antitumoral Activity and the Cytotoxicity on Renal Cells of Ethanolic Extracts from the Leaves of Four Varieties of *Olea europaea* L. Grown in Morocco. *Analytical Chemistry Letters*, Vol. 1, No. 1, pp. 63 – 69, ISSN 2229-7928

Erdoğan, T.F. (2009). Brine Shrimp Lethality Bioassay of *Fumaria densiflora* Dc. and *Fumaria officinalis* L. Extracts. *Hacettepe University Journal of the Faculty of Pharmacy*, Vol. 28, No. 2, pp. 125-132, ISSN 1300-0608

Evans, W.C. (2009). *Trease and Evans' Pharmacognosy* (16th Edition), Saunders, ISBN 978-0-7020-2933-2, London.

Franssen, F.F.J., Sweijsters, L.L.J., Berger, I. & Medinilla Aldana, B.E. (1997). *In vivo* and *In vitro* Antiplasmodial Activities of some plants traditionally used in Guatemala aginst Malaria. Antimicrobial Agents and Chemotherapy, Vol. 41, No. 7, pp. 1500-1503, ISSN 0066-4804

Gleeson, P.A. & Clarke, A.E. (1979). Structural studies on the major component of *Gladiolus* style mucilage, an arabinogalactan-protein. Biochemical Journal, Vol. 181, No. 3, pp. 607–621, ISSN 0264-6021

Goda, F.E. & Badria, F.A. (2005). Synthesis and Biological Evaluation of Certain New Substituted Pyrido[2,3-D]Pyrimidin-4(1h)-One and Pyrido [2,3-D]Triazolo[3,4-B]Pyrimidine Analogs. *Saudi Pharmaceutical Journal*, Vol. 13, No. 2-3, pp. 65-73, ISSN 1319-0164

Gudej, J. and Czapski, P. (2009). Components of the petroleum ether and chloroform extracts of *Chrysosplenium alternifolium*. *Chemistry of Natural Compounds*. Vol. 45, No. 5, pp. 717-719. ISSN 0009-3130

Guarrera, P.M. (2003). Food medicine and minor nourishment in the folk traditions of Central Italy (Marche, Abruzzo and Latium), *Fitoterapia*, Vol. 74, pp. 515-544. ISSN 0367-326X

Gulia, G. (1855). *Repertorio Botanico Maltese*, Ex Libris Publii, Malta.

Harborne, J.B. (1984). *Phytochemical Methods* (Second Edition), Chapman and Hall, ISBN 0-412-25550-2, London and New York.

Hultin, E. & Torssell, K. (1965). Alkaloid-screening of Swedish plants. *Phytochemistry*, Vol. 4, No. 3, pp. 425-433, ISSN 0031-9422

Isbilir, S.S., Ozcan, H.M. & Yagar, H. (2008). Some Biochemical Properties of Lipase from Bay Laurel (*Laurus nobilis* L.) Seeds. *Journal of the American Oil Chemists' Society*, pp. 227-233, ISSN 0003-021X

Jaki, B., Orjala, J., Burgi, H.R. & Sticher, O. (1999). Biological screening of cyanobacteria for antimicrobial and molluscicidal activity, brine shrimp lethality and cytotoxicity. *Pharmaceutical Biology*, Vol. 37, pp. 138-143, ISSN 1388-0209

Javidnia, K, Miri, R, Najifi, RB & Jagromi, NK (2003). A preliminary study on the Biological Activiy of *Daphne mucronata* royle. *DARU Journal of the School of Pharmacy*, Vol 11, pp. 28-31, ISSN 1560-8115

Kanegusuku, M., Benassi, J.C., Pedrosa, R.C., Yunes, R.A., Filho, V.C., Maia, A.A., de Sousa, M.M., Delle Monache, F. & Niero, R. (2001). Cytotoxic, Hypoglycemic Activity and Phytochemical Analysis of *Rubus imperialis* (Rosaceae), *Zeitschrift für Naturforschung*, Vol. 57c, pp. 272-276, ISSN 0932-0784

Kim, E.J., Tian, F. & Woo, M.H. (2000). Asitrocin, (2,4)-cis- and trans-asitrocinones: novel bioactive mono-tetrahydrofuran acetogenins from *Asimina triloba* seeds, *Journal of Natural Products*, Vol. 63, No. 11, pp. 1503-1506, ISSN 0163-3864

King, G.A., Woollard, D.C., Irving, D.E. & Borst, W.M. (1990). Physiological changes in asparagus spear tips after harvest, *Physiologia Plantarum*, Vol. 80, No. 3, pp. 393–400, ISSN 0031-9317

Konning, G.H., Agyare, C. & Ennison, B. (2003). Antimicrobial activity of some medicinal plants from Ghana, *Fitoterapia*, Vol. 75, pp. 65-67, ISSN 0367-326X

Koukoulitsa, E., Skaltsa, H., Karioti, A., Demetzos, C. & Dimas, K. (2002). Bioactive Sesquiterpene Lactones from *Centaurea* Species and their Cytotoxic/Cytostatic Activity Against Human Cell Lines *in vitro, Planta Medica*, Vol. 68, No. 7, pp. 649-652, ISSN 0032-0943

Krey, A.K. & Hahn, F.E. (1975). Studies on the methyl green-DNA complex and its dissociation by drugs. *Biochemistry*, Vol. 14, No. 23, pp. 5061 - 5067, ISSN 0006-2960

Kumarasamy Y., Fergusson M.E., Nahar L. & Sarker S.D. (2002) Bioactivity of Moschamindole from *Centaurea moschata. Pharmaceutical Biology*, Vol. 40, No. 4, pp. 307 - 310, ISSN 1388-0209

Kurnick B. & Foster M. (1950). Methyl green. III. Reaction with desoxyribonucleic acid: Stoichiometry and behavior of the reaction product, *Journal of General Physiology*, Vol. 34, pp. 147-159, ISSN 0022-1295

Kurnick, N. (1950) The determination of desoxyribonuclease activity by methyl green: Application to Serum, Archives of Biochemistry, Vol. 29, pp. 41-53, ISSN 0570-6963

Lanfranco, G. (1975). *Duwa u Semm il-Ħxejjex Maltin*. Edizzjoni Klabb Kotba Maltin, Malta.

Lanfranco, G. (1980). Some Recent Communications on the Folk Medicine of Malta, *L-Imnara*, Vol. 3

Lanfranco, G. (1993). *Ħxejjex mediċinali u oħrajn fil-Gżejjer Maltin*. Media Centre Publications, Malta

Loukis, A. & Philianos, S. (1980). Phytochemical investigation of *Acanthus mollis* L. *Fitoterapia*, Vol. 51, No. 4, pp. 183-185, ISSN 0367-326X

Maiza-Benabdesselam, F., Chibane, M., Madani, K., Max, H. & Adach, S. (2007). Determination of isoquinoline alkaloids contents in two Algerian species of *Fumaria* (*Fumaria capreolata* and Fumaria *bastardi*), *African Journal of Biotechnology*, Vol. 6, No. 21, pp. 2487-2492, ISSN 1684-5315

Mangion Randon, A. & Attard, E (2007). The *in vitro* Immunomodulatory Activity of Oleuropein, a Secoiridoid Glycoside from *Olea europaea* L. *Natural Product Communications*, Vol. 2, No. 5, pp. 515-519, ISSN 1934-578X

Martin, C., Ellis, N. & Rook F. (2010). Do Transcription Factors Play Special Roles in Adaptive Variation? *Plant Physiology*, Vol. 154, No. 2, pp. 506-511, ISSN 0032-0889

Martin, M.J., Alarcón de la Lastra, C., Marhuenda, E., Delgado, F. & Torreblanca J. (1988). Anti-ulcerogenicity of the flavonoid fraction from *Dittrichia viscosa* (L.) W. Greuter in rats. *Phytotherapy Research.* Vol. 2, No. 4, pp. 183–186, ISSN 0951-418X

Meyer, B.N., Ferrigni, N.R., Putnam, J.E., Jacobsen, L.B., Nichols, D.E. & McLaughlin, J.L. (1982). Brine Shrimp: A convenient general bioassay for active plant constituents. *Planta Medica*, Vol. 45, pp. 31-34, ISSN 0032-0943

Nagegowda, D.A., Gutensohn, M., Wilkerson, C.G. & Dudareva N. (2008). Two nearly identical terpene synthases catalyze the formation of nerolidol and linalool in snapdragon flowers. *The Plant Journal*, Vol. 55, No. 2, pp. 224–239, ISSN 0960-7412

Nayak, S., Nalabothu, P., Sandiford, S., Bhogadi, V. & Adogwa, A. (2006). Evaluation of wound healing activity of *Allamanda cathartica*. L. and *Laurus nobilis*. L. extracts on rats. *BMC Complementary and Alternative Medicine*, Vol. 6, p. 12, ISSN 1472-6882

Negi, J.S., Singh, P., Joshi, G.P., Rawat, M.S. & Bisht, V.K. (2010). Chemical constituents of *Asparagus*. *Pharmacognosy Review*, Vol. 4, No. 8, pp. 215-220, ISSN 0973-7847

Papagiannopoulos, M., Wollseifen, H.R., Mellenthin, A., Haber, B. & Galensa, R. (2004). Identification and Quantification of Polyphenols in Carob Fruits (*Ceratonia siliqua* L.) and Derived Products by HPLC-UV-ESI/MS. *Journal of Agricultural and Food Chemistry*, Vol. 52, No. 12, pp. 3784–3791, ISSN 0021-8561

Peebles, K.A., Baker, R.K., Kurz, E.U., Schneider, B.J. & Kroll, D.J. (2001). Catalytic inhibition of human DNA topoisomerase IIα by hypericin, a naphthodianthrone from St. John's wort (*Hypericum perforatum*). *Biochemical Pharmacology*. Vol. 62, No. 8, pp. 1059-1070. ISSN 0006-2952

Penza, C. (1969). *Flora Maltija Mediċinali*, Progress Press Co. Ltd., Malta

Punjani, B.L. & Kumar, V. (2003) Ethnomedicinal plants specially used for liver disorders in the Aravalli ranges of Gujarat, India. *Journal of Natural Remedies*, Vol. 3, No. 2, pp. 195-198, ISSN 0972-5547

Rajendran, R. & Krishnakumar, E. (2010). Hypolipidemic Activity of Chloroform Extract of *Mimosa pudica* Leaves. *Avicenna Journal of Medical Biotechnology*. Vol. 2, No. 4, pp. 215-221, ISSN 2008-4625

Rehecho, S., Hidalgo, O., García-Iñiguez de Cirano, M., Navarro, I., Astiasarán, I., Ansorena, D., Cavero, R.Y. & Calvo, M.I. (2011). Chemical composition, mineral content and antioxidant activity of *Verbena officinalis* L. *LWT- Food Science and Technology*, Vol. 44, No. 4, pp. 875-882, ISSN 0023-6438

Rodriguez-Lopez, V, Salazar, L & Estrada, S. (2003). Spasmolytic activity of several extracts obtained from some Mexican medicinal plants. *Fitoterapia*, Vol. 74, pp. 725-728, ISSN 0367-326X

Rossi, B. & Attard, E. (2011). The Haemagglutination potential of extracts from *Urtica dubia* plant parts. *Journal of Natural Remedies*, Vol. 11, No. 1, pp. 76-78, ISSN 0972-5547

Sabeh, F., Wright, T. & Norton, S.J. (1993). Purification and characterization of a glutathione peroxidase from the *Aloe vera* plant. *Enzyme & Protein*, Vol. 47, No. 2, pp. 92-98, ISSN 1019-6773

Shamsa, F., Monsef, H., Ghamooshi, R. & Verdian-rizi, M. (2008). Spectrophotometric determination of total alkaloids in some Iranian medicinal plants. Thai J. Pharm. Sci. Vol. 32, pp. 17-20, ISSN 0125-4685

Shao, Y., Chin, C.K., Ho, C.T., Ma, W., Garrison, S.A. & Huang, M.T. (1996). Anti-tumor activity of the crude saponins obtained from asparagus. *Cancer Letters*, Vol. 104, No. 1, pp. 31-36, ISSN 0304-3835

Soušek, J., Guédon, D., Adam, T., Bochořáková H., Táborská E., Válka I. & Šimánek V. (1999). Alkaloids and organic acids content of eight *Fumaria* species. *Phytochemical Analysis*. Vol. 10, No. 1, pp. 6–11, ISSN 0958-0344

Steinberg, D.M., Sokoll, L.J., Bowles, K.C., Nichols, J.H., Roberts, R., Schultheis, S.K. & O'Donnell, C.M. (1997). Clinical evaluation of Toxi-Prep™: A semiautomated solid-phase extraction system for screening of drugs in urine. *Clinical Chemistry*, Vol. 43, pp. 2099-2105, ISSN 0009-9147

Sun, T., Powers, J.R. & Tang, J. (2007). Evaluation of the antioxidant activity of asparagus, broccoli and their juices. *Food Chemistry*. Vol. 105, No. 1, pp. 101-106, ISSN 0308-8146

Tawara, J.N., Blokhin, A., Foderaro, T. A., Stermitz, F. R. & Hope, H. (1993). Toxic piperidine alkaloids from pine (*Pinus*) and spruce (*Picea*) trees. New structures and a biosynthetic hypothesis. *Journal of Organic Chemistry*, Vol. 58, No. 18, pp. 4813–4818, ISSN 0022-3263

Vaya, J. & Mahmood, S. (2006). Flavonoid content in leaf extracts of the fig (*Ficus carica* L.), carob (*Ceratonia siliqua* L.) and pistachio (*Pistacia lentiscus* L.). *BioFactors*, Vol. 28, No. 3-4, pp. 169-175, ISSN 0951-6433

Waller, G.R., Mangiafico, S. & Ritchey, C.R. (1978). A Chemical Investigation of Aloe barbadensis Miller. *Proceedings of the Oklahoma Academy of Science*, Vol. 58, pp. 69-76, ISSN: 0078-4303.

Williams, R.D. & Ellis, B.E. (1989). Age and tissue distribution of alkaloids in *Papaver somniferum*. Phytochemistry, Vol. 28, No. 8, pp. 2085-2088, ISSN 0031-9422

Zidorn, C. & Stuppner, H. (2001). Evaluation of chemosystematic characters in the genus *Leontodon* (Asteraceae). *Taxon*, Vol. 50, pp. 115-133, ISSN 0040-0262

6

Phytochemicals Components as Bioactive Foods

Aicha Olfa Cherif
*Laboratoire de Biochimie, des Lipides et des Protéines,
Département de Biologie,
Faculté des Sciences de Tunis, Tunis,
Tunisia*

1. Introduction

Phytochemicals in plant material have raised interest among scientists, food manufacturing and pharmaceutical industry, as well as consumers for their roles in the maintenance of human health. Phytochemicals are the bioactive, non-nutrient, and naturally occurring plant compounds found in fruits, vegetables, and whole grains. They can be categorized into various groups, i.e., polyphenols, organosulfur compounds, carotenoids, alkaloids, and nitrogen-containing compounds (Lampe & Chang, 2007).

Many phytochemicals are potent effectors of biologic processes and have the capacity to influence disease risk via several complementary and overlapping mechanisms (Lampe 2007).Further some phytochemicals undergo bacterial modification to produce metabolites that are more biologically active than the parent compounds (Lampe & Chang, 2007).

At present, one of the main objectives of the industry is to identify plant matrices rich in these compounds.

The goal of this chapter is devoted to the description of four classes of phytochemical compounds founded in oil-seeds such as: Sterols, Aliphatic alcohols (e.g. Policosanol), Squalene, Phenolic acids (e.g. resveratrol) and their content in oil-seeds. We will also evoke the physiological impact of these nutraceuticals on human health.

2. The main phytochemical compounds: structures and sources

The chemical compounds of oilseeds can be divided into two groups: the saponifiable fraction, which accounts for almost the entire weight of the oil (98–99% of total weight) and the nonsaponifiable fraction, which represents 0.5–2.0% of the total weight and is constituted of diverse components that are of great importance in terms of its biological value (Samaniego-Sanchez, 2010).

This fraction is used when we wish to study the characteristics and authenticity of oil or fat, due to its varied composition, including phytosterols, policosanol, hydrocarbons, polyphenols, tocopherols, triterpenics alcohol and volatile products.

2.1 Phytosterols

Structure

Phytosterols (plants sterols) are a group of naturally substances occurring in plants as bioactive minor constituents (up to 5%). They are derived from 3-hydroxylated polycyclic isopentanoids which have a 1,2-cyclopentanophenthrene structure with a 5,6- double bond (Fig. 1) (Abidi, 2004, 2001). These compounds contain a total of 27-30 carbon atoms (the number of carbon atoms in the biosynthetic precursor squalene oxide) and that of the side chain attached at the carbon-17 position can be equal to or greater than seven (Abidi, 2004).In addition to the free form (FS), phytosterols occur as four types of "conjugates" in which the 3β-OH group is esterified to a fatty acid (SE) or a hydroxycinnamic acid (HSE), or glycosylated with a hexose (SG) or a 6-fatty-acyl hexose (ASG) (Moreau et al., 2002). In free phytosterols (FS), the 3β-OH group on the A-ring is underivatized, whereas in the four conjugates the OH is covalently bound with another constituent. In the case of SE, the OH group is ester-linked with a fatty acid and linked with a 1-O - β-glycosidic bond with a hexose (most commonly glucose). In ASG, there is an addition of a fatty acid esterified to the 6-OH of the hexose moiety. In the fourth group the sterol 3β-OH group is esterifid to ferulic or *p*-coumaric acid especially in rice and corn seeds (Moreau et al., 2002).

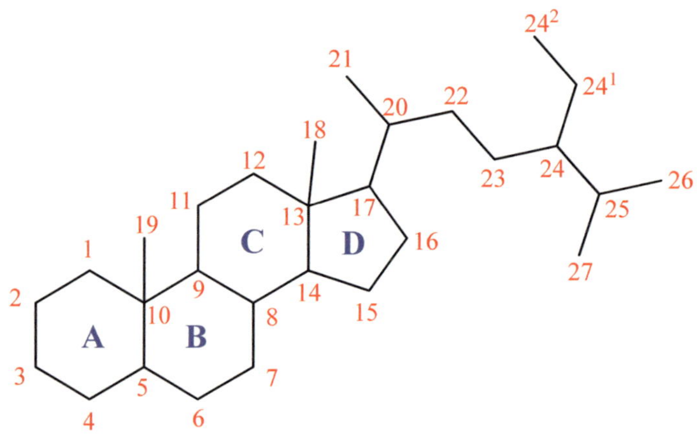

Fig. 1. Structure of a steroid numbered.

Phytosterols have been recognized into three subclasses (Fig 2); on the basis of the number of methyl groups at the C_4 position: none (4-desmethylsterols or sterols), one (4α-monomethylsterols) and two (4,4'-dimetylsterols or triterpenes alcohols (Cherif, 2011a; Moreau, 2002; Benveniste, 2002) (Fig. 2.). These later two groups are metabolic intermediates in the biosynthetic pathway leading to the end-product, 4-desmethylsterols, but they are usually present at lower levels than 4-desmethylsterols in most plant tissues (Cherif, 2011a; Moreau, 2002; Grunnwald, 1975). According to the position of the double bond at C_5 or C_7 in A ring (Fig. 1.); 4-desmethylsterols are present in two groups which are Δ_5-desmethylsterols and Δ_7-desmethylsterols. The most proportion of 4-desmethylsterol is Δ_5-desmethylsterol which contained mainly β-sitosterol, Δ_5- avenasterol, campesterol and stigmasterol (Pardo, 2007).

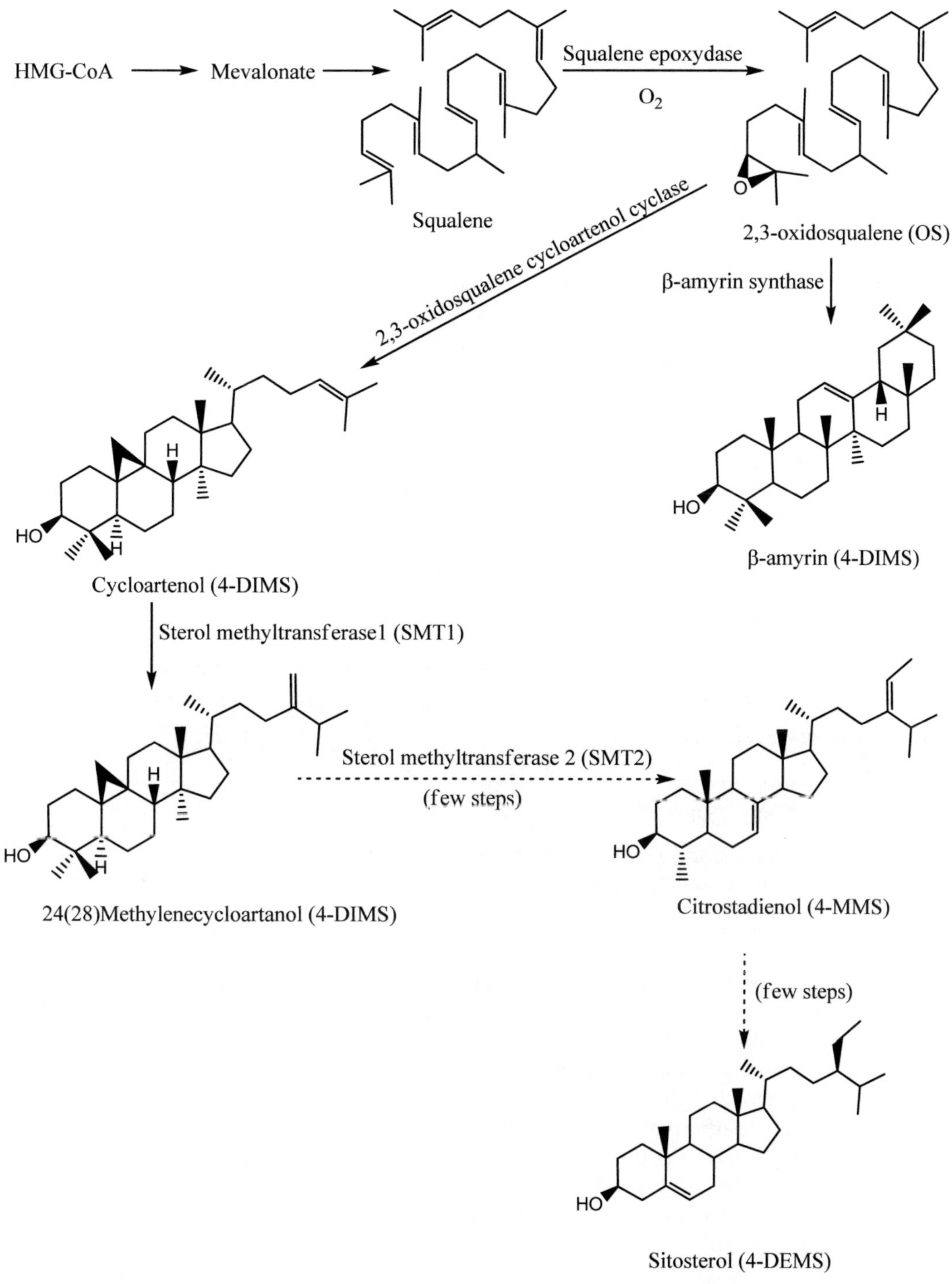

Fig. 2. The sterol pathway for higher plants.

Indeed, 250 types of phytosterols are actually reported in the literature, nutrition research has focused mostly upon the unsaturated *β* -sitosterol (24α-ethylcholest-5en-3β-ol), campesterol (24α-methyl-5-cholesten-3β-ol), stigmasterol (5,22-cholestadien-24α-ethyl-3β-ol) and Δ^5- avenasterol (24-ethyl-cholesta-5,24 (28)Z-dien-3β-ol) (Kochar, 1983).

Compounds 4-DEMS	MW	Mains fragmentation ions (M/Z) and others
Campesterol	472	382, 343, 255, 129
Stigmasterol	484	394, 255, 175, 129, 83
β-sitosterol	486	396, 381, 357, 255, 129, 73
Δ5-avenasterol	484	469, 386, 379, 355,296, 129, 55
Fucosterol	484	469, 386, 296, 129, 55
Δ7-sitosterol	486	303, 255, 229, 213
Δ7-avenasterol	486	386, 343, 255, 213

MW: Molecular Weight (g/mol)

Table 1. Retention time and mass spectrometric data for trimethylsilyl derivatives of 4-desmethylsterols identified by GC-MS (Cherif, 2011a)

Compounds 4-DIMS and 4-MMS	MW	Mains fragmentation ions (M/Z) and others
Obtusifoliol	498	.498 ; 483 ; 393 ; 109
β-amyrin	498	483 ; 408 ; 393 ; 218 ; 203.
α-amyrin	498	483 ; 408 ; 393 ; 218 ; 203.
Gramisterol	484	469 ; 393 ; 357 ; 254 ; 206 ; 83 ; 41.
Cycloartenol	498	483 ; 408 ; 393 ; 365 ; 271 ; 189 ; 69
28-methyleneobtusifoliol	512	497 ; 407 ; 309 ; 295 ; 281 ; 255 ; 55
24-methylenecycloartanol	512	497 ; 422 ; 407 ; 379 ; 353 ; 255 ;73.
Citrostadienol	498	400 ; 357 ; 264 ; 250 ; 83 ; 47.

MW: Molecular Weight (g/mol)

Table 2. Retention time and mass spectrometric data for trimethylsilyl derivatives of 4,4'-dimethyl and 4α-monomethylsterols identified by GC-MS (Cherif, 2011a)

Effects

Phytosterols exist in all foods of plant origin and are known to have several bioactive properties with possible benefits for human health (Cherif et al.,2010a).They contribute to lowering serum cholesterol levels (Cherif, 2010a), and are also considered to have anti-inflammatory, anti-bacterial, anti-artherosclerotic, anti-oxidative, anti-ulcerative, anti-tumor properties in humans (Lagarda, 2006; Moreau, 2002; Beveridgs, 2002), as well as contributing to the oxidative and thermal stability and shelf-life of vegetable oils (Przybylski, 2006). Additional, they are useful emulsifiers for cosmetic manufacturers and supply the majority of steroidal intermediates and precursors for the production of hormone pharmaceuticals (Grunnwald, 1975). Phytosterols might also prevent the development of colon cancer and benign prostatic hyperplasia (Awad, 2000). Among different plant sterols, *β*-sitosterol has been most intensively investigated and has been shown to exhibit anti-inflammatory; antineoplastic, antipyretic, and immunomodulating activities (Careri, 2006). Also, *β*-sitosterol, campesterol and stigmasterol exert antioxidant effects. Indeed, Δ_5- avenasterol has an essential antipolymerization effect, which could protect oils from oxidation during heating, exposure to ionizing radiation, light, chemical catalysts, or enzymatic processes (Nasar, 2007).

Titerpenes compounds and 4α-monomethylsterols are also important bioactive secondary metabolites, due to the wide range of their biological activities. They show mainly antimicrobial, cytotoxic, antitumoral, antiviral, anti-inflammatory, hepatoprotective, antifeedant and insecticidal activities (Alvarenga, 2005). These methylsterols have been used as markers to characterize and to detect admixture of vegetable oils (Cert, 1997; Jimenez, 1996).

It is noteworthy that the compositional distributions of phytosterols in certain vegetable oils have been used for their identification (Abidi, 2001). Hence, phytosterols and other non-saponifiable compounds in oils are often used as markers for the assessment of adulterated oils (Abidi, 2001). Recently, plant sterols have been added to margarine and vegetable oils as examples of successful functional foods and used as food ingredients in modern formulations (Fernandes, 2007). Reported phytosterols data for some oilseeds have shown that (Lin, 2004)

Vegetable oils	PS totaux	ß-sitosterol	Campesterol	Stigmasterol	Δ5avénasterol
peanut	315	203	52	28	22,8
Linseed	471	226	120	38	70,7
Olive	177	141	9	4	22,9
corn	843	519	184	56	41,4
grapes	215	169	24	24	nd

nd : not detected

Table 3. The major phytosterols components content in selected vegetable oils (mg/100g of oil) (Lin, 2004)

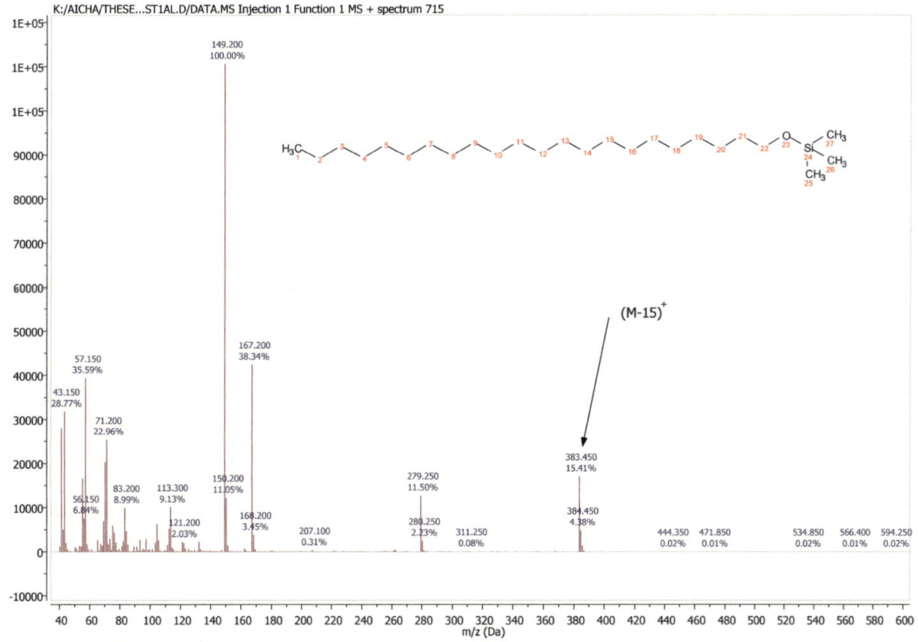

Fig. 3. Mass spectrum of Docosanol (Cherif, 2011b)

2.2 Aliphatic alcohols (e.g. Policosanol)

Structure

POLICOSANOL (PC) is a trivial name of a mixture of high molecular weight (HMW) aliphatic primary alcohols (C_{20} to C_{36}), originally isolated from sugar cane (*Saccharum officinarum* L.) (Cherif, 2010b).

It is also found from a diversity of other natural substances, such as bee wax, rice bran and wheat germ (Lin, 2004). These plants represent good sources of PC with its health-enhancing components. PC is present also in the fruits, leaves, and surfaces of plants and whole seeds (peanut seeds) (Cherif, 2010b). It is containing mainly docosanol (C_{22}), tetracosanol (C_{24}), hexacosanol (C_{26}), octacosanol (C_{28}) and triacontanol (C_{30}) (Irmak, 2006).

The analysis of individual policosanol components required mass spectrometric for tentative identification of the chromatographic peaks (Cherif, 2010b). Several components have been identified in the literature.The majorities of them are saturated n-alcohols, but we also note the presence of some unsaturated alcohols as in the case of peanut (Cherif, 2010b).

M[b]	$[M-15]^+$ (m/z)	Alcohol[1]
286	271	Tetradecan-1-ol
300	285	Pentadecan-1-ol
314	299	Hexadecan-1-ol
328	313	Heptadecan-1-ol
340	325	(Z) Octadec-9-en-1-ol
342	327	Octadecan-1-ol
356	341	Nonadacan-1-ol
368	353	Eicosen-1-ol
370	355	Eicosan-1-ol
382	367	Heneicosen-1-ol
384	369	Heneicosan-1-ol
396	381	Docosen-1-ol
398	383	Docosan-1-ol
412	397	Tricosan-1-ol
424	409	Tetracosen-1-ol
426	411	Tetracosan-1-ol
440	425	Pentacosan-1-ol
454	439	Hexacosan-1-ol
468	453	Heptacosan-1-ol
482	467	Octacosan-1-ol
510	495	Triacontan-1-ol

[b]Mass of the trimethylsilylated alcohol. In all cases the mass spectrum exihibited a major peak due to CH_3 loss, [M-15], and a peak characteristic of the Trimethylsilyl group on a terminal ether site, m/z =103 $[(CH_3)_3SiOCH_2]^+$
[1]Compounds tentatively identified.

Table 4. Retention indices and mass spectrometric data for trimethylsilyl derivatives of aliphatic alcohols identified by GC-MS (Cherif, 2010b).

Beneficial effects of policosanol

Several researchers have reported the biological effects of active compounds extracted from sugar cane crude wax (CW) such as long chain *n*-alcohols, fatty acids or ethanolic extracts, which have application to artherosclerotic vascular, coronary heart diseases, and dermatologic diseases (Lucas, 2007).

In fact, policosanol has been shown to decrease platelet aggregation, endothelial damage, and foam cell formation. The effectiveness of policosanol as a lipid-lowering agent, in several different populations has been extensively (Irmak, 2006). PC is supposed to downregulate the cellular expression of hydroxymethylglutamyl coenzyme Z (HMG-CoA) reductase; the rate-limiting enzyme in the cholesterol synthesis, rather inhibit the enzyme activity (Lin, 2004). So inhibiting cholesterol biosynthesis and enhancing low-density lipoprotein (LDL) decatabolism (Menendez, 1994). Similarly, PD improves protection of lipoproteins against lipid peroxidation, both in the lipid and the protein moieties (Menendez, 1999).However, Franci-Pesenti et al (Francini-Pesenti, 2008) have reported that the mechanisms by which PC improves plasma lipid profile are unclear, and there is a continuing debate about the exact effect of PC. Nevertheless, PC was successful worldwide, and it is sold as a lipid-lowering supplement in more than 40 countries (Cherif, 2010b). The majority of these supplements are prepared from bees wax or sugar cane extracts.

Marcelleti et al. reported that docosanol inhibits replication of herpes viruses in vitro and in vivo. While, octacosanol might be oxidized and degraded to fatty acids via β-oxidation in mammals (Menendez, 2005).

Samples	C_{22}	C_{24}	C_{26}	C_{28}	C_{30}	PC
Wheat germ (mg/kg)	2,8	1,4	nd	2,9	2,5	10,0
Beeswax (g/kg)	0,06	2,6	1,7	2,0	5,7	12,0
Sugar cane (mg/kg)	0,92	1,68	0,9	10,0	1,0	17,4
Policosanol ™ (mg/comprimé)	7,1	14,8	8,5	8,8	8,3	53,6

Policosanol ™ : commercial dietary supplement; nd : non détecté.

Table 5. Policosanol content of some natural sources rich in PC in compared with that PC supplement (Cherif, 2011b)

2.3 Squalene

Structure

In virgin oil, the major hydrocarbon is the squalene (2,6,10,15,19,23-hexamethyl-2,6,10,14,18,20-tetracosahexaene) ($C_{30}H_{50}$), a terpenoid hydrocarbon occurring in high concentrations (800-12000 mg/kg which can constitute up to 90% of the hydrocarbon fraction of olive oil and pumpkin oils (Fig .4) (Tuberoso, 2007). It is also present in all plant oils and fats except flaxseed, grapeseed, and soybean oils (Tuberoso, 2007). It is accompanied by *n*-alkanes in the range of C_8-C_{35}, being the more abundant the comprehended between C_{21} and C_{35}, in which alkanes with an odd number of carbon atoms predominated over those of even numbers (Cert, 2000).

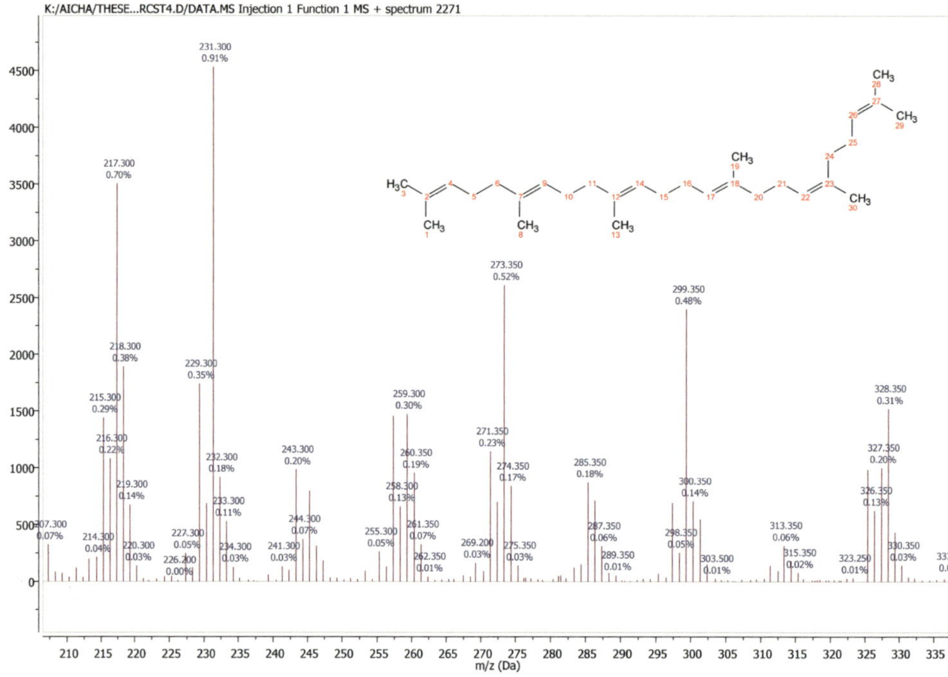

Fig. 4. Mass spectrum of squalene

Squalene is built up from a universal C5 building block isopentenyl diphosphate (IDP or IPP). The IPP in the classical Bloch-Lynen pathway; is formed from three molecules of acetyl-CoA via the mevalonate (MVA pathway). Then the squalene epoxidase catalyzes the epoxidation of squalene to 2,3-oxidosqualene, which is the substrate for formation of sterols and a wide range of triterpenoids (Volkman, 2005).

In humans, squalene is synthesized in the liver and the skin, transported in the blood by very low density lipoproteins (VLDL) and low density lipoproteins (LDL), and secreted in large quantities by the sebaceous glands (Reddy, 2009).

Beneficial effects of squalene

Squalene is also regarded as one of the compounds responsible for the beneficial effects against certain type of cancers (Tuberoso, 2007).Antioxidant activity of squalene is demonstrated against polyunsaturated fatty acid (PUFA), and it is secondary to that of phenols and tocopherols (Tuberoso, 2007). Its antioxidant activity can reinforce the endogenous antioxidant system against oxidative damage (Tuberoso, 2007). Together with other components of the non-saponifiable fraction, it prevents also the autooxidation process and thus contributes to the stability of the oil and its aroma and flavor characteristics (Tuberoso, 2007). It is normally used in its natural or hydrogenated form (squalene) as a moisturizing or emollient agent in cosmetic preparations (Moreda, 2001). Squalene is widespread in nature, especially among olives, liver oil, wheat germ and rice bran.

Oilseeds	Squalene
peanut	1276.0±27.8
olive	5990.0±95.1
maize	338.7±11.5
sunflower	170.5±6.4
pumpkin	3529.9±61.4
rapeseed	437.4±18.3

Table 6. Squalene content of selected vegetable oils (mg/kg, mean±SD) (Tuberoso, 2007)

2.4 Polyphenols (e.g. resveratrol)

The polyphenols are some of the most studied compounds and can be further divided into flavonoids (including flavonols, flavones, catechins, flavanones, anthocyanidins, and isoflavones), phenolic acids, stilbenes, coumarins, and tannins (Lampe, 2007).

Structure

Trans-Resveratrol or Res (trans-3,5,4'-trihydroxystilbene) (Fig.5) (Lin 2007) and its many derivatives (pterostilbene, piceatannol) are naturally occurring phytoalexins; a class of antibiotic compounds, produced in a select number of plant species as part of the plant's defense system (Bolivar, 2007).The terminal enzyme in the production of resveratrol is resveratrol synthase, which condenses *p*-coumaroyl-coenzyme A and three malonyl-coenzyme A molecules to form resveratrol (Bolivar, 2007).This enzyme is highly regulated by elicitors and general plant defense compounds in an effort to protect the plant. Resveratrol exist as both the *trans*- and *cis*-isomers but the most active for is the *trans* one.

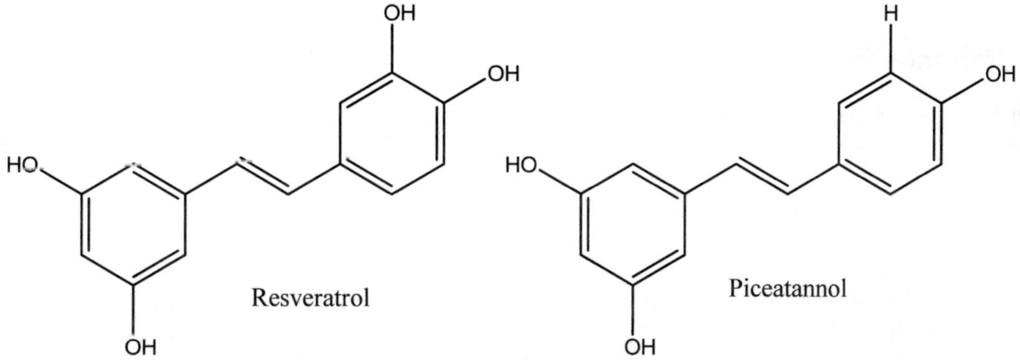

Fig. 5. The chemical structure of *trans*-resveratrol and *trans*-piceatannol (Lin, 2007)

Resveratrol and effects

Res and its derivatives like piceatannol, has similar structure (Fig Lin, 2007), but piceatannol has much potent biological activities than resveratrol. Piceatannol is more efficient inducer of apoptosis (Lin, 2007). Other reports, suggested that both piceatannol and resveratrol are able to induce apoptosis in many cancer cell lines, but to different extent (Lin 2007).Lin et al. reported that piceatannol is more effective in cancer prevention and could be an anticancer compound while resveratrol is a chemoprotective one. In fact, resveratrol and piceatannol become promising natural compounds in cancer treatments (Lin, 2007), they blocks the carcinogenesis stages of initiation, promotion and progression (Lu, 2009).

In plants, the amount of piceatannol is much lower than that of Res. Lu et al reported that roots can produce higher levels of phytoalexins in response to environmental stimulations like injury or fungal attack (Lu, 2009).

Besides, its strong anitcarcinogenic effect, Res decreased coronary heart diseases mortality (Lu, 2009), modulates lipid metabolism, protects low-density lipoproteins against oxidative and free radical damage (Lu, 2009), and inhibits platelets activation and aggregation (Lu, 2009), and anti-aging benefits (Bolivar, 2007)

A number of taxonomically unrelated plant families (72 plant species) have been reported to produce marked levels of resveratrol including: peanuts, several types of berries, some pine trees and most recently tomato fruit skin (Ragab, 2006).

The highest level of piceatannol and resveratrol was detected in roots due to their consistent exposure to the micoorganisms in soil.

3. Conclusion

Phytochemicals in plant material have raised interest among scientist, producers, and consumers for their roles in the maintenance of human health and in assessing the protective status of people from chronic degenerative disorders. Given the importance of dietary habit and food components to health, the provision of phytochemical information of a range of foods is vital to support the future work in assessing the protective status of people from chronic degenerative disorders. Food-based approaches would be essential for sustainable solutions to combat the alarming prevalence of chronic cancer, coronary heart diseases and diabetes. The health benefits of these foods may prompt research onto the assessment and determination of potential rich sources of phytochemicals compounds in agricultural produce.

4. References

Abidi, S.L. (2004). Capillary electrochromatography of sterols and related steryl esters derived from vegetable oils. *Journal of chromatography A*, Vol.1059, (10/2004), pp.199-208, ISSN: 0021-9673

Abidi, S.L. (2001). Chromatographic analysis of plant sterols in foods and vegetable oils. *Journal of chromatography A*, Vol. 935, (11/2001), pp. 173-201, ISSN: 0021-9673

Alvarenga, N. & Esteban, A. (2005). Bioactives triterpenes and related compounds from celastraceae. *Stud. Nat. Prod. Chem.*Vol. 30, (08/2005), pp. 635-702, DOI:10.1016/S1572-5995(05)80044-4.

Awad, A.B.; Chan, K.C.; Downie, A.C.& Fink, C.S.(2000). Peanuts as a source of β-sitosterol, a sterol with anticancer properties. *Nutr Cancer.*, Vol.36, No.2, (09/2001), pp.238-41, ISSN: 0163-5581.

Benveniste, P. (2002).*The Arabidopsis book,* Retrieved from <www;aspb.org/publications>.

Beveridge, T.H.J.; Li, T.S.C. & Drover, J.C.G. (2002). Phytosterols content in American ginseng seed oil. *J. Agric. Food Chem.*, Vol.50, No. 4, (2/2002), pp. 744-750, ISSN: 00218561.

Careri, M.; Elviri, L. & Mangia, A. (2006).Liquid chromatography-UV determination and liquid chromatography-atmospheric pressure chemical ionization mass spectrometric characterization of sitosterol and stigmasterol in soybean oil. *Journal of chromatography A*, Vol.935, ( ), pp.249-257, ISSN: 1363-1950.

Cert, A.; Moreda, W & Garcia-Moreno, J. (1997). Determinación de esteroles y alcohols triterpénicos en aceite de oliva mediante separación de la fracción por cromatografia liquida de alta efficacia y análisis por cromatografia de gases, Estandarización del método analítico. *Grasas Aceites,* Vol. 48, No. 4, (07/1997), pp. 207-218, ISSN: 0017-3495.

Cert, A. ; Moreda, W. & Pérez-Camino , M. C. (2000). Chromatographic analysis of minor constituents in vegetable oils. Journal of Chromatography A, Vol.881, No.1-2, (09/ 2000), pp.131-148, ISSN : 0021-9673.

Cherif, A.O.; Trabelsi, H.; Ben Messaouda, M.; Kâabi, B.; Pellerin, I.; Boukhchina, S.; Kallel, H. & Pepe, C. (2010a).Gas chromatography-mass spectrometry screening for phytochemical 4-desmethylsterols accumulated during development of Tunisian peanut kernels (Arachis hypogaea L.). J Agric Food Chem.,Vol. 58, No.15, (08/2010), pp.8709-14, ISSN: 0021-8561.

Cherif, A. O.; Ben Messaouda, M.; Kaabi, B.; Boukhchina, S.; Pepe, C. & Kallel, H. (2010b). Comparison of the concentrations of long-chain alcohols (policosanol) in three Tunisian peanut varieties (*arachis hypogaea* L.). *J.Agric. Food Chem.,* Vol.58, (10/2010), pp.12143–12148, DOI: 10.1021/jf1030345.

Cherif, A.O.; Trabelsi, H.; Ben Messaouda, M. ; Kaabi B. ; Pellerin I. ; Boukhchina, S. & Kallel,H . (2011a). Characteristics and pathways of bioactive 4-desmethylsterols, triterpene alcohols and 4α-monomethylsterols, from developing Tunisian cultivars and wild peanut (Arachis hypogaea L.).*Plant Physiology and Biochemistry,* Vol.49, No. 7, ( ), pp. 774-81, PMID: 21356594.

Cherif A.O. (PhD Thesis) (2011b)

De Lucas A.; Garcia, A.; Alvarez, A. & Gracia, I. (2007). Supercritical extraction of long chain n-alcohols from sugar cane crude wax. *Journal of supercritical fluids,* vol. 41, No. 2, pp. 267-271, ISSN: 0896-8446.

Fernandes, P. & Cabral, J.M.S. (2007). Phytosterols: applications and recovery methods. *Bioresour. Technol.,* Vol. 98, ( ), pp. 2335-2350, ISSN: 0960-8524.

Francini-Pesenti, F.; Brocadello, F.; Beltramolli, D.; Nardi, M. & Caregaro, L. (2008). Sugar cane Policosanol failed to lower plasma cholesterol in primitive, diet-resistant hypercholesterolaemia: a double blind, controlled study. *Compl. Ther. Med.,* Vol.16, (04/2008), pp.61-65, PMID: 18514906.

Grunnwald, C. (1975). Plant Sterols. *Annual review of plant physiology,* Vol. 26, ( ) pp.209-236, ISSN: 0300-9483.

Irmak, S.; Dunford, N. T. & Milligan, J.(2006). Policosanol contents of beeswax, sugar cane and wheat extracts. *Food Chem.,* Vol. 95, ( ), pp.312-318, ISSN

Jiménez, O. & Del Valle, A. (1996). Determination of sterols by capillary column gas chromatography. Differentiation among different types of olive oil, virgin, refined and solvent-extracted. *J. Am. Chem. Soc.,* Vol. 73, No.12, ( ), pp.1685-1689, ISSN

Kochhar, S.P. (1983) Influence of processing on sterols of edible vegetable oils. *Prog. Lipid Res.,* Vol. 22, ( ), pp.161–188, ISSN

Lagarda, M.J.; Garcia-Liatas, G. & Farre, R. (2006). Analysis of phytosterols in foods. *J. Pharm. Biomed. Anal.,* Vol.41, ( ), pp. 1486–1496, ISSN

Lampe, J.W. & Chang, J-L.(2007). Interindividual differences in phytochemical metabolism and disposition. *Seminars in cancer biology,* Vol. 17, No. 5, ( ), pp. 347-353, ISSN: 1044-579X.

Lin, Y.; Rudrum, M.; Van Der Wielen, R. P.J; Trautwein, E. A. M..; McNeill, G.; Sierksma, A. & Meijer, G.W. (2004). Wheat germ policosanol failed to lower plasma cholesterol in subjects with normal to mildly elevated cholesterol concentrations. *Metabolism Clinical And Experimental,* Vol.53, No.10, (10/2004), pp.1309-1314, ISSN 0026-0495.

Lin, L.L.; Lien, C.Y.; Chen, Y.C. & Ku, K.L. (2007). An effective sample preparation approach for screening the anticancer compound piceatannol using HPLC coupled with UV and fluorescence detection. J. Chromatogr., B: Anal. *Technol. Biomed. Life Sci.*, Vol. 853, No. 1-2, ( ), pp.175-182, ISSN

Lu, Z.; Cheng, B.; Hu, Y.; Zhang,Y. & Zou, G. (2009). Complexation of resveratrol with cyclodextrins: Solubility and antioxidant activity. Food Chemistry. Vol. 113, No.1, (03/1999), pp.17-20, ISSN

López-Martínez, M.C.(2010). β-Carotene, squalene and waxes determined by chromatographic method in picual extra virgin olive oil obtained by a new cold extraction system. *Journal of food composition and analysis*, Vol. 23, No. 7, (11/2010), pp. 671–676, ISSN

Medina-Bolivar, F.; Condori, J.; Rimando, A.M.; Hubstenberger, J.; Shelton, K.; O'Keefe, S.F.; Bennett, S. & Dolan, M. C. (2007). Production and secretion of resveratrol in hairy root cultures of peanut. *Phytochemistry*, Vol.68, No.14, ( ), pp.1992-2003, ISSN: 00319422

Menéndez, R.; Fernandez, S.I. ; Del Rio, A.; Gonzalez, R.M. ; Fraga, V.; Amor, A.M. & Mas, R.M. (1994). Policosanol inhibits cholesterol biosynthesis and enhances low density lipoprotein processing in cultured human fibroblasts. *Biol Res.*, Vol.27, No. 3-4, ( ), pp.199-203, ISSN

Menéndez, R.; Fraga, V.; Amor, A. M.; González, R. M. & Mas R. (1999). Oral Administration of Policosanol Inhibits In Vitro Copper Ion-Induced Rat Lipoprotein Peroxidation. *Physiology & Behavior*, Vol.67, No.1, (08/1999), pp.1-7, ISSN

Menendez, R.; Marrero, D.; Mas, R.; Fernandez, I.; Gonzalez, L. & Gonzalez, R. M. (2005). In vitro and in vivo study of octacosanol metabolism. *Arch. Med. Res.*, Vol.36, ( ), pp.113-119, ISSN

Moreau, R.A.; Whitaker, B.D. & Hicks, K.B. (2002). Phytosterols, phytostanols, and their conjugates in foods: structural diversity, quantitative analysis, and health-promoting uses. *Progress in Lipid Rsearch*, Vol.41, ( ), pp. 457-500, ISSN

Nasari, N.; Fady, B & Triki, S. (2007). Quantification of sterols and aliphatic alcohols in Mediterranean stone pine (Pinus pinea L.) populations. *J. Agric. Food Chem.*, Vol.55, ( ), pp.2251–2255, ISSN

Pardo, J.E.; Cuesta M.A.; Alvarruiz, A.; Granell, J.D. & Álvarez-Ortí, M. (2007). Evaluation of potential and real qualities of virgin olive oil from the designation of origin (DO) "Aceite Montes de Alcaraz" (Albacete, Spain). *Food chemistry*, Vol. 100, ( ), pp. 977-984, ISSN

Przybylski, R. & Eskin, N.A.M. (2006). Minor components and the stability of vegetable oils. *Inform*, Vol. 17, ( ), pp. 187-189, ISSN

Ragab, A. S.; Van Fleet, J.; Jankowski, B.; Park, J-H. & Bobzin S.C.(2006). Detection and Quantitation of Resveratrol in Tomato Fruit (*Lycopersicon esculentum* Mill.) *J. Agric. Food Chem.*, Vol.54, No. 19, ( ), pp. 7175–7179, ISSN

Reddy, L. H. & Couvreur, P. (2009). Squalene: A natural triterpene for use in disease management and therapy. *Adv Drug Deliv Rev.*, Vol. 61, No.15, (12/2009), pp.1412-26, ISSN

Samaniego-Sánchez, C.; Quesada-Granados, J.J.; De la Serrana, H.L-G.; Tuberoso, C.I.G.; Kowalczyk, A.; Sarritzu, E. & Cabras, P. (2007). Determination of antioxidant compounds and antioxidant activity in commercial oilseeds for food use. *Food Chemistry*, Vol.103, No.4, ( ), pp. 1494-1501, ISSN 03088146

Volkman, J. (2005). Sterols and other triterpenoids: source specificity and evolution of biosynthetic pathways. *Organic Geochemistry*, Vol.36, No. 2, ( ), pp.139-159, ISSN: 01466380

7

Diosgenin, a Steroid Saponin Constituent of Yams and Fenugreek: Emerging Evidence for Applications in Medicine

Jayadev Raju[1] and Chinthalapally V. Rao[2]
[1]*Toxicology Research Division, Bureau of Chemical Safety, Health Products and Food Branch, Health Canada,*
[2]*Department of Medicine, Hematology-Oncology Section, University of Oklahoma Health Sciences Center*
USA

1. Introduction

Phytochemicals found in foods and spices are progressively gaining popularity over conventional synthetic drugs mainly because they act *via* multiple molecular targets that synergize to efficiently prevent or treat chronic illnesses. Phytochemicals are also safe (with minimal or no toxic or side effects) with better bioavailability. Food saponins have been used in complimentary and traditional medicine against a variety of diseases including several cancers. Diosgenin, a naturally-occurring steroid saponin is found abundantly in legumes (*Trigonella* sp.) and yams (*Dioscorea* sp.). Diosgenin is a precursor of various synthetic steroidal drugs that are extensively used in the pharmaceutical industry. Over the past two decades, a series of pre-clinical and mechanistic studies have been independently conducted to understand the beneficial role of diosgenin against metabolic diseases (hypercholesterolemia, dyslipidemia, diabetes and obesity), inflammation and cancer. In experimental models of obesity, diosgenin decreases plasma and hepatic triglycerides and improves glucose homeostasis plausibly by promoting adipocyte differentiation and inhibiting inflammation in adipose tissues. A limited number of experiments have been conducted to understand the pre-clinical efficacy of diosgenin as a chemopreventive/therapeutic agent against cancers of several organ sites. Mechanistic studies using *in vitro* models suggest that diosgenin suppresses cancer cell growth through multiple cell signaling events associated with proliferation, differentiation, apoptosis, inflammation and oncogenesis. This chapter provides a comprehensive review of the biological activity of diosgenin that contributes to several diseases in its role as a health beneficial phytochemical by citing new studies. In addition, diosgenin's safety with regards to its potential toxicity is also critically discussed. Altogether, the findings from pre-clinical and mechanistic studies strongly implicate the use of diosgenin as a novel multi-target based chemopreventive or therapeutic agent against several chronic diseases.

1.1 Background of origin

Diosgenin is a major bioactive constituent of various edible pulses and roots, well characterized in the seeds of fenugreek (*Trigonella foenum graecum* Linn) as well as in the root tubers of wild yams (*Dioscorea villosa* Linn) (No authors listed, 2004; Taylor et al., 2000). Reference to the ethnobotanical use of fenugreek seeds appears in the Egyptian Ebers papyrus (*c.* 1500 BC) as a medicine to induce childbirth. Fenugreek seeds were referred as a "soothing herb" by the Greek physician *Hippocrates* (5th century BC) and *Dioscorides* (1st century AD) suggested its use in the treatment of gynaecological inflammation (Chevalier, 2000). Wild yam tubers on the other hand have been used traditionally as a pain reliever by the ancient *Aztec* and *Mayan* people in the Americas (Chevalier, 2000). Data available from various traditional medical practices indicate that fenugreek seeds and wild yam tubers have been purported to be used as a preventive or therapeutic medicine against several ailments including arthritis, cancer, diabetes, gastrointestinal disorders, high cholesterol, and inflammation suggesting a variety in its use (Memorial Sloan-Kettering Cancer Center).

1.2 Chemistry, structure-function and bioavailability

Structurally, diosgenin [(25*R*)-spirost-5-en-3b-ol] is a spirostanol saponin consisting of a hydrophilic sugar moiety linked to a hydrophobic steroid aglycone (Figure 1). Diosgenin is structurally similar to cholesterol and other steroids. Since its discovery, diosgenin is the single main precursor in the manufacture of synthetic steroids in the pharmaceutical industry (Djerassi et al., 1952). In a recent study it was shown that spirostanol compounds, especially diosgenin glycosides exhibited inducible or inhibitory activity in rat uterine contraction based on (a) the number, length and position of sugar side chains attached by a glycoside, and (b) related to the structure of the aglycone (Yu et al., 2010). The structure-related functions of diosgenin have been extensively tested using cancer cells *in vitro*. In comparison to two-structurally-related saponins, hecogenin and tigogenin, only diosgenin caused a cell cycle arrest associated with strong apoptosis *in vitro* (Corbiere et al., 2003).) The biological activities of diosgenin and other structurally-related steroid saponins and alkaloids were tested *in vitro* (Trouillas et al., 2005). By using molecular modelling, the spatial conformation and electron transfer capacity were calculated in relation to the structural characteristics of diosgenin necessary to elicit its effect on proliferation rate, cell cycle distribution and apoptosis; and the anti-cancer bioactivity of diosgenin was shown to be related to the presence of a hetero-sugar moiety and the 5,6-double bond in its structure (Trouillas et al., 2005). Moreover, structural conformation at C-5 and C-25 carbon atoms was shown to be important for diosgenin's biological activity (Trouillas et al., 2005). Further studies are warranted to assess the structure-function relationship of diosgenin and to understand whether and how synthetic changes brought about could augment its biological activity in favour of its role as a therapeutic agent. Rodent studies on the disposition of diosgenin revealed that diosgenin was poorly absorbed and underwent extreme biotransformation (Cayen et al., 1979). In the same study, 1 μg/mL of diosgenin was recovered from the serum of human subjects receiving an oral dose of 3 g diosgenin per day for 4 weeks suggesting poor absorption and possibly active biotranformation (Cayen et al., 1979).

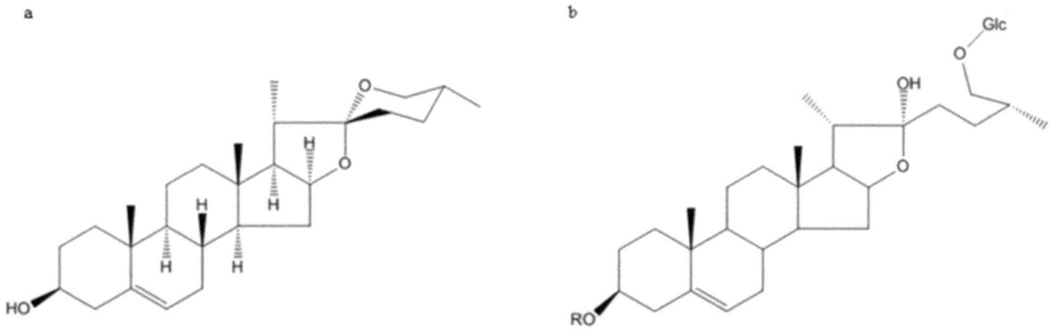

Fig. 1. Structure of diosgenin: Diosgenin (a) and its analogue protodioscin (b) are steroid saponins consisting of a hydrophilic sugar moiety linked to a hydrophobic steroid aglycone

2. Metabolic diseases

Fenugreek seeds and *Dioscorea* sp. yam tubers together with their constituent diosgenin have been shown to have biological activity against several metabolic diseases (Ulbricht et al., 2007; Raju & Rao, 2009). In the following sections, studies that have used the active constituent diosgenin in both experimental models of metabolic diseases and human clinical studies are reviewed. A list of studies evaluating the effects of diosgenin against different metabolic diseases is summarised in Table 1.

Disease/ Effect	**Experimental model**	**Benificial potency Yes (Y) or No (N)**	**References**
Dyslipidemia/obesity			
Cholesterol-lowering	Cholesterol-fed rats	Y	Cayen and Dvornik, 1979 Juarez-Oropeza et al., 1987 Son et al., 2007
	Cholesterol-fed chickens	Y	Cayen and Dvornik, 1979
	Cholesterol-fed rabbits	Y	Cayen and Dvornik, 1979
Adipocyte-	Normal rats	N	Cayen and Dvornik, 1979
differentiation/ inflammation	3T3-L1 (Mouse embryonic fibroblast - adipose like cells)	Y	Uemura et al., 2010
Diabetes			
Blood glucose	Streptozotocin-induced diabetic rats	Y	McAnuff et al., 2005
Liver function			
Cholestasis	FVB mice	Y	Kosters et al., 2005
	Wistar rats	Y	Nibbering et al., 2001 Nervi et al., 1998
	NPC1L1-knockout (L1KO) and wild-type mice	Y	Temel et al., 2009

Table 1. Effect of diosgenin (purified) on metabolic and related diseases

2.1 Dyslipidemia and obesity

The lipid-lowering potential of diosgenin has been demonstrated by several experimental studies (Sauvaire et al., 2000). Diosgenin decreased the elevated cholesterol in serum LDL and HDL fractions in cholesterol-fed rats, and had no effect on serum cholesterol in normocholesterolemic rats. In addition, diosgenin inhibited cholesterol absorption, and suppressed its uptake in serum and liver, and its accumulation in the liver (Cayen and Dvornik, 1979). Diosgenin lowered plasma cholesterol in diet-induced hypercholesterolemic rats, chicken and rabbits when administered orally or parenterally (Juarez-Oropeza et al., 1987). Recently, it was shown that diosgenin (at a oral dose of 0.1% or 0.5% in the diet for 6 weeks) decreased total cholesterol levels and increased the plasma high-density lipoprotein (HDL) cholesterol level in both plasma and livers of diet-induced hypercholesterolemic rats (Son et al., 2007). In a study that evaluated the anti-obesity role of diosgenin-rich *Dioscorea nipponica* Makino, a related species to *Dioscorea villosa,* Sprague-Dawley rats fed a diet containing 40% beef tallow and 5% freeze-dried extract of the yam gained less body weight and adipose tissue than those that received only the 40% beef tallow diet (Kwon et al., 2003). In the same study it was shown that diosgenin suppressed the time-dependent increase of blood triacylglycerol levels when orally administered with corn oil to ICR mice, suggesting an inhibitory potential against fat absorption (Kwon et al., 2003).

An evidence-based systemic review clearly suggests that fenugreek seeds (rich in diosgenin content) have an important role in the control of metabolic diseases such as diabetes and obesity (Ulbricht et al., 2007). Fenugreek decreased the size of adipocytes in diabetic obese KK-Ay mice suggesting an increased differentiation of adipocytes leading to decreased adipocyte lipid accumulation (Uemura et al., 2010). These results were further validated with molecular data that showed that fenugreek increased the mRNA expression levels of differentiation-related genes in adipose tissues (Uemura et al., 2010). Furthermore, *in vitro* experiments using 3T3-L1 adipocytes showed that diosgenin, the major saponin in fenugreek, promoted 3T3-L1 adipocyte differentiation to enhance insulin-dependent glucose uptake (Uemura et al., 2010). Two clinical studies were recently published showing the anti-obesity properties of fenugreek seeds. First, a double-blind randomized placebo-controlled three-period (14 days) cross-over trial with twelve healthy male volunteers, demonstrated that fenugreek seed extract selectively reduced spontaneous fat consumption compared to placebo controls (Chevassus et al., 2009). However, there was no effect on body weight, normal and fasting glucose levels, insulin and lipid profile, and visual analogue scale scores of appetite/satiety in subjects receiving the fenugreek seed extract (Chevassus et al., 2009). In the second study, a 6-week double-blind randomized placebo-controlled parallel trial with thirty-nine healthy overweight male volunteers, showed decreased dietary fat consumption in subjects that received a fixed dose of a fenugreek seed extract compared to those that received the placebo (Chevassus et al., 2010). In addition, subjects that received the fenugreek seed extract also demonstrated a decrease in the insulin/glucose ratio in the serum of fasted subjects (Chevassus et al., 2010). Put together, these two clinical studies provided evidence to support that fenugreek seeds may potentially regulate fat consumption in humans. Whether diosgenin *per se* can mimic these results at appreciable doses in human subjects need to be addressed.

2.2 Diabetes

There are several reports suggesting that diosgenin-rich food sources such as fenugreek seeds and yam tubers contribute to anti-diabetic effects in experimental models (Basch et al., 2003; Omoruyi, 2008). Evidence from human clinical trials clearly suggests that fenugreek seeds improve blood glucose and other metabolic parameters leading to treatment of diabetes (Basch et al., 2003).) Diosgenin significantly decreased plasma glucose in streptozotocin-induced diabetic rats by comparison to the diabetic controls suggesting its anti-diabetic properties (McAnuff et al., 2005). These results were further strengthened by the fact that several hepatic rate-limiting enzymes commonly involved in glucose metabolism altered in the diabetic state were normalized by treatment with diosgenin (McAnuff et al., 2005). While there is ample evidence (including clinical trials) suggesting that fenugreek seeds may be used as an alternative medicine to treat diabetes and associated complications, more experimental studies are warranted to address if diosgenin can be efficaciously used in the control of diabetes and to understand the mechanism(s) of action.

2.3 Liver function, liver disease and bile secretion

There is a plethora of information that suggests that both fenugreek seeds and yam tubers influence several metabolic diseases directly affecting a number of molecular targets involved in enzyme metabolism as well as signal transduction pathways in the liver suggesting that their active compounds such as diosgenin may plausibly modulate liver function and may aid in the therapeutic control of liver diseases. A lyophilized fraction of *Dioscorea* sp. yam tubers attenuated CCl_4-induced hepatic fibrosis in rats in a dose-dependent manner (Chan et al., 2010). On the other hand, aqueous extract of fenugreek seeds contributed to a significant histopathological protection against ethanol-induced liver toxicity in rats (Thirunavukkarasu et al., 2003). Furthermore, the authors reported that this protection against ethanol-induced toxicity was by modulating lipid peroxidation and the antioxidant status (Thirunavukkarasu et al., 2003). Powdered fenugreek seeds administered in the diet at a dose of 5% (wt/wt) reduced the liver weight and alleviated hepatic steatosis in Zucker obese (*fa/fa*) rats (Raju and Bird, 2006). The main mechanism of fenugreek seeds in controlling hepatic steatosis was through lowering plasma tumor necrosis factor (TNF)-α, a proinflammatory cytokine and by decreasing total fat and triglycerides in the liver (Raju and Bird, 2006). Specifically, there are no reports demonstrating the therapeutic potency of diosgenin against liver disease. It is postulated that diosgenin feeding causes cholesterol excretion in the stool of experimental animals, mainly by cholesterol secretion from the bile (Cayen and Dvornik, 1979). Diosgenin has been shown to increase cholesterol secretion five- to seven-fold in the bile of rats without altering the output of bile salts and phospholipids (Kosters et al., 2005; Nervi et al., 1988; Nibbering et al., 2001). Recently, it was shown that the biliary cholesterol secretion stimulated by diosgenin and leading to fecal cholesterol excretion is independent of intestinal cholesterol absorption (Temel et al., 2009).

3. Cancer

3.1 *In vivo* studies

There are limited experimental studies addressing the *in vivo* tumor modulating potential of diosgenin (summarised in Table 2). Diosgenin inhibited the formation of colon aberrant crypt foci (ACF), putative precancerous lesions induced by azoxymethane (AOM) in F344 rats. In this study, administration of diosgenin in the diet at a dose of 0.1% and 0.05% (wt/wt) either during initiation/post-initiation or promotion stages significantly suppressed AOM-induced colon ACF (Raju et al., 2004). The demonstrated ability of diosgenin to inhibit both the total number of ACF and large ACF (those with crypt multiplicity of four or more) suggests that it could effectively prevent, retard and cease the appearance and growth of precancerous lesions in the colon (Raju et al., 2004). Furthermore the lower dose of 0.05% was as effective as the higher dose of 0.1% in blocking ACF formation (Raju et al., 2004). In a double-blind study designed to assess the tumor-modulating potential of diosgenin using the AOM-injected F344 rats, Malisetty et al. (2005) reported that 0.1% of diosgenin suppressed the incidence of both invasive and non-invasive colon adenocarcinomas by up to 60% (Malisetty et al., 2005). In addition, diosgenin decreased colon tumor multiplicity (adenocarcinomas/rat) compared to Controls. In part, these *in vivo* effects were shown to be related to a lower proliferating cell nuclear antigen (PCNA) index in colon tumors suggesting that diosgenin attenuates tumor cell proliferation (Malisetty et al., 2005).

Organ site Pathological target	**Experimental model**	**Inhibition* Yes (Y) or No (N)**	**References**
Colon			
Aberrant crypt foci	AOM-induced rats	Y	Raju et al., 2004
Tumors	AOM-induced rats	Y	Malisetty et al., 2005
Ulcers/tumors	AOM/DSS-induced ICR mice	Y	Miyoshi et al., 2011
Breast			
MCF-7 tumor xenografts	Nude (*nu/nu*) mice	Y	Srinivasan et al., 2009
MDA 231 tumor xenografts	Nude (*nu/nu*) mice	Y	Srinivasan et al., 2009
Lung			
LA795 ectopic tumors	T739 mice	Y	Yan et al., 2009

*Inhibition of either (a) tumor incidence [number of tumor-bearing animals], (b) tumor multiplicity [number of tumors per tumor-bearing rats], or (c) tumor size.

Table 2. *In vivo* anticancer effects of diosgenin (purified)

Diosgenin has been shown to attenuate inflammatory process in relevant animal models. For instance, diosgenin dose-dependently attenuated sub-acute intestinal inflammation and normalized bile secretion in indomethacin-induced intestinal inflammation in rats (Yamada et al., 1997). The role of chronic inflammation on carcinogenesis is vital (Dinarello, 2006); thus the study by Yamada et al. (1997) demonstrating the ability of diosgenin to effectively treat inflammation could be extrapolated to its prospective chemopreventive action against cancers. Recently, the efficacy of diosgenin against AOM/dextran sodium sulphate (DSS)-induced inflammation-associated colon carcinogenesis in ICR mice was reported (Miyoshi N et al., 2011). Diosgenin at doses of 20, 100 and 500 mg/kg (wt/wt) in the diet reduced AOM/DSS induced ulcers to 53%, 46% and 40%, respectively in comparison to control (Miyoshi et al, 2011). While diosgenin did not alter the incidence of colon tumors (adenoma + adenocarcinoma), it reduced the tumor multiplicity significantly at all the three tested doses (Miyoshi N et al., 2011). Furthermore, it was shown that diosgenin's potency against experimentally-induced inflammation-associated colon carcinogenesis was in part mediated by the alteration of lipid metabolism (reduced serum triglyceride levels by up-regulation of lipoprotein lipase), and the modulation of genes associated with inflammation and multiple signaling pathways (Miyoshi N et al., 2011).

With regards to breast cancer, the effect of diosgenin on the ectopic growth of human breast cancer MCF-7 and MDA 231 tumor xenografts was studied in nude mice (Srinivasan et al., 2009). It was reported that diosgenin (10 mg/kg body weight administered intra-tumorally) significantly inhibited the growth of tumor xenografts of both MCF-7 and MDA 231 compared to vehicle-treated controls, with no toxicity to any of the vital organs in the experimental mice (Srinivasan et al., 2009). To test the anti-aging properties of diosgenin in relation to hormonal-effects *in vivo*, Tada et al. (2009) assessed the effect of diosgenin-rich *Dioscorea* Sp. yam tuber extract on the ectopic growth of estradiol-dependent human breast cancer (MCF-7) in ovarectomized nude mice for 12 weeks. Diosgenin containing extracts was shown to repress the size of the tumors compared to sham controls (Tada et al., 2009). Yan et al. (2009) reported that oral administration of diosgenin at a dose of 200 ppm (p.o.) significantly inhibited the growth mouse LA795 lung adenocarcinoma tumors by 33.94% in T739 inbred mice.

3.2 *In vitro* studies

The anti-cancer effects of diosgenin *in vitro* through different mechanisms are discussed in the following sub-sections. Many molecular candidates critical to tumorigenesis are affected by diosgenin (Raju and Mehta, 2009; Raju and Rao, 2009). The *in vitro* anticancer effects of diosgenin and its cellular/molecular effects is summarised in Table 3.

3.2.1 Colon cancer

Diosgenin inhibited the growth of HT-29 and HCT-116 human colon adenocarcinoma cells (Lepage et al., 2010; Raju and Bird, 2007; Raju et al., 2004). Diosgenin induced apoptosis in HT-29 cells, in part by inhibition of bcl-2 and by induction of caspase-3 protein expression (Raju et al., 2004). Lepage et al. (2010) reported that in HT-29 cells, diosgenin at 40 μM caused delayed apoptosis together with an increase in cyclooxygenase (COX)-2 expression and activity, higher 5-lipooxygenase (LOX) expression and enhanced leukotriene B4 production. COX-2 inhibition by NS-398 strongly sensitized HT-29 cells to diosgenin-induced apoptosis (Lepage et al., 2010). Furthermore, diosgenin was shown to sensitize HT-29 cells to TRAIL-induced apoptosis (Lepage et al., 2011). In HCT-116 cells, diosgenin was shown to induce apoptosis by the cleavage of the 116 kDa poly (ADP-ribose) polymerase (PARP) protein to the 85kDa fragment (Raju and Bird, 2007). In addition, it was shown that diosgenin significantly lowered the expression of HMG-CoA reductase at both mRNA and protein levels, suggesting the involvement of the cholesterol biosynthetic pathway in diosgenin's efficacy as an anti-cancer agent (Raju and Bird, 2007).

3.2.2 Breast cancer

Diosgenin arrested the growth of HER2 oncoprotein-overexpressing AU565 human breast adenocarcinoma cells at sub-G_1 phase (Chiang et al., 2007). Selective apoptosis induced by diosgenin in these cells was found to be through PARP cleavage involving the down-

Organ site	Cancer cell type	Cellular/molecular targets	References
Colon	HT-29	Apoptosis/ bcl-2, caspase-3, COX-2, 5-LOX	Raju et al., 2004 Lepage et al., 2010; 2011
	HCT-116	Apoptosis/ PARP, COX-2, 5-LOX Lipid metabolism/ HMG-CoA reductase	Raju et al., 2007 Lepage et al., 2010; 2011 Raju et al., 2007
Breast	AU565	Apoptosis/ PARP, mTOR, JNK Lipid metabolism/FAS	Chiang et al., 2007
	MCF-7	Growth-proliferation/ Akt, p53 Apoptosis/ NF-κB, Bcl-2, survivin	Srinivasan et al., 2009
	MDA 231	Growth-proliferation/ ERK Apoptosis/caspase-3, NF-κB, Bcl-2, survivin	Srinivasan et al., 2009
Prostate	PC-3	Growth-proliferation/ PI3K, Akt, ERK, JNK, NF-κB Angiogenesis/ VEGF	Chen et al., 2011
	DU145	Growth-invasion/ HGF, mdm2, vimentin, Akt, mTOR	Chang et al., 2011
Cervix	CaSki	Growth-proliferation	Fernández-Herrera et al., 2010
Liver	HCC	Apoptosis/caspase-3, PARP Transcription/ STAT3, cSrc	Li et al., 2010
Bone/blood	1547 osteosarcoma	Apoptosis/ NF-κB, p53, PPAR-γ, COX-2	Corbiere et al., 2003; 2004a Moalic et al., 2001
	RAW-264.7	Growth-proliferation/ NF-κB, RANK-L	Shishodia and Aggarwal, 2006
	KBM-5	Growth-proliferation/ NF-κB, IκBα, cyclin-D1,	Shishodia and Aggarwal, 2006
	HEL	Apoptosis/ PARP, caspase-3, p21 Eicosanoid biosynthesis/ COX-2, 5-LOX/cPLA2	Leger et al., 2004a; 2006 Leger et al., 2004b; Napez et al., 1995
	K562	Apoptosis/ PARP, caspase-3, NF-κB, COX-2, p38 MAPK	Liagre et al., 2005
Larynx	HEp-2	Apoptosis/ p53	Corbiere et al., 2004b
Skin	M4Beu	Apoptosis/ p53	Corbiere et al., 2004b

Table 3. *In vitro* anticancer activities of diosgenin (purified)

regulation of phospho-Akt and phospho- mammalian target of rapamycin (mTOR), and up-regulation of phospho- c-Jun N-terminal kinase (JNK) independent of p38 and extracellular signal regulating kinase (ERK) phosphorylations (Chiang et al., 2007). In the same cell-line (AU565 cells), diosgenin inhibited the expression of fatty acid synthase (Chiang et al., 2007). The anti-cancer mechanism of diosgenin was shown to be different in human breast cancer cells based on the status of estrogen receptor (ER) expression (Srinivasan et al., 2009). In ER-positive MCF-7 human breast cancer cells, diosgenin induced p53 tumor suppressor protein; while the pro-apoptotic mechanism of diosgenin in ER-negative MDA human breast carcinoma cells involved the activation of caspase-3 and down-regulation of bcl-2 (Srinivasan et al., 2009).

3.2.3 Prostate cancer

Diosgenin inhibited proliferation of PC-3 human prostate cancer cells in a dose-dependent manner (Chen et al., 2011). At non-toxic doses, diosgenin suppressed cell migration and invasion by reducing the activities and mRNA expression of matrix metalloproteinase (MMP) -2 and MMP-9 (Chen et al., 2011). Diosgenin abolished the expression of vascular endothelial growth factor (VEGF) in PC-3 cells and tube formation of endothelial cells (Chen et al., 2011). In addition, diosgenin downregulated the phosphorylation of phosphatidylinositide-3 kinase (PI3K), Akt, ERK and JNK proteins and significantly decreased the nuclear level of nuclear factor (NF)-κB, suggesting that diosgenin inhibited NF-κB activity (Chen et al., 2011). Another study using DU145 human prostate cancer cells found that diosgenin abrogated hepatocyte growth factor (HGF)-induced cell scattering and invasion, together with inhibition of Mdm2 and vimentin through down-regulation of phosphorylated Akt and mTOR (Chang et al., 2011).

3.2.4 Cervical cancer

Recently, Fernández-Herrera et al. (2010) reported the synthesis of a novel 26-hydroxy-22-oxocholestanic steroid from diosgenin and its anticancer activity against human cervical cancer CaSki cells. Mainly this diosgenin-derivative caused apoptosis at non cytotoxic doses activation of caspase-3 along. Furthermore, they report that antiproliferative doses of this compound observed in cancer cells did not affect the proliferative potential of normal fibroblasts from cervix and peripheral blood lymphocytes (Fernández-Herrera et al., 2010).

3.2.5 Liver cancer

Diosgenin was shown to inhibit the proliferation of hepatocellular carcinoma (HCC) cells in a dose and time-dependent manner (Liu et al., 2005). Diosgenin caused arrest of HCC cells at the G_1 phase of the cell cycle and induced apoptosis through caspase-3 activation leading to PARP cleavage (Li et al., 2010). In these cells, diosgenin inhibited both constitutive and inducible activation of signal transducers and activators of transcription (STAT)3 with no effect on STAT5, and suppressed the activation of c-Src, Janus-family tyrosine kinases (JAK)1 and JAK2 implicated in STAT3 activation (Li et al., 2010).

3.2.6 Other cancers

Cytotoxic effects of diosgenin were reported in human cancer cell lines of various other organ types: osteosarcoma (Corbiere et al., 2003, Moalic et al., 2001), leukemia (Liu et al.,

2005) and erythroleukemia (Leger et al., 2004a). The growth of 1547 human osteosarcoma cells was inhibited through G_1 phase cell cycle arrest and induction of apoptotic demise; and the main the mechanism involved the activation of p53 and binding of NFκB to DNA independent of PPAR-γ (Corbiere et al., 2003, 2004a). Interestingly, diosgenin's effect in suppressing osteoclastogenesis in RAW-264.7 cells was reported to follow a pro-apoptotic mechanism through receptor activated NFκB ligand (RANK-L) induction (Shishodia and Aggarwal, 2006). Moalic et al. (2001) demonstrated that diosgenin inhibited COX-2 activity and expression in human osteosarcoma 1547 cells.

Diosgenin arrested chronic myelogenous leukemia KBM-5 cells of human origin at sub-G_1 phase of cell cycle arrest (Shishodia and Aggarwal, 2006). This cell cycle arrest was correlated to the inhibition of tumor necrosis factor (TNF)-dependent NF-κB activation and TNF-induced degradation and phosphorylation of IκBα (the inhibitory subunit of NF-κB) (Shishodia and Aggarwal, 2006). Diosgenin downregulated TNF-induced cyclin D1 in KBM-5 cells (Shishodia and Aggarwal, 2006). Furthermore it abolished both basal and TNF-induced COX-2 gene products in a time-dependent manner (Shishodia and Aggarwal, 2006). Diosgenin controlled the growth of human erythroleukemia TIB-180 (HEL) cells by arresting cells at G_2/M cell cycle and inducing apoptosis through PARP cleavage, activation of caspase-3 and up-regulation of p53-independent p21 (Leger et al., 2004a, 2004b, 2006). Diosgenin treatment to HEL cells induced cytosolic phospholipase (cPL)A2 activation through translocation to the cellular membrane together with an increase in COX-2 expression (Leger 2004b). In a study by Nappez et al. (1995), it was reported that diosgenin treatment in HEL cells did not affect 5-LOX mRNA or 5-LOX activating protein (FLAP) mRNA at the transcriptional level. However, when HEL cells undergoing differentiation were incubated with diosgenin in the presence of indomethacin (a COX inhibitor), the growth inhibitory effect of diosgenin was reversed and an exponential growth kinetic of undifferentiated cells was observed (Nappez et al., 1995). Taken together, these studies provide an insight into the role of 5-LOX in diosgenin's modulation of growth and differentiation in HEL cells. Leger et al. (2004b) demonstrated that diosgenin increased the synthesis of arachidonic acid in HEL cells leading to COX-2 overexpression, which was accompanied by apoptosis induction. The anticancer activity of diosgenin was also shown in human erythroleukemia K562 cells through caspase-3-activation dependent PARP-mediated pro-apoptotic effects (Liagre et al., 2005). Diosgenin induced COX-2-independent apoptosis through activation of the p38 MAP kinase signalling pathway and inhibition of NFκB binding in COX-2 deficient K562 cells (Liagre et al., 2005). The anticancer mechanism of diosgenin was also shown in laryngocarcinoma HEp-2 and melanoma M4Beu cells through a p53-dependent cell death meachnism (Corbiere et al., 2004b).

4. Other diseases and ailments

A clinical study by Turchan-Cholewo et al. (2006) reported that diosgenin may have therapeutic potential against an increased risk of developing dementia in opiate abusers with HIV infection. Recently, the effect of diosgenin on hepatitis C virus (HCV) replication was reported (Wang et al., 2011). Based on a reporter-based HCV subgenomic replicon system, diosgenin was found to inhibit HCV replication at low μM concentrations *in vitro* (Wang et al., 2011). Furthermore, a combination of diosgenin and interferon-α exerted an additive effect on the resultant anti-HCV activity (Wang et al., 2011). The neuroprotective effect of diosgenin against d-galactose-induced senescence in mice by improving cognitive abilities as assessed through the Morris water maze test and mediated by enhancing endogenous antioxidant enzyme activities (Chiu et al., 2011). Diosgenin induced apoptosis in non-cancerous human rheumatoid arthritis synoviocytes (RAS) through the overexpression of COX-2 protein and concomitant increase in the level of prostaglandin (PG)-E_2 (Liagre et al., 2004, 2007). Diosgenin may be an effective inhibitor of hyperpigmentation, commonly seen in skin disorders and inhibits melanogenesis by activating the PI3K pathway and (Lee et al., 2007). A novel effect of diosgenin in restoration of keratinocyte proliferation in aged skin in an animal model suggests that diosgenin may have a potential in slowing the aging process in the skin commonly associated with climacteric (Tada et al., 2009). Recent data support the possibility that some diosgenin-glycoside derivatives may represent a new type of contractile agonist for the uterus and their synergism may be responsible for their therapeutic effect against abnormal uterine bleeding (Yu et al., 2010).

5. Safety

There is a claim that diosgenin has an endocrine effect (estrogen-like or progesterone-like activity) in humans, however there is no scientific evidence to its validation (Djerassi et al., 1952; No authors listed, 2004). Diosgenin is neither synthesized nor metabolically converted into steroid by-products in the mammalian body. Toxicology studies using relevant experimental models have established that even at an upper concentration of 3.5% (wt/wt), diosgenin was safe and failed to cause systemic toxicity, genotoxicity, or estrogenic activity (63). Qin et al. (2009) reported that ethanol extracts of *Dioscorea* sp. containing 28.34% (wt/wt of lyophilized powder) did not cause any signs of acute toxicity in mice at an upper tested dose of 562.5 mg/kg/d, and did not significantly change toxicological parameters up to a dose of 255 mg/kg/d. No acute renal or hepatic toxicity associated with the administration of extracts of *Dioscorea villosa* at an oral dose of 0.79 g/kg/d (Wojcikowski et al., 2008). However, an increase in fibrosis in the kidneys and in inflammation in livers when rats were on the dose for 28 days was reported in the same study (Wojcikowski et al., 2008). Thus it was concluded that these toxicology effects be considered when consuming these extracts on a long-term basis, especially in people with compromised renal or hepatic function (Wojcikowski et al., 2008). On the other hand, in a 90-day subchronic study, rats fed fenugreek seeds, at doses between 1% and 10% in pure diet, had no toxic effects (Muralidhara et al., 1999). Typically, fenugreek seeds are known to contain ~0.42% to 0.75% diosgenin depending on the cultivars and seed quality (Taylor et al., 2000). Fenugreek seed extract evaluated using the standard battery of tests (reverse mutation assay, mouse lymphoma forward mutation assay and mouse micronucleus assay) recommended by US Food and Drug Administration (FDA) for food ingredients came negative and thus rendered safe for consumption at the therapeutic doses tested (Flammang et al., 2004). A recent study using human sera indicated that fenugreek seed powder contains several proteins that potentially act as allergens (Faeste et al., 2009); however, it remains unclear if diosgenin in interaction with any proteins would test positive in these allergen tests. More studies are warranted to understand the toxicological effects of diosgenin at both levels present in common foods as well as therapeutic doses. Although there is toxicology data with regards to diosgenin-rich botanicals such as *Dioscorea* sp. yam tubers and fenugreek seeds, there is a clear lack of data studying the safety of diosgenin *per se*. Some of the important aspects for future studies assessing the toxicology of diosgenin include those related to developmental toxicity, neurotoxicity and allergenicity.

6. Conclusions

With changing lifestyle patterns such as diet and physical activity combined with factors such as genetic predispositions and smoking, the incidences of metabolic diseases including diabetes and obesity and certain kinds of cancers are increasing worldwide and hence are a public health concern with major economic impacts. While the pathogenesis of these diseases is different, there appears to be one or more molecular candidates that are commonly up- or down-regulated leading to the notion that these could be common molecular targets in prevention or therapeutic interventions of diseases. Ethnomedicine has been instrumental in providing important clues as to the role herbs and foods and their bioactive constituents in disease prevention and therapy; however, rigorous experimental-based evidence in support of ethnomedicine-derived notions would lead to the development of products relevant to and drug development. Several naturally-occurring compounds such as those in edible plants or spices are known to target multiple molecular pathways of signalling, thus bestowing them a broad preventive/therapeutic potential against several diseases. For example, curcumin from turmeric, resveratrol from grapes and epigallocatechin gallate (EGCG) from green tea have shown excellent pre-clinical potency against a wide range of diseases (reviewed in Epstein et al., 2010; Marques et al., 2009; Saito et al., 2009). These natural compounds have also been tested in clinical trials as potential therapeutics against several diseases. One emerging natural compound of interest with similar potency as curcumin, resveratrol and EGCG is diosgenin. In the above sub-sections, we have discussed in detail, the health promoting effects of diosgenin and diosgenin-rich

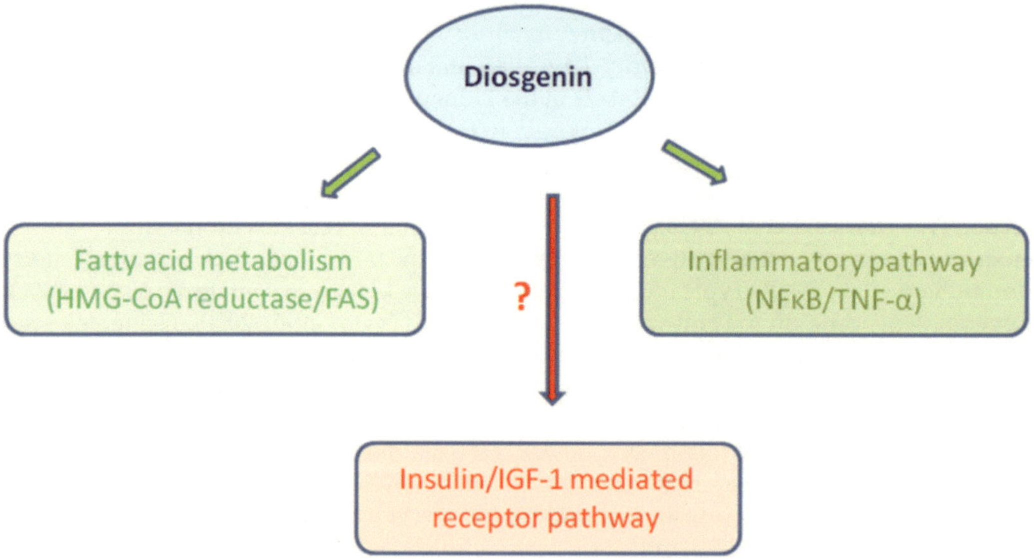

Fig. 2. Schematic representation depicting the molecularmode of action of diosgenin in the control of metabolic pathway. Diosgenin plausibly regulates signaling molecules in fatty acid metabolism and inflammatory pathway. Insulin and IGF-1 mediated signalling pathways may also be regulated by diosgenin and are thus candidates for future studies

sources: (a) *Dioscorea* sp. yam tubers and (b) *Trigonella* sp. (fenugreek) seeds. In addition, we have summarised the toxicology data pertaining to the safe use of diosgenin either in a pure form (where data was available) or in extracts. The health promoting effects of diosgenin can be broadly divided according to the differential molecular mechanisms it elicits. First, there is a growing body of experimental evidence suggesting the use of diosgenin in the treatment of metabolic diseases. Much of this is rendered through diosgenin's capacity to lower lipids in the blood and perhaps in tissues such as liver and adipose tissue. To date, there is some evidence that implicates both inflammatory pathway-associated NFκB and fatty acid metabolism-associated HMG-CoA reductase and FAS as potential molecular targets of diosgenin (Chiang et al., 2007; Raju and Bird, 2007), and these may be extended to its role as a therapeutic against metabolic diseases (Figure 2). Pathways associated with insulin and insulin-like growth factor (IGF)-1 may be of relevance in understanding the molecular mechanism of diosgenin's action in the control of metabolic diseases (Figure 2). Second, the role of diosgenin in modulating cancers has been substantially addressed; most of these data are related to the growth and proliferation of human cancer cell types and its potential mechanism(s) of action *in vitro*. Several molecular candidates associated with fatty acid metabolism (Chiang et al., 2007; Raju and Bird, 2007), inflammatory pathway (Leger et al., 2006; Liagre et al., 2005; Shishodia and Aggarwal, 2006), eicosanoid biosynthesis (Leger et al., 2004; Lepage et al., 2010; 2011; Moalic et al., 2001; Napez et al., 1995), cell proliferation and growth (Chiang et al., 2007; Leger et al., 2006; Srinivasan et al., 2009), apoptosis (Corbiere et al., 2004; Leger et al., 2006; Lepage et al., 2010; 2011; Raju and Bird, 2007; Raju et al., 2004), and regulation of transcription (Chiang et al., 2007; Li et al., 2010) are affected (up- or down-regulated) by diosgenin leading to tumor cell death (Figure 3).

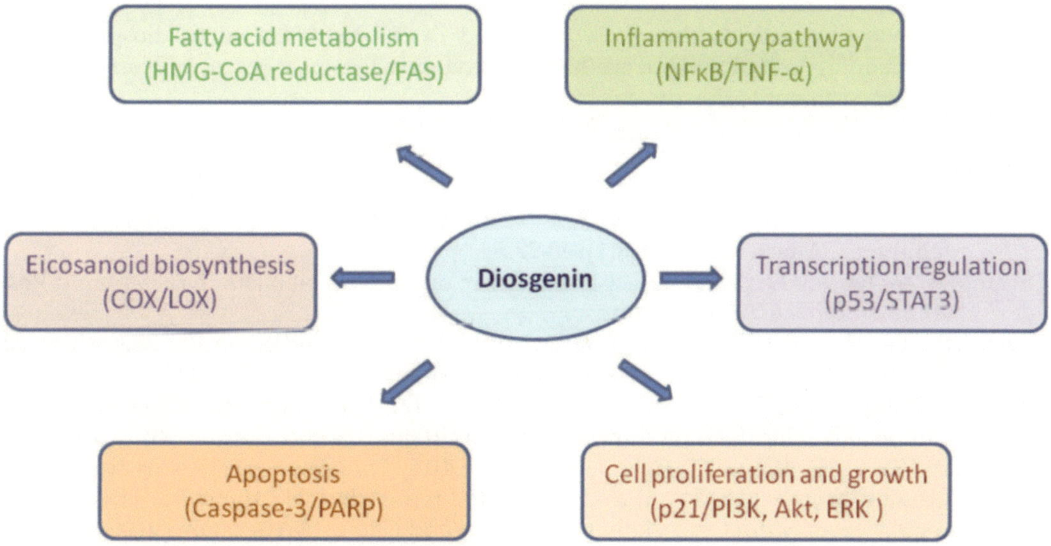

Fig. 3. Schematic representation of plausible mechanism of action(s) of diosgenin at the cellular level as a cancer chemopreventivel/therapeutic agent. Diosgenin up- or down-regulates several molecular candidates associated with cell proliferation and growth, apoptosis, regulation of transcription, fatty acid metabolism, inflammatory pathway and eicosanoid biosynthesis leading to tumor cell death.

While there are ample *in vivo* studies available to implicate the beneficial effects of diosgenin against metabolic disease, more studies to understand the specific modes of action at the molecular level are warranted. On the contrary, substantial *in vitro* evidence exists to understand the molecular mechanism of action of diosgenin against several cancers. More *in vivo* studies are thus essential to understand the physiological relevance of such data in controlling cancers. Moreover, there is excellent opportunity to address whether diosgenin plays a role in chemoprevention versus therapy, or both, in cancers of various organ sites using relevant models. The health beneficial effects of diosgenin are further extended to its potential role to treat other ailments such as HIV and hepatitis-C infections as well as liver diseases. There is little information regarding the bioavailability, pharmacokinetics and pharmacodynamics of diosgenin in relation to its health beneficial effects. Diosgenin and diosgenin-containing products are emerging in the market and are being promoted as natural health products. The scientific knowledge in this area is limited and hence extensive pre-clinical and clinical research should be carried out prior to advocating the safe and efficacious use of diosgenin and diosgenin-rich plant extracts against the prevention and control of diseases. Furthermore, such research will assist in the development of evidence-based regulation of diosgenin and disogenin-containing products as they become increasingly popular and enter the market.

7. Grant information

This work was in part supported by PHS NIH/NCI R01CA 094962 and the Kerley-Cade Endowment.

8. Acknowledgements

We acknowledge all authors that have published in the field related to diosgenin and diosgenin-containing botanicals, but we have quoted only the most recent publications and original articles pertinent to this review.

9. References

Basch E, Ulbricht C, Kuo G, Szapary P & Smith M. (2003). Therapeutic applications of fenugreek. Altern Med Rev. 8(1): 20-27.

Cayen MN, & Dvornik D. (1979). Effect of diosgenin on lipid metabolism in rats. J Lipid Res. 20: 162–174.

Cayen MN, Ferdinandi ES, Greselin E, & Dvornik D. (1979). Studies on the disposition of diosgenin in rats, dogs, monkeys and man. Atherosclerosis 33: 71-87.

Chan YC, Chang SC, Liu SY, Yang HL, Hseu YC, & Liao JW. (2010) Beneficial effects of yam on carbon tetrachloride-induced hepatic fibrosis in rats. J Sci Food Agric. 90(1): 161-167.

Chang HY, Kao MC, Way TD, Ho CT, & Fu E. (2011) Diosgenin suppresses hepatocyte growth factor (HGF)-induced epithelial-mesenchymal transition by down-regulation of Mdm2 and vimentin. J Agric Food Chem. 59(10): 5357-5363.

Chen PS, Shih YW, Huang HC, & HW. (2011) Diosgenin, a Steroidal Saponin, Inhibits Migration and Invasion of Human Prostate Cancer PC-3 Cells by Reducing Matrix Metalloproteinases Expression. PLoS One. 6(5): e20164.

Chevallier A. (2000) The encyclopedia of herbal medicine. 2nd edition Dorling Kindersley, Ltd. London.

Chevassus H, Molinier N, Costa F, Galtier F, Renard E, & Petit P. (2009) A fenugreek seed extract selectively reduces spontaneous fat consumption in healthy volunteers. Eur J Clin Pharmacol. 65(12): 1175-1178.

Chevassus H, Gaillard JB, Farret A, Costa F, Gabillaud I, Mas E, Dupuy AM, Michel F, Cantié C, Renard E, Galtier F, & Petit P. (2010) A fenugreek seed extract selectively reduces spontaneous fat intake in overweight subjects. Eur J Clin Pharmacol. 66(5): 449-455.

Chiang CT, Way TD, Tsai SJ, & Lin JK. (2007) Diosgenin, a naturally occurring steroid, suppresses fatty acid synthase expression in HER2-overexpressing breast cancer cells through modulating Akt, mTOR and JNK phosphorylation. FEBS Lett. 581(30): 5735-5742.

Corbiere C, Liagre B, Bianchi A, Bordji K, Dauca M, Netter P, & Beneytout JL. (2003) Different contribution of apoptosis to the antiproliferative effects of diosgenin and other plant steroids, hecogenin and tigogenin, on human 1547 osteosarcoma cells. Int J Oncol. 22, 899-905.

Corbiere C, Battu S, Liagre B, Cardot PJ, & Beneytout JL (2004a) SdFFF monitoring of cellular apoptosis induction by diosgenin and different inducers in the human 1547 osteosarcoma cell line. J Chromatogr B Analyt Technol Biomed Life Sci. 808, 255-262.

Corbiere C, Liagre B, Terro F, & Beneytout JL. (2004b) Induction of antiproliferative effect by diosgenin through activation of p53, release of apoptosis-inducing factor (AIF) and modulation of caspase-3 activity in different human cancer cells. Cell Res. 14(3): 188-196.

Chiu CS, Chiu YJ, Wu LY, Lu TC, Huang TH, Hsieh MT, Lu CY, & Peng WH. (2011) Diosgenin ameliorates cognition deficit and attenuates oxidative damage in senescent mice induced by D-galactose. Am J Chin Med. 39(3): 551-563.

Dinarello CA. (2006) The paradox of pro-inflammatory cytokines in cancer. Cancer Metastasis Rev. 25: 307-313.

Djerassi C, Rosenkranz G, Pataki J, Kaufmann S. (1952) Steroids, XXVII. Synthesis of allopregnane-3~, 11 beta, 17-, 20~, 21-pentol from cortisone and diosgenin. J Biol Chem. 194: 115-118.

Epstein J, Sanderson IR, & Macdonald TT. (2010) Curcumin as a therapeutic agent: the evidence from in vitro, animal and human studies. Br J Nutr. 103(11): 1545-1557.

Faeste CK, Namork E, & Lindvik H. (2009) Allergenicity and antigenicity of fenugreek (Trigonella foenum-graecum) proteins in foods. J Allergy Clin Immunol. 123(1): 187-194.

Fernández-Herrera MA, López-Muñoz H, Hernández-Vázquez JM, López-Dávila M, Escobar-Sánchez ML, Sánchez-Sánchez L, Pinto BM, & Sandoval-Ramírez J. (2010) Synthesis of 26-hydroxy-22-oxocholestanic frameworks from diosgenin and hecogenin and their in vitro antiproliferative and apoptotic activity on human cervical cancer CaSki cells. Bioorg Med Chem. 18(7): 2474-2484.

Flammang AM, Cifone MA, Erexson GL, & Stankowski LF Jr. (2004) Genotoxicity testing of a fenugreek extract. Food Chem Toxicol. 42(11): 1769-1775.

Juarez-Oropeza MA, Diaz-Zagoya JC, & Rabinowitz JL. (1987) In vivo and in vitro studies of hypocholesterolemic effects of diosgenin in rats. Int J Biochem. 19: 679-683.

Kosters A, Frijters RJ, Kunne C, Vink E, Schneiders MS, Schaap FG, Nibbering CP, Patel SB, & Groen AK. (2005) Diosgenin-induced biliary cholesterol secretion in mice requires Abcg8. Hepatology. 41(1): 141-150.

Kwon CS, Sohn HY, Kim SH, Kim JH, Son KH, Lee JS, Lim JK, & Kim JS. (2003) Anti-obesity effect of Dioscorea nipponica Makino with lipase-inhibitory activity in rodents. Biosci Biotechnol Biochem. 67, 1451-1456.

Lee J, Jung K, Kim YS, & Park D. (2007) Diosgenin inhibits melanogenesis through the activation of phosphatidylinositol-3-kinase pathway (PI3K) signaling. Life Sci. 81(3): 249-254.
Leger DY, Liagre B, Cardot PJ, Beneytout JL, & Battu S. (2004a) Diosgenin dose-dependent apoptosis and differentiation induction in human erythroleukemia cell line and sedimentation field-flow fractionation monitoring. Anal Biochem. 335: 267-278.
Leger DY, Liagre B, Corbiere C, Cook-Moreau J, & Beneytout JL. (2004b) Diosgenin induces cell cycle arrest and apoptosis in HEL cells with increase in intracellular calcium level, activation of cPLA2 and COX-2 overexpression. Int J Oncol. 25: 555-562.
Leger DY, Liagre B, & Beneytout JL. (2006) Role of MAPKs and NF-kappaB in diosgenin-induced megakaryocytic differentiation and subsequent apoptosis in HEL cells. Int J Oncol. 28: 201-207, 2006.
Lepage C, Liagre B, Cook-Moreau J, Pinon A, & Beneytout JL. (2010) Cyclooxygenase-2 and 5-lipoxygenase pathways in diosgenin-induced apoptosis in HT-29 and HCT-116 colon cancer cells. Int J Oncol. 36(5): 1183-1191.
Lepage C, Léger DY, Bertrand J, Martin F, Beneytout JL, & Liagre B. (2011) Diosgenin induces death receptor-5 through activation of p38 pathway and promotes TRAIL-induced apoptosis in colon cancer cells. Cancer Lett. 301(2): 193-202.
Li F, Fernandez PP, Rajendran P, Hui KM, & Sethi G. (2010) Diosgenin, a steroidal saponin, inhibits STAT3 signaling pathway leading to suppression of proliferation and chemosensitization of human hepatocellular carcinoma cells. Cancer Lett. 292(2): 197-207.
Liagre B, Vergne-Salle P, Corbiere C, Charissoux JL, & Beneytout JL. (2004) Diosgenin, a plant steroid, induces apoptosis in human rheumatoid arthritis synoviocytes with cyclooxygenase-2 overexpression. Arthritis Res Ther. 6: R373-R383.
Liagre B, Bertrand J, Leger DY, & Beneytout JL. (2005) Diosgenin, a plant steroid, induces apoptosis in COX-2 deficient K562 cells with activation of the p38 MAP kinase signalling and inhibition of NF-kappaB binding. Int J Mol Med. 16: 1095-1101.
Liagre B, Leger DY, Vergne-Salle P, & Beneytout JL. (2007) MAP kinase subtypes and Akt regulate diosgenin-induced apoptosis of rheumatoid synovial cells in association with COX-2 expression and prostanoid production. Int J Mol Med. 19: 113-122.
Liu MJ, Wang Z, Ju Y, Wong RN, & Wu QY. (2005) Diosgenin induces cell cycle arrest and apoptosis in human leukemia K562 cells with the disruption of Ca2+ homeostasis. Cancer Chemother Pharmacol. 55: 79-90.
Malisetty VS, Patlolla JMR, Raju J, Marcus LA, Choi CI, & Rao CV. (2005) Chemoprevention of colon cancer by diosgenin, a steroidal saponin constituent of fenugreek. Proc Amer Assoc Cancer Res 46 : 2473.
Marques FZ, Markus MA, & Morris BJ. (2009) Resveratrol: cellular actions of a potent natural chemical that confers a diversity of health benefits. Int J Biochem Cell Biol. 41(11): 2125-2128.
McAnuff MA, Omoruyi FO, Morrison EY, & Asemota HN. (2005) Changes in some liver enzymes in streptozotocin-induced diabetic rats fed sapogenin extract from bitter yam (Dioscorea polygonoides) or commercial diosgenin. West Indian Med J. 54(2): 97-101.
Memorial Sloan-Kettering Cancer Center. About herbs, botanicals and other products: http://www.mskcc.org/mskcc/html/11570.cfm
Moalic S, Liagre B, Corbiere C, Bianchi A, Dauca M, Bordji K, & Beneytout JL. (2001) A plant steroid, diosgenin, induces apoptosis, cell cycle arrest and COX activity in osteosarcoma cells. FEBS Lett. 506: 225-230.

Miyoshi N, Nagasawa T, Mabuchi R, Yasui Y, Wakabayashi K, Tanaka T, & Ohshima H. (2011) Chemoprevention of azoxymethane/dextran sodium sulfate-induced mouse colon carcinogenesis by freeze-dried yam sanyaku and its constituent diosgenin. Cancer Prev Res. 4(6): 924-934.

Muralidhara, Narasimhamurthy K, Viswanatha S, & Ramesh BS. (1999) Acute and subchronic toxicity assessment of debitterized fenugreek powder in the mouse and rat. Food Chem Toxicol. 37: 831-838.

Nappez C, Liagre B, & Beneytout JL. (1995) Changes in lipoxygenase activities in human erythroleukemia (HEL) cells during diosgenin-induced differentiation. Cancer Lett. 96: 133-140.

Nervi F, Marinovic I, Rigotti A, & Ulloa N. (1988) Regulation of biliary cholesterol secretion. Functional relationship between the canalicular and sinusoidal cholesterol secretory pathways in the rat. J Clin Invest. 82: 1818–1825.

Nibbering CP, Groen AK, Ottenhoff R, Brouwers JF, vanBerge-Henegouwen GP, & van Erpecum KJ. Regulation of biliary cholesterol secretion is independent of hepatocyte canalicular membrane lipid composition: a study in the diosgenin-fed rat model. J Hepatol 2001; 35: 164–169.

No authors listed. (2004) Final report of the amended safety assessment of Dioscorea Villosa (Wild Yam) root extract. Int J Toxicol. 23: 49-54.

Omoruyi FO. (2008) Jamaican bitter yam sapogenin: potential mechanisms of action in diabetes. Plant Foods Hum Nutr. 63(3): 135-140.

Qin Y, Wu X, Huang W, Gong G, Li D, He Y, & Zhao Y. (2009) Acute toxicity and sub-chronic toxicity of steroidal saponins from Dioscorea zingiberensis C.H.Wright in rodents. J Ethnopharmacol. 126(3): 543-650.

Raju J, & Bird RP. (2007) Diosgenin, a naturally occurring steroid [corrected] saponin suppresses 3-hydroxy-3-methylglutaryl CoA reductase expression and induces apoptosis in HCT-116 human colon carcinoma cells. Cancer Lett. 255(2): 194-204.

Raju J, & Bird RP. (2006) Alleviation of hepatic steatosis accompanied by modulation of plasma and liver TNF-alpha levels by Trigonella foenum graecum (fenugreek) seeds in Zucker obese (fa/fa) rats. Int J Obes. 30(8): 1298-1307.

Raju J, & Mehta R. (2009) Cancer chemopreventive and therapeutic effects of diosgenin, a food saponin. Nutr Cancer. 61(1): 27-35.

Raju J & Rao CV. (2009) Molecular Targets and Therapeutic uses of Fenugreek (Diosgenin). In: Molecular Targets and Therapeutic uses of Spices: Modern Uses for Ancient Medicine Aggarwal BB and Kunnumakkara AB (Eds.) pp 173-196, World Scientific Publishing Company Inc., Hackensack, New Jersey.

Raju J, Patlolla JM, Swamy MV, & Rao CV. (2004) Diosgenin, a steroid saponin of Trigonella foenum graecum (Fenugreek), inhibits azoxymethane-induced aberrant crypt foci formation in F344 rats and induces apoptosis in HT-29 human colon cancer cells. Cancer Epidemiol Biomarkers Prev. 13: 1392-1398.

Saito ST, Gosmann G, Pungartnik C, & Brendel M. (2009) Green tea extract-patents and diversity of uses. Recent Pat Food Nutr Agric. 1(3): 203-215.

Sauvaire Y, Petit P, Baissac Y, & Ribes G. (2000) Chemistry and pharmacology of fenugreek. In: Herbs, botanicals and teas. Mazza G and Oomah BD (Eds.) pp 107–129, Technomic Pub. Co., Lancaster, Pensylvannia.

Shishodia S, & Aggarwal BB. (2006) Diosgenin inhibits osteoclastogenesis, invasion, and proliferation through the down-regulation of Akt, I kappa B kinase activation and NF-kappa B-regulated gene expression. Oncogene. 25: 1463-1473.

Srinivasan S, Koduru S, Kumar R, Venguswamy G, Kyprianou N, & Damodaran C. (2009) Diosgenin targets Akt-mediated prosurvival signaling in human breast cancer cells. Int J Cancer. 125(4): 961-967.

Son IS, Kim JH, Sohn HY, Son KH, Kim JS, & Kwon CS. (2007) Antioxidative and hypolipidemic effects of diosgenin, a steroidal saponin of yam (Dioscorea spp.), on high-cholesterol fed rats. Biosci Biotechnol Biochem. 71: 3063-3071.

Tada Y, Kanda N, Haratake A, Tobiishi M, Uchiwa H, & Watanabe S. (2009) Novel effects of diosgenin on skin aging. Steroids. 74(6): 504-511.

Taylor WG, Elder JL, Chang PR, & Richards KW. (2000) Microdetermination of diosgenin from fenugreek (Trigonella foenum-graecum) seeds. J Agric Food Chem. 48: 5206-5210.

Temel RE, Brown JM, Ma Y, Tang W, Rudel LL, Ioannou YA, Davies JP, & Yu L. (2009) Diosgenin stimulation of fecal cholesterol excretion in mice is not NPC1L1 dependent. J Lipid Res. 50(5): 915-23.

Thirunavukkarasu V, Anuradha CV, & Viswanathan P. (2003) Protective effect of fenugreek (Trigonella foenum graecum) seeds in experimental ethanol toxicity. Phytother Res. 17(7): 737-43.

Trouillas P, Corbiere C, Liagre B, Duroux JL, & Beneytout JL. (2005) Structure-function relationship for saponin effects on cell cycle arrest and apoptosis in the human 1547 osteosarcoma cells: a molecular modelling approach of natural molecules structurally close to diosgenin. Bioorg Med Chem. 13, 1141-1149.

Turchan-Cholewo J, Liu Y, Gartner S, Reid R, Jie C, Peng X, Chen KC, Chauhan A, Haughey N, Cutler R, Mattson MP, Pardo C, Conant K, Sacktor N, McArthur JC, Hauser KF, Gairola C, & Nath A. (2006) Increased vulnerability of ApoE4 neurons to HIV proteins and opiates: protection by diosgenin and L-deprenyl. Neurobiol Dis. 23: 109-119.

Uemura T, Hirai S, Mizoguchi N, Goto T, Lee JY, Taketani K, Nakano Y, Shono J, Hoshino S, Tsuge N, Narukami T, Takahashi N, & Kawada T. (2010) Diosgenin present in fenugreek improves glucose metabolism by promoting adipocyte differentiation and inhibiting inflammation in adipose tissues. Mol Nutr Food Res. 54(11): 1596-1608.

U lbricht C, Basch E, Burke D, Cheung L, Ernst E, Giese N, Foppa I, Hammerness P, Hashmi S, Kuo G, Miranda M, Mukherjee S, Smith M, Sollars D, Tanguay-Colucci S, Vijayan N, & Weissner W. (2007) Fenugreek (Trigonella foenum-graecum L. Leguminosae): an evidence-based systematic review by the natural standard research collaboration. J Herb Pharmacother. 7: 143-177.

Wang YJ, Pan KL, Hsieh TC, Chang TY, Lin WH, & Hsu JT. (2011) Diosgenin, a plant-derived sapogenin, exhibits antiviral activity in vitro against hepatitis C virus. J Nat Prod. 74(4): 580-584.

Wojcikowski K, Wohlmuth H, Johnson DW, & Gobe G. (2008) Dioscorea villosa (wild yam) induces chronic kidney injury via pro-fibrotic pathways. Food Chem Toxicol. 46(9): 3122-3131.

Yamada T, Hoshino M, Hayakawa T, Ohhara H, Yamada H, Nakazawa T, Inagaki T, Iida M, Ogasawara T, Uchida A, Hasegawa C, Murasaki G, Miyaji M, Hirata A, & Takeuchi T. (2009) Dietary diosgenin attenuates subacute intestinal inflammation associated with indomethacin in rats. Am J Physiol. 273: G355-G364.

Yan LL, Zhang YJ, Gao WY, Man SL, & Wang Y. (2009) In vitro and in vivo anticancer activity of steroid saponins of Paris polyphylla var. yunnanensis. Exp Oncol. 31(1): 27-32.

Yu ZY, Guo L, Wang B, Kang LP, Zhao ZH, Shan YJ, Xiao H, Chen JP, Ma BP, & Cong YW. (2010) Structural requirement of spirostanol glycosides for rat uterine contractility and mode of their synergism. J Pharm Pharmacol. 62: 521-529.

8

Polyphenols as Adaptogens – The Real Mechanism of the Antioxidant Effect?

David E. Stevenson
The New Zealand Institute for Plant & Food Research Limited
New Zealand

1. Introduction

It is well-established from numerous population-based observational studies, that consumption of polyphenol-rich foods, principally fruits and vegetables is beneficial to health, reducing mortality rates and the incidence of the major diseases of modern civilisation, cancer and cardiovascular disease (Stevenson & Hurst, 2007). Until relatively recently, it was widely believed that these health benefits were mediated by free radical-scavenging antioxidants, i.e., vitamins C and E and polyphenols, all compounds with high antioxidant capacity when measured by in vitro chemical tests such as "ORAC". A large body of research, however, has not found a conclusive link between the apparent health benefits of polyphenols and their antioxidant capacity. In addition, supplementation with vitamins C and E, which are thought to operate in the body by radical scavenging, has been the subject of intensive research and large-scale intervention trials. The overall conclusion of this work is that there is no consistent evidence that supplementation of these vitamins above normal dietary intakes is of any benefit to health (Bjelakovic et al., 2008). This suggests that the health benefits of vitamins C and E and polyphenols are not related to their antioxidant capacity. More recent research is, nevertheless, linking polyphenols to other biological effects that have the same end-result as chemical antioxidants were thought to have, i.e., a sustained decrease in free radicals in the body, resulting from enhanced endogenous antioxidant defences and/or reduced production in the mitochondria, the main source of free radical generation. In subsequent sections, the evidence for this is discussed.

2. Relevance of mitochondria to antioxidant effects of polyphenols

Mitochondria are the major producers of free radicals or reactive oxygen species (ROS) in the body and some of the adaptive effects of polyphenols that modulate oxidative stress appear to act through the mitochondria. It is beyond the scope of this review to cover mitochondrial biology in depth, but there is an excellent and comprehensive book on the subject (Scheffler, 2008). For the purposes of this review, an appreciation of the essentials of mitochondrial function will be sufficient to allow interpretation of studies on how polyphenols interact with mitochondria.

2.1 Mitochondria generate metabolic energy and ROS

Mitochondria are responsible for the bulk of cellular energy production (Scheffler, 2008), with only a small proportion being accounted for by the glycolytic pathway. The "electron transport chain" (ETC - Figure 1) oxidises NADH, one output from the TCA acid cycle (Brookes, 2005). This generates electrons, which are transferred through the various components of the ETC, ultimately reducing oxygen to water. In the process, a membrane potential (or proton gradient) is generated by the five ETC complexes pumping protons across the mitochondrial membrane. The return flow of protons through ATP synthase drives ATP synthesis from ADP. The ATP produced during this process is the main energy source used by cells and tissues.

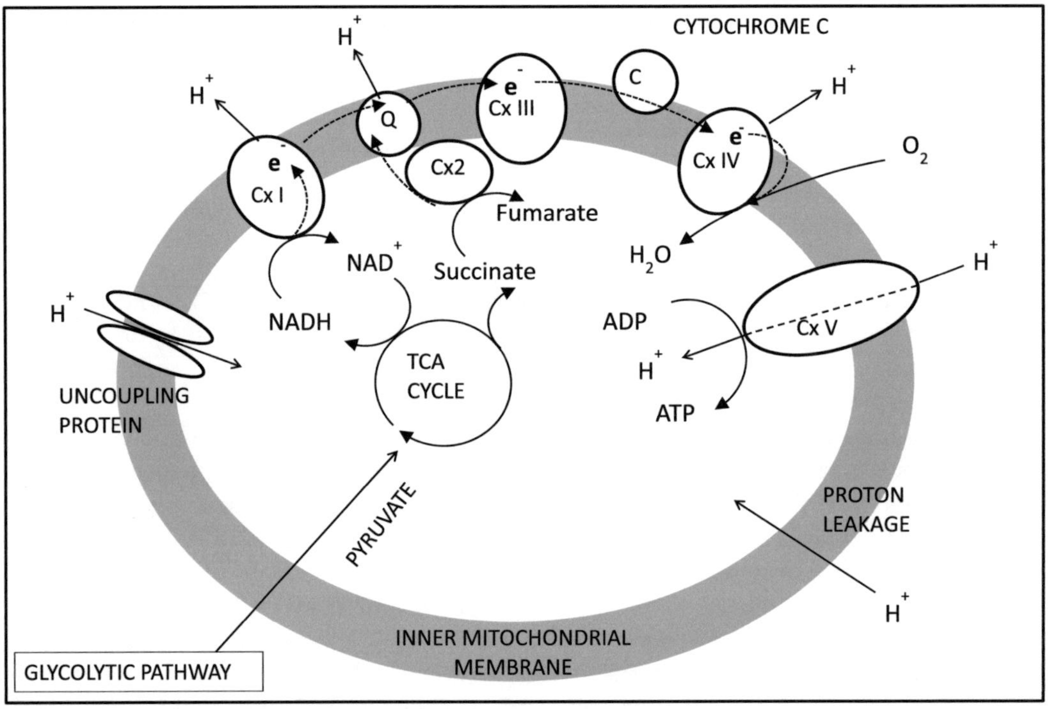

Fig. 1. Schematic summarising the main features of mitochondrial metabolism (Brookes, 2005). Electrons (e-) from the NADH to NAD^+ transition are transferred between electron donors and acceptors, in the process generating energy to pump protons outside the inner membrane. The resulting proton gradient can leak back through the membrane or through uncoupling proteins, but most flow through Complex V (ATP synthase) and power ATP synthesis. Complex I (Cx I, NADH dehydrogenase) passes electrons to Complex III (Cx III, cytochrome bc1) via Q (ubiquinone). Complex II (Cx II, succinate dehydrogenase) delivers more electrons via Q, while Complex IV (Cx IV, cytochrome C oxidase) accepts electrons from Cx III, carried by cytochrome C and uses them to reduce oxygen to water.

The ETC is not 100% efficient and some oxygen molecules are incompletely reduced into the free radical (or reactive oxygen species - ROS) superoxide (Scheffler, 2008; Dorta et al., 2006). Superoxide can in turn generate other ROS species. The production of ROS by muscle cells is greatest during exercise, and the condition arising when ROS increase to damaging levels, is termed "oxidative stress" (Powers & Jackson, 2008). Mitochondria are the major source (approx. 90%, the remainder coming from immune system action and the environment) of ROS in the body (Ristow et al., 2009), but in healthy and especially, physically fit individuals, the mitochondria are also well-equipped with antioxidant enzymes to inactivate ROS before they can do more than minor damage to DNA or other vital cellular components (Hu et al., 2007).

The mitochondrial form of the antioxidant enzyme superoxide dismutase (SOD), Manganese , or MnSOD, converts superoxide into hydrogen peroxide, which is not in itself a radical, but easily forms one (Hu et al., 2007). This is, in turn, reduced to water by a mitochondrial form of another enzyme, glutathione peroxidase (GPX) (Dorta et al., 2006). The cell cytosol has a different form of SOD (Copper Zinc, or CuZnSOD) and a different enzyme, catalase, is primarily responsible for removing hydrogen peroxide (Dinkova-Kostova & Talalay, 2008). Under most circumstances, mitochondria in healthy cells leak only a tiny proportion of ROS into the cytoplasm. ROS generation and leakage increase markedly in unhealthy cells during e.g., exhaustive exercise, because the ETC becomes much less efficient when working close to its maximum capacity.

2.2 Mitochondrial adaptation to oxidative stress

It is well established that exercise increases the mitochondrial content of muscle fibres (known as mitochondrial biogenesis or MB) and consequently their respiratory capacity (Holloszy & Coyle, 1984; Hood et al., 2006; Huang & Hood, 2009). More recently, the increase in ROS generation during exercise has been found to be the primary signal for this adaptive effect of exercise (Ji et al., 2008). The benefit to the organism of MB is greater energy generation capacity and reduced ROS generation for a given energy output. Although it might be expected that increases in mitochondrial/ETC density would lead to increased respiration and ROS production, the opposite actually appears to be the reality. ROS are primarily produced when the flow of electrons through the ETC is limited later in the chain (Barros et al., 2004; Kushnareva et al., 2002). Under these conditions, electrons back up and start to leak out of the complexes earlier in the chain, thereby generating ROS. Under conditions of rigorous exercise, for example, oxygen, the final electron acceptor, would be in limited supply, thus flow of electrons from Complex IV to oxygen would be limited and leakage would occur, primarily from Complex I (Brookes, 2005). There is strong supporting evidence for the link between limited electron flow and ROS generation. Compounds that inhibit any of the ETC complexes cause backing-up of electrons and increased ROS production (Cadenas & Boveris, 1980). The Complex III inhibitor antimycin A increased superoxide production in an in vitro cell model (Dairaku et al., 2004). Inhibition slows the flow of electrons through the ETC and increases the probability of incomplete reduction of oxygen, thereby making superoxide generation more likely.

Moderate regular exercise is reported to induce a low level of ROS, which is thought to up-regulate antioxidant/repair enzymes and consequently to reduce ROS-associated diseases (heart disease, type 2 diabetes, rheumatic arthritis, Alzheimer's and Parkinson's diseases, and certain cancers) (Radak et al., 2008; Ji et al., 2008; Jackson, 2008). Another complementary benefit is that increased mitochondrial respiration capacity and/or MB should reduce resting ROS generation and reduce the effects of aging (Lopez-Lluch et al., 2006). This comes about because ROS generation is highest when the flow of electrons through the ETC is limited. Increased respiratory capacity permits faster electron flow and lowers basal ROS generation. High basal ROS generation is thought to be the main factor causing aging (Cadenas & Davies, 2000), through damage to mitochondrial DNA. Whereas nuclear DNA is heavily protected from damage by ROS, mitochondrial DNA is located in the inner mitochondrial membrane, close to the ETC complexes and very exposed to damage from ROS. It is thought that damage to mitochondrial DNA leads to synthesis of defective ETC protein subunits and thereby, defective ETCs, which generate less energy and more ROS. A negative feedback loop then results in further increase in ROS generation and DNA damage, to both mitochondrial and nuclear DNA (Huang & Hood, 2009; Droge, 2002).

2.3 Mitochondrial adaptation - a new mechanism of antioxidant action?

It is reasonable to assume that, if exercise-induced oxidative stress is the primary signal leading to mitochondrial adaptation and consequently, increased respiratory capacity and decreased basal ROS production, then other sources of oxidative stress could generate similar adaptations. This is an excellent example of the principle of hormesis (Calabrese, 2008), i.e., a non-linear, adaptive, dose response to a toxin. High doses of ROS are clearly harmful, but low doses appear to be essential to initiate the signalling pathways that lead to beneficial adaptive responses. A hypothesis has been proposed recently to explain how oxidative stress induces mitochondrial adaptation to improve efficiency of energy generation, thereby improving physical fitness and general health, ameliorating health issues such as metabolic syndrome and diabetes and above all, increasing life span (Nunn et al., 2009, 2010). Oxidative stressors that are proposed to induce mitochondrial adaptation include exercise, calorie restriction, ionising radiation and most relevant to this discussion, phytochemical "pro-oxidants" (Nunn et al., 2009; Ristow & Zarse, 2010). The ways in which exercise and polyphenols generate oxidative stress are discussed below. Ionising radiation generates ROS directly, from any molecule encountered (Harman, 1956), thereby causing oxidative stress. Calorie restriction stimulates increased respiration that also leads to oxidative stress (Guarente, 2008; Tapia, 2006).

2.4 Signalling pathways that control mitochondrial adaptation

It is thought that mitochondrial adaptation to exercise is primarily brought about by a complex signalling cascade, which is initiated by increased generation of ROS (Droge, 2002) generated by the mitochondria during exercise. The most important aspect of this adaptation is MB i.e., an increase in the number and mass of mitochondria and/or an increase in the density of ETC complexes (Hoppeler et al., 1973; Baar et al., 2002; Holloszy & Coyle, 1984). Most mitochondrial proteins, including those that make up the ETC, are actually encoded by nuclear genes (Scheffler, 2008) and these are regulated by nuclear respiratory factors (Nrf) including Nrf-1 and Nrf-2 (Hawley & Holloszy, 2009). These Nrfs activate genes that encode mitochondrial respiratory chain proteins. Nrf-1 also up-regulates expression of mitochondrial transcription factor A (TFAM), which is transported into the mitochondria and regulates transcription of the mitochondrial genome (Hawley & Holloszy, 2009). Expression of mitochondrial fatty acid oxidation enzymes is regulated by peroxisome-proliferator coactivator 1-α (PGC1-α) (Baar et al., 2002; Lopez-Lluch et al., 2006; Poderoso et al., 2000). Sirtuin1 (a regulatory protein deacetylase, is discussed further in Section 5.1) is thought to be involved in deacetylating and thus activating PGC-1α, which, in turn, co-activates peroxisome-proliferator activated receptor-γ (PPAR-γ).

PPAR-γ is primarily a receptor for fatty acids, which regulates fatty acid oxidation, but it can apparently also be activated by a number of natural products, including some polyphenols (Huang et al., 2005). The anti-diabetic drugs "glitazones" are known to activate PPAR-γ and have also been shown in vitro to induce MB and reduce mitochondrial ROS production (Fujisawa et al., 2009). Polyphenols isolated from red wine, particularly ellagic acid and epicatechin gallate (ECG), were able to activate PPARγ in vitro with similar affinity to the reference pharmaceutical compound rosiglitazone (Zoechling et al., 2011). A number of studies on resveratrol, another polyphenol found in red wine, suggest that many of its purported beneficial effects are mediated by its stimulation of PGC1-α signalling (Tan et al., 2008). Interactions with PPARγ therefore appear to be a possible means for polyphenols to influence mitochondrial adaptation. These interactions may be mediated through direct binding to and activation of PPARγ, or indirectly through its co-activator PGC1-α.

2.5 How do ROS interact with signalling pathways?

One uncertainty in our knowledge of the MB signalling pathway is how an increase in ROS generation initiates signalling. One possible mechanism involves oxidised lipids and the Electrophile (or Antioxidant) Response Element (ERE, or ARE). Mitochondria are primarily composed of membranes into which the ETC complexes are embedded. The lipids in these membranes should be highly susceptible to peroxidation by superoxide generated in their immediate vicinity. One species of breakdown products known to arise from lipid peroxidation is a number of conjugated aldehydes such as 4-hydroxy-2-nonenal (HNE) (Uchida et al., 1999). Conjugated aldehydes and ketones are also potent activators of the ERE (Dinkova-Kostova & Talalay, 2008). The ERE itself is a regulatory region in nuclear DNA that controls the expression of a series of cytoprotective proteins, including a number of antioxidant enzymes, cytochrome P-450 xenobiotic hydroxylases and xenobiotic conjugative enzymes (Dinkova-Kostova & Talalay, 2008). The transcription factor that controls the ERE is Nrf2, which is normally bound to the sensory protein Keap1. Binding of an inducer, such as HNE, or phytochemicals such as curcumin, some polyphenols or sulphoraphane releases Nrf2, which activates the ERE and the proteins it regulates (Dinkova-Kostova & Talalay, 2008). It is possible that the ERE and Nrfs are a link between lipid peroxidation by ROS and the signalling pathway for MB. It appears from this discussion that one of the potential mechanisms for the adaptive effects of polyphenols and other phytochemicals is direct interaction with the MB signalling pathway, through direct activation of either PPAR receptors or the ERE, through interaction with its regulatory protein Keap1.

3. Effect of exercise on mitochondria

This area of science has been subjected to intensive research for at least two decades and is now well understood. The mechanisms of action of exercise in mitochondrial adaptation would reasonably be expected to be very similar to those of other adaptogens, such as polyphenols, if they work through generation of oxidative stress. Evidence that polyphenols can have a hormetic effect through generation of oxidative stress is discussed below. Exercise science should, therefore, be a good source of insights into the mechanistic details of how polyphenols should interact with mitochondria, as well as providing validated assays to monitor these effects both in vitro and in vivo.

3.1 Macroscopic effects of exercise

The well-known benefits of exercise in weight management have been explored by a comparison of mitochondrial metabolism between trained athletes and sedentary individuals (Befroy et al., 2008). The athletes had a 53% higher resting TCA cycle flux, but the same ATP synthesis rate as the sedentary individuals. Essentially, the athletes appeared to have much higher mitochondrial respiration capacity, which "wasted" energy in the resting state, thereby raising their metabolic rate. As discussed above (Section 3.2), it would be reasonable to expect that the athletes' mitochondria would generate less ROS than the sedentary controls in a resting state, because of greater mitochondrial capacity and efficiency, in spite of their higher metabolic rate.

3.2 Antioxidants may inhibit exercise-induced mitochondrial adaptation

If the mechanism underlying the adaptive effects of exercise is initiated by increased oxidative stress, i.e., ROS production, then logically, radical-scavenging antioxidants may be expected to at best have no effect, or at worst hinder adaptations. A number of studies on the use of radical-scavenging antioxidants, i.e., vitamins C and E, appear to support this hypothesis. In a comparison between "Ironman" triathletes and untrained controls, the triathletes had higher resting plasma levels of glutathione peroxidase (GPX), catalase, and superoxide dismutase (SOD), plus lower malondialdehyde (MDA, a biomarker of lipid peroxidation). Participation in the Ironman event then lowered the athletes' antioxidant enzymes and raised MDA. Triathletes who took antioxidant supplements had greater increases in MDA than those that did not (Knez et al., 2007). This suggests that training-level exercise up-regulates antioxidant defences, but competition-level exercise suppresses them. Antioxidant supplements taken during training may cause further suppression of endogenous antioxidant defences. Supplementation of both trained and untrained subjects during a one-month training programme revealed that the supplements suppressed several early biomarkers of mitochondrial adaptation, including expression of PGC1-α, PPAR-γ, SOD2 and GPX1 (Ristow et al., 2009). It appears, however, that there is no overall inhibition of exercise adaptation resulting from antioxidant supplementation because no effect on markers of oxidative stress or on increases in training-induced muscle performance was identified (Theodorou et al., 2011).

It appears reasonable to suggest that exercise is an antioxidant in itself, because it leads to significant up-regulation of antioxidant enzymes in humans (Gomez-Cabrera et al., 2006; Gomez-Cabrera et al., 2008). Similarly, SOD2, the specific mitochondrial form of the enzyme, was induced in rodents by exercise (Higuchi et al., 1985). Although antioxidant supplementation appears to be of no benefit to most sports training, it may be useful if applied in a well-planned and timely manner, to protect untrained individuals from the most damaging effects of high ROS production at the start of a fitness programme (Vincent et al., 2006). These findings are consistent with the hormetic hypothesis of polyphenol-stimulated mitochondrial adaptation. It seems reasonable to conclude that if radical-scavenging antioxidants inhibit the signalling of mitochondrial adaptive effects, but polyphenols promote them, then polyphenols are not primarily acting as radical-scavenging antioxidants in vivo.

4. Evidence that polyphenols can induce mitochondrial adaptation

4.1 Polyphenols may be able to regulate Sirtuins

"Sirtuins" are a family of regulatory protein deacetylases, coded by SIRT genes. Sirtuin1 is thought to play a role in regulation of MB (see above). SIRT1 activation by a synthetic activator was found to up-regulate lipid oxidation (a pathway located in the mitochondria), suggesting potential in treatment of obesity, diabetes and metabolic disorders (Feige et al., 2008). Mice over-expressing SIRT1 showed a phenotype resembling calorie restriction, supporting the involvement of the SIRT1 pathway (and by implication, MB) in adaptations to calorie restriction (Bordone et al., 2007).

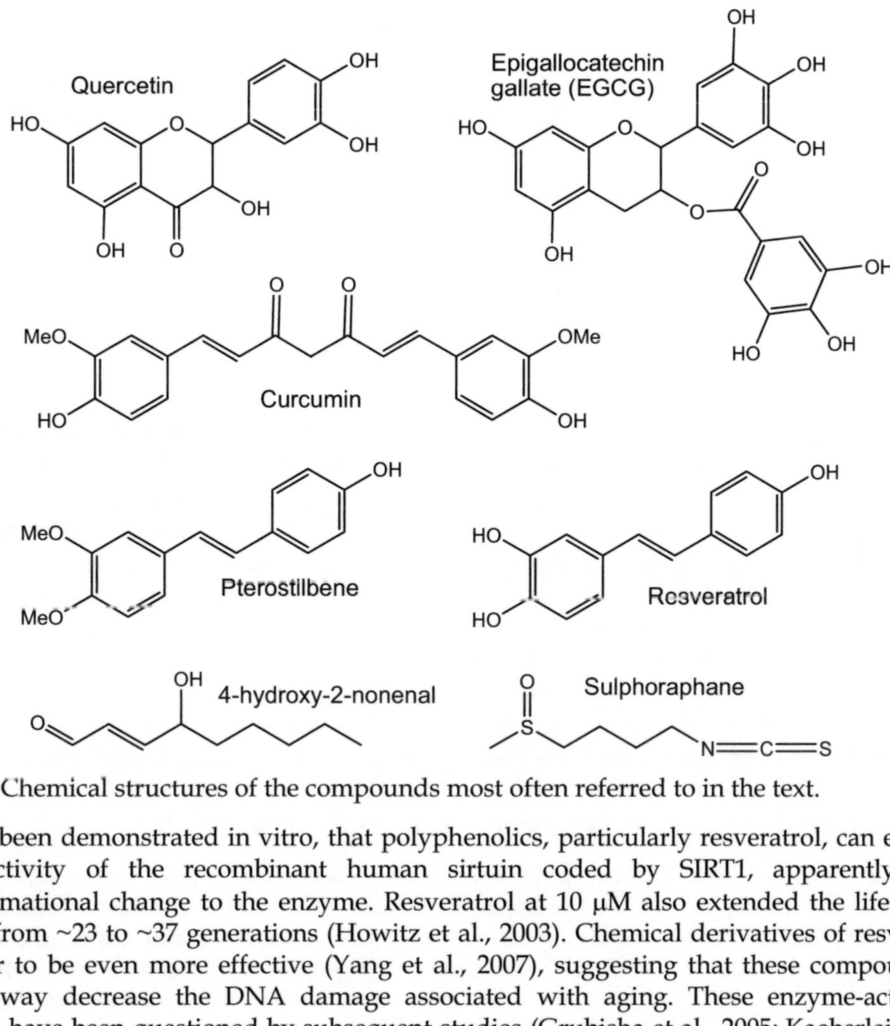

Fig. 2. Chemical structures of the compounds most often referred to in the text.

It has been demonstrated in vitro, that polyphenolics, particularly resveratrol, can enhance the activity of the recombinant human sirtuin coded by SIRT1, apparently by a conformational change to the enzyme. Resveratrol at 10 μM also extended the lifespan of yeast from ~23 to ~37 generations (Howitz et al., 2003). Chemical derivatives of resveratrol appear to be even more effective (Yang et al., 2007), suggesting that these compounds in some way decrease the DNA damage associated with aging. These enzyme-activation results have been questioned by subsequent studies (Grubisha et al., 2005; Kaeberlein et al., 2005) on the grounds that resveratrol required highly supra-physiological concentrations (a 3-fold activation at 20 μM) and a non-physiological substrate to have a measurable effect. Observations that the plasma concentration of resveratrol from a realistic dose is in the nanomolar range and that it exists in vivo almost entirely as conjugates, rather than as free resveratrol (Goldberg et al., 2003) cast further doubt on sirtuin activation as a key mechanism in vivo. It appears more likely that direct sirtuin activation is only a very minor mechanism of MB stimulation by polyphenols in vivo.

4.2 Inhibition of the ETC by polyphenols

It is well-established that inhibitors of the ETC increase ROS generation (Cadenas & Boveris, 1980). It has been shown, in vitro, that flavonoids can inhibit specific mitochondrial functions, including NADH oxidase (Hodnick et al., 1986), F1-ATPase (Gledhill et al., 2007) and the membrane permeability transition (Santos et al., 1998). Other in vitro studies found that polyphenols inhibited overall mitochondrial respiration (Hodnick et al., 1987) and the closely related rate of ATP generation (Dorta et al., 2005). The former study also detected a burst of ROS generation associated with the inhibition of respiration. A wide range of compounds was tested in these studies, to the extent that structure-activity relationships were established. The two best classes of compound appeared to be stilbenes (e.g., resveratrol) and flavonols (e.g., quercetin). These findings suggest that polyphenols, if they were able to access the mitochondria in vivo, could directly but transiently increase ROS generation, thereby inducing beneficial adaptations in a similar way to exercise.

4.3 Can polyphenols access mitochondria to exert biological effects?

The ability of a compound to inhibit mitochondrial metabolism strongly suggests, but does not prove, that it can access the interior of the mitochondria. Several in vitro studies, however, have provided indirect evidence to support the potential of polyphenols to access the interior of mitochondria in vivo. In a study of the effects of treatment with EGCG on rat neuronal cells in vitro, in which the cells were fractionated to isolate the mitochondria, 90-95% of the detectable EGCG was present in the mitochondrial fraction (Schroeder et al., 2009). Similarly, quercetin was rapidly and extensively absorbed by Jurkat cells and their isolated mitochondria, as well as by the mitochondria of preloaded cells (Fiorani et al., 2010). When isolated rat kidney mitochondria were treated with quercetin, various changes consistent with access of quercetin to the interior of the mitochondria were observed, including increased mitochondrial membrane permeability and oxygen consumption, but decreased membrane potential and oxidative phosphorylation (Ortega & Garcia, 2009). It thus appears that mitochondria would be easily able to absorb significant concentrations of polyphenols, provided the intracellular concentrations around them were high enough.

4.4 Bioavailability and access of polyphenols to mitochondria *in vivo*

Studies in vitro can only indicate potential for in vivo effects; to date there is very little direct evidence to support "mitochondrial bioavailability" in vivo. The many hundreds of polyphenol bioavailability studies done in vivo have only measured concentrations of polyphenols and their metabolites in plasma and/or urine; this proves only that the compound or compounds got as far as the circulatory system (Stevenson et al., 2008). A radioactive tracer approach is also unable to resolve the intracellular location of the radioactivity or the specific chemical compound involved. Studies on animals find radioactivity in all tissues in the body, but cannot distinguish between the original polyphenol, a conjugate or some much simpler breakdown product (Stevenson et al., 2008). This approach is also unable to resolve the intracellular location of the radioactivity.

Polyphenol feeding studies on pigs have found polyphenols at micromolar concentrations in a variety of tissues and organs (Bieger et al., 2008; Kalt et al., 2008; Kalt et al., 2007), but one concern with these studies is that entrained blood may not have been completely removed, thus casting doubt on the actual concentrations in the tissues. On balance, it seems probable that polyphenols can access tissues and therefore cells in vivo, but probably in the form of conjugated metabolites or breakdown products, rather than the unconjugated forms tested in vitro. We therefore have no solid evidence of the mitochondrial bioavailability in vivo of the polyphenols tested in vitro. A number of in vivo trials (discussed in later sections) have successfully detected physiological changes consistent with mitochondrial adaptation, linked to dosing with polyphenols, suggesting that polyphenols or their metabolites can in some way stimulate mitochondrial adaptation, but these trials give little information on how these effects could be mediated.

4.5 *In vitro* evidence for mitochondrial adaptation by polyphenols

The in vitro studies reported to date have nearly all been carried out on the polyphenols resveratrol and hydroxytyrosol. Resveratrol, at a supra-physiological concentration of 50 μM, was found to induce MB significantly and greatly up-regulate antioxidant enzyme synthesis including MnSOD in both mouse and human cell cultures (Robb et al., 2008). The critical importance of MnSOD to health and life itself has been demonstrated by several studies. Genetically modified mice that over-express this enzyme have a modestly extended lifetime (Hu et al., 2007), whereas MnSOD-knockout mice die within a few days of birth (Y. Li et al., 1995). Recombinant lactobacilli over-expressing the antioxidant enzymes SOD and CAT demonstrated greatly enhanced resistance to oxidative stress and significantly increased longevity compared with normal bacteria (An et al., 2011).

Resveratrol treatment of isolated human vascular endothelial cells up-regulated many biomarkers of mitochondrial adaptation, including PPAR-α, Nrf1, TFAM, mitochondrial DNA, ETC proteins and MB. Endothelial nitric oxide synthase (eNOS) was also up-regulated, but if NO synthesis was blocked, MB and the other adaptations were also blocked (Csiszar et al., 2009). These findings support the regulatory effects of eNOS/NO on mitochondria, at least in vascular cells. NO itself is well-established as an important factor in mitochondrial regulation (Cadenas et al., 2000).

Hydroxytyrosol (HT), a polyphenol found in olives and olive oil, at concentrations as low as 1 μM significantly stimulated MB and ETC complex synthesis, concomitant with up-regulation of the MB-signalling molecules PGC1-α and Nrf-1 and-2 (Hao et al., 2010). Very similar results were obtained from ARPE-19 cells, a human retinal pigment epithelial line, challenged with acrolein and in addition, HT increased expression of ERE-regulated phase II detoxifying enzymes (Lu et al., 2010). These in vitro studies provide considerable evidence that polyphenols could stimulate adaptive effects in vivo, provided they could accumulate in the cell or mitochondria at sufficient concentrations. Adaptations mediated by eNOS/NO would only require access to the vascular system, which is well-proven by numerous plasma bioavailability studies.

4.6 Other potential adaptogenic effects of polyphenols

Other adaptive effects, not necessarily related to mitochondria, have been associated with polyphenols. Quercetin glycosides stimulated glucose uptake in C2C12 mouse muscle cells in vitro (Eid et al., 2010), an effect that should be beneficial in treating type 1 diabetes, a condition thought to involve mitochondrial dysfunction (Fujisawa et al., 2009). The glycolytic pathway for ATP generation in the cytosol converts glucose to lactate (Scheffler, 2008). Lactate is converted to pyruvate, which is a major input into the TCA cycle in the mitochondria (Figure 1). Treatment with elevated concentrations of pyruvate stimulates MB in both L6E9 myoblasts and C2C12 cells (Duguez et al., 2004; Wilson et al., 2007). Induction of MB by increased pyruvate supply in vitro suggests that there could be a similar effect in vivo. Stimulation of glucose uptake by muscle cells may increase glycolysis and indirectly stimulate MB and other mitochondrial adaptations. In other words, this may be an additional mechanism for stimulation of mitochondrial adaptation by polyphenols.

4.7 Animal trials linking polyphenols with mitochondrial adaptation

Support for the in vivo effects of polyphenolics being closely related to those of exercise on mitochondria has been provided by two trials in mice, which found that high doses of dietary resveratrol (400 and 20 mg/kg/day respectively) reversed all the harmful biological changes (in particular, a shortened lifespan) induced by a high calorie diet, apart from weight gain (Lagouge et al., 2006; Baur et al., 2006). Both trials found increased activity of the mitochondrial signalling molecules SIRT1 and PGC1-α, as well as increased insulin sensitivity. Although 400 mg/kg/day is far from a practical intake for humans, the absence of any ill-effects to the test animals strongly suggests that this compound should have no toxicity in humans at any realistic dietary intake. A subsequent trial found significant increases in the major antioxidant enzymes in mice dosed with resveratrol as part of a high fat diet (Robb et al., 2008). Of particular interest was a doubling of the activity of MnSOD in brain and kidney tissue, in agreement with the observations from in vitro trials of resveratrol.

Resveratrol and its methylated analogues were found to be effective in an in vitro cellular model of oxidative stress. One of these analogues, the naturally-occurring dimethylated derivative of resveratrol, pterostilbene, was subsequently found to reduce neuro-degeneration, a major contributor to age-related cognitive decline, in a long-term rat trial (Joseph et al., 2008). Mitochondrial dysfunction has been implicated in and may be a primary cause of most common neurodegenerative conditions, including those related to aging (Scheffler, 2008). Although these trials do not provide a definitive link between the observed health benefits and resveratrol-induced MB, the results are consistent with such a link and certainly lend support to the link between polyphenols and human health benefits.

4.8 *In vivo* evidence for mitochondrial adaptation by polyphenols

Highly significant augmentation of exercise performance resulted from dietary supplementation with quercetin in a mouse model (Davis et al., 2009). Groups of mice were fed 0, 12.5 or 25 mg/kg/day of quercetin (approximately equivalent to a realistic dose of 1 or 2 g/day for an 80 kg human) for 7 days. Increases (relative to placebo) were observed in gene expression of PCG-1α and SIRT1 by up to 2 fold in muscle and brain, whilst levels of cytochrome C (a marker of mitochondrial mass) increased by 23% in muscle and 18% in brain. Mitochondrial DNA also increased up to 2 fold (Davis et al., 2009). This suggests that the numbers of mitochondria approximately doubled and their overall respiration capacity increased by around 20%. The importance of these results is the clear link between quercetin consumption, increases in biomarkers for mitochondrial adaptation, and MB itself. This trial is therefore, the first to demonstrate unequivocally mitochondrial adaptive effects of a common polyphenol, administered orally. Exercise trials were done on other, similarly dosed mice, in the same study. Forced treadmill running time to exhaustion increased by 37% at both doses of quercetin. Voluntary wheel running activity also increased, both in speed and in time spent. Total distance covered increased by ~45% by the end of the 7-day treatment period and was sustained for the following 7 days (Davis et al., 2009).

Although these performance improvements appear spectacular, they are not unexpected. Laboratory animals are over-fed, chronically under-exercised and lack social interaction and environmental stimulation, being confined to single cages for most of their lives (Cressey, 2010). Although such animals may be poor models of human responses in most cases, they would be expected to be excellent models of obese, unfit and depressed humans who could benefit most from exercise and a healthy, high-polyphenol diet. In this light, the physical performance improvements observed in the trial undertaken by Davis and colleagues would not be expected to be reproduced in humans; much smaller changes in human fitness would be expected from the same treatment. The salient point here is that the performance-enhancing effects of the quercetin are of minor relevance to human health, compared with the clear demonstration of its adaptive effects on mitochondria. In another study, resveratrol supplementation (0.2% w/w) for 12 weeks increased exercise performance in a mouse model of senescence, whereas performance declined in the control group (Murase et al., 2009). Polyphenols therefore, may have potential to ameliorate age-related physical decline in humans.

One aspect of the Davis et al. (2009) study that cannot be easily explained by mitochondrial adaptation is the large increase in voluntary wheel running. Davis and colleagues suggested that this resulted from an entirely different property of quercetin, namely that, in vitro, it is an adenosine A_1 receptor antagonist, as are caffeine and some other common flavonoids (Alexander, 2006). Caffeine is both psycho-stimulatory and ergogenic and this may explain the apparently increased motivation for the mice to exercise.

There is also solid evidence from human trials for adaptive effects of quercetin. A supplementary combination of quercetin (1 g), isoquercetin, EGCG and polyunsaturated fatty acids was tested on *trained* cyclists undergoing 3 hours of cycling on each of 3 days (Nieman et al., 2009). Significant decreases in inflammatory biomarkers were detected relative to the control (placebo), but no change was observed in performance, or any marker of exercise or mitochondrial adaptation. The latter finding is not unexpected in trained athletes, who would be expected to have minimal capacity for increased performance or additional exercise-induced adaptation. In a further trial, 1 g/day of quercetin for two weeks was tested on *untrained* male test subjects (Nieman et al., 2010). Distance travelled in 12 minutes on a treadmill was determined. Relative to placebo, a small but significant increase in distance was observed, accompanied by slight increases in RNA coding for the MB biomarkers PGC-1α, sirtuin 1, citrate synthase and cytochrome C oxidase (Complex IV) (Nieman et al., 2010). Similar results were obtained when Davis et al. (2009) undertook a human trial to examine whether they could replicate the effects previously observed in mice. Twelve untrained volunteers were given 500 mg of quercetin twice daily for 7 days, dissolved in a drink. After treatment, both VO_2max and ride time to fatigue on an exercise bike were determined. The observed increases in VO_2max and ride time to fatigue were

3.9% and 13.2%, respectively, compared with the control (placebo). Whilst no mitochondrial biomarkers were measured in this trial, the enhancement of endurance capacity observed, in the absence of any physical training, is entirely consistent with mitochondrial adaptation.

One should bear in mind that the physical performance aspects of polyphenol-stimulated mitochondrial adaptation are of minor importance in the context of human health. In this respect, mitochondrial dysfunction is of much higher importance, given that it is implicated in some way in both the major diseases of modern civilisation (CVD, cancer and neuro-degeneration) and the aging process (Huang & Hood, 2009). Mitochondrial adaptation, rather than antioxidant capacity, is emerging as the primary mode of action of the health benefits of dietary polyphenols. Whilst there is, to date, no evidence that polyphenol consumption can increase human lifespan, there is good evidence from animal trials (Baur et al., 2006; Lagouge et al., 2006). This suggests that humans may benefit similarly, even if only through reduction in the incidence of life-threatening diseases. It is unlikely that dietary polyphenols could have a major effect on the maximum life-span of humans, but they do appear to have great potential to increase the proportion of people who attain all or most of the maximum lifespan.

4.9 Polyphenolics, mitochondria and apoptosis

Mitochondria are the instigators of programmed cell death, or apoptosis (Dorta et al., 2006). If mitochondria are sufficiently damaged by oxidative stress and DNA damage to become dysfunctional and lose their capacity to adapt to oxidative stress, they initiate a signalling pathway leading to apoptosis, or programmed death, of the host cell and thus the demise of the defective mitochondria. This mechanism has been proposed to explain the "chemo-preventive" effects of polyphenolics (Roy et al., 2009; Juan et al., 2008), based on the observation that cancer cells in vitro are more sensitive to mitochondrial-induced apoptosis than normal cells. Therefore, polyphenols may promote apoptosis of cancerous cells in vivo. The ability to induce apoptosis was demonstrated in vitro for pterostilbene, a natural methylated derivative of resveratrol (Pan et al., 2007), resveratrol itself (Shakibaei et al., 2009), kaempherol, a flavonol similar to quercetin (Marfe et al., 2009), EGC (W. Li et al., 2009) and catechin (Iwasaki et al., 2009). This property of polyphenols may explain at least part of the putative anti-cancer effect of polyphenol-rich foods (see Introduction).

4.10 Does the antioxidant capacity of polyphenols have any role in health?

Polyphenol concentrations achieved in plasma from a realistic dietary intake are both transient and at most, ~2-4% of the small-molecule antioxidants normally present in the plasma; antioxidant enzymes contribute a large additional endogenous antioxidant capacity (Clifford, 2004; Stevenson & Lowe, 2009; Stevenson et al., 2009). In comparison, polyphenols are clearly insignificant in the overall context of resistance to oxidative stress. They could make a contribution at sites within the body where localised concentrations are much higher than the average. One example of this may be in the gastrointestinal (GI) tract, where polyphenol concentrations have been demonstrated to be many times that achieved in plasma (Stevenson et al., 2009), a consequence of the low proportions of most polyphenols that are absorbed from the GI tract. The cells of the GI tract are thus exposed to concentrations that should be more than sufficient for a significant radical-scavenging antioxidant effect. Another possible example is in cell membranes, where in vitro studies found that up to 75% of polyphenols spiked into blood samples can end up bound to the membranes of the blood cells (Biasutto et al., 2010; Koren et al., 2010). This may allow them a significant and direct role in prevention of lipid peroxidation. If this membrane-binding phenomenon translates to the in vivo environment and is common to other cells (and to mitochondria) in the body, polyphenols may have a significant whole-body protective effect from lipid peroxidation.

5. The role of homeostasis in polyphenol action in the body

A good question to ask is why so many trials of antioxidants have failed to demonstrate any benefit and why polyphenol-induced mitochondrial adaptation appears only to be readily detected and manifested as an augmentation of exercise-induced adaptation. The answer may lie in the principle of homeostasis (van Ommen et al., 2009). Homeostasis is the normal state of a healthy cell or organism, where all biochemicals and enzymes are regulated to their optimal concentrations. When an organism is in homeostasis, dietary or pharmaceutical intervention has no particular benefit, because there is no "problem" to rectify. This may go some way towards explaining the apparent 'failure' of intervention trials with antioxidants. If the concentrations of endogenous antioxidants are tightly regulated, then addition of large amounts of exogenous antioxidants would result in down-regulation of endogenous synthesis to restore homeostasis. Van Ommen and colleagues propose that any search for biomarkers of the effects of interventions must be undertaken with simultaneous perturbation of homeostasis, so the intervention can assist its restoration. This is not a major consideration for pharmaceutical interventions, which are typically designed to treat disease, in which homeostasis has already been perturbed. Dietary interventions, in contrast, are usually aimed at optimisation of health, rather than treatment of disease. The search for health benefits of either dietary antioxidants or adaptogens will almost inevitably fail unless tested on subjects with pre-existing or applied oxidative stress. Oxidative stress may be applied to animals by treatment with toxins, enforced exercise, or the use of animal models of suitable disease states. For humans, the options are restricted to the use of test subjects with pre-existing conditions that elevate oxidative stress, such as metabolic syndrome, or the performance of endurance exercise by healthy subjects. If oxidative stress is applied during a trial, appropriate intervention reduces the magnitude of the perturbation (i.e., the stress) and accelerates the restoration of homeostasis.

6. Conclusion

A large body of evidence has now been accumulated to support the concept that polyphenols are primarily adaptogens rather than radical-scavenging antioxidants. This does not negate their potent capacity to reduce oxidative stress; rather it indicates that the mechanism is far more complex and subtle than previously realised. Several in vivo trials have clearly linked polyphenol interventions with actual mitochondrial adaptation, or macroscopic effects consistent with adaptation, specifically mitochondrial biogenesis (MB) and up-regulation of MB-signalling molecules and antioxidant enzymes as the main biomarkers established for detection of mitochondrial adaptation. In vitro trials have been entirely consistent in demonstrating up-regulation of the same biomarkers that provide clues to possible mechanisms of action for polyphenols. These are direct activation of the components of the MB signalling pathway (e.g., sirtuin 1 and PPARγ); direct activation of the ERE via binding to its regulatory protein Keap1; stimulation of glycolysis and glucose uptake, which increases the supply of nutrients to the mitochondria; stimulation of NO synthesis, which is a known signal for MB; and generation of a mild oxidative stress in the mitochondria through inhibition of the ETC or other mechanisms.

Since mitochondrial dysfunction is implicated in aging and major diseases such as cancer, CVD and neuro-degeneration, any means of improving mitochondrial function, or inducing destruction of the most dysfunctional mitochondria, should be highly beneficial to healthy aging and maintenance of good health. Dietary polyphenols are almost certainly a good means of achieving these ends.

7. List of abbreviations and definitions

ORAC : Oxygen radical absorbance capacity; an in vitro measure of relative antioxidant power. **ROS**: Reactive oxygen species; another term for free radicals. **ETC**: Electron transport chain; a group of mitochondrial proteins that generates **ATP** (adenosine triphosphate) by reduction of oxygen to water. **NADH**: Nicotinamide adenine dinucleotide; a biochemical reducing agent. **MnSOD** or **SOD2**: Mitochondrial form of the antioxidant enzyme, manganese superoxide dismutase. **CuZnSOD** or **SOD1**: Cytosolic form of superoxide dismutase. **MB**: Mitochondrial biogenesis; the increase of mitochondrial numbers within cells. **Complex III**: One of the five components of the mitochondrial electron transport chain (ETC). **Nrf-1** and **Nrf-2**: Nuclear respiratory factors; transcription factors involved in control of adaptive responses. **TFAM**: Mitochondrial transcription factor A; transcription factor involved in control of adaptive responses. **PGC-1α**: Peroxisome proliferator-activated receptor gamma coactivator 1-alpha. **PPAR-γ**: Peroxisome-proliferator activated receptor-γ; receptor involved in control of adaptive responses. **ERE/ARE**: Electrophile (or Antioxidant) Response Element; gene promoter controlling antioxidant enzyme gene expression. **HNE**: 4-hydroxy-2-nonenal; product of lipid peroxidation and likely activator of the ERE. **Keap1**: Kelch-like ECH-associated protein 1; a sensing protein linked to the ERE. **TCA cycle**: Tricarboxylic acid cycle; ATP-generating metabolic pathway in mitochondria. **eNOS**: Endothelial nitric oxide (**NO**) synthase enzyme. **GPX**: glutathione peroxidase; antioxidant enzyme. **MDA**: malondialdehyde; a commonly used plasma biomarker of lipid peroxidation. **SIRT**: silent mating type information regulation 2 homolog; gene coding for a sirtuin, or regulatory protein deacetylase. **EGCG**: epigallocatechin gallate; a flavonoid polyphenol mainly found in green tea.

8. References

Alexander, S.P.H. (2006). Flavonoids as antagonists at A(1) adenosine receptors. *Phytotherapy Research*, Vol. 20, Issue 11, pp. 1009-1012, ISSN 0951-418X.

An, H.; Zhai, Z.; Yin, S. et al. (2011). Coexpression of the Superoxide Dismutase and the Catalase Provides Remarkable Oxidative Stress Resistance in Lactobacillus rhamnosus. *Journal of Agricultural and Food Chemistry*, Vol. 59, Issue 8, pp. 3851-3856, ISSN 0021-8561.

Baar, K.; Wende, A.R.; Jones, T.E. et al. (2002). Adaptations of skeletal muscle to exercise: rapid increase in the transcriptional coactivator PGC-1. *FASEB J.*, Vol. 16, Issue 14, pp. 1879-1886.

Barros, M.H.; Bandy, B.; Tahara, E.B. et al. (2004). Higher respiratory activity decreases mitochondrial reactive oxygen release and increases life span in Saccharomyces cerevisiae. *Journal of Biological Chemistry*, Vol. 279, Issue 48, pp. 49883-49888, ISSN 0021-9258.

Baur, J.A.; Pearson, K.J.; Price, N.L. et al. (2006). Resveratrol improves health and survival of mice on a high-calorie diet. *Nature*, Vol. 444, Issue 7117, pp. 337-342, ISSN 0028-0836.

Befroy, D.E.; Petersen, K.F.; Dufour, S. et al. (2008). Increased substrate oxidation and mitochondrial uncoupling in skeletal muscle of endurance-trained individuals. *Proceedings of the National Academy of Sciences*, Vol. 105, Issue 43, pp. 16701-16706.

Biasutto, L.; Marotta, E.; Garbisa, S. et al. (2010). Determination of Quercetin and Resveratrol in Whole Blood—Implications for Bioavailability Studies. *Molecules*, Vol. 15, Issue 9, pp. 6570-6579, ISSN 1420-3049.

Bieger, J.; Cermak, R.; Blank, R. et al. (2008). Tissue Distribution of Quercetin in Pigs after Long-Term Dietary Supplementation. *J. Nutr.*, Vol. 138, Issue 8, pp. 1417-1420.

Bjelakovic, G.; Nikolova, D.; Ll, G. et al. (2008). Antioxidant supplements for prevention of mortality in healthy participants and patients with various diseases. *Cochrane Database of Systematic Reviews*, Vol. 2, Issue 2, pp. 1-252, ISSN 1469-493X.

Bordone, L.; Cohen, D.; Robinson, A. et al. (2007). SIRT1 transgenic mice show phenotypes resembling calorie restriction. *Aging Cell*, Vol. 6, Issue 6, pp. 759-767, ISSN 1474-9718.

Brookes, P.S. (2005). Mitochondrial H+ leak and ROS generation: An odd couple. *Free Radical Biology and Medicine*, Vol. 38, Issue 1, pp. 12-23, ISSN 0891-5849.

Cadenas, E. & Boveris, A. (1980). Enhancement of hydrogen peroxide formation by protophores and ionophores in antimycin-supplemented mitochondria. *Biochem. J.*, Vol. 188, Issue 1, pp. 31-37.

Cadenas, E. & Davies, K.J.A. (2000). Mitochondrial free radical generation, oxidative stress, and aging. *Free Radical Biology and Medicine*, Vol. 29, Issue 3-4, pp. 222-230, ISSN 0891-5849.

Cadenas, E.; Poderoso, J.J.; Antunes, F. et al. (2000). Analysis of the pathways of nitric oxide utilization in mitochondria. *Free Radical Research*, Vol. 33, Issue 6, pp. 747-756, ISSN 1071-5762.

Calabrese, E.J. (2008). Hormesis: Why it is important to toxicology and toxicologists. *Environmental Toxicology and Chemistry*, Vol. 27, Issue 7, pp. 1451-1474, ISSN 0730-7268.

Clifford, M.N. (2004). Diet-derived Phenols in plasma and tissues and their implications for health. *Planta Medica*, Vol. 70, Issue 12, pp. 1103-1114.

Cressey, D. (2010). Fat rats skew research results; Overfed lab animals make poor subjects for experiments. *Nature*, Vol. 464, 19.

Csiszar, A.; Labinskyy, N.; Pinto, J.T. et al. (2009). Resveratrol induces mitochondrial biogenesis in endothelial cells. *American Journal of Physiology-Heart and Circulatory Physiology*, Vol. 297, Issue 1, pp. H13-H20, ISSN 0363-6135.

Dairaku, N.; Kato, K.; Honda, K. et al. (2004). Oligomycin and antimycin A prevent nitric oxide-induced opoptosis by blocking cytochrome C leakage. *Journal of Laboratory and Clinical Medicine*, Vol. 143, Issue 3, pp. 143-151, ISSN 0022-2143.

Davis, J.M.; Murphy, E.A.; Carmichael, M.D. et al. (2009). Quercetin increases brain and muscle mitochondrial biogenesis and exercise tolerance. *American Journal of Physiology-Regulatory Integrative and Comparative Physiology*, Vol. 296, Issue 4, pp. R1071-R1077, ISSN 0363-6119.

Dinkova-Kostova, A.T. & Talalay, P. (2008). Direct and indirect antioxidant properties of inducers of cytoprotective proteins. *Molecular Nutrition & Food Research*, Vol. 52, S128-S138, ISSN 1613-4125.

Dorta, D.J.; Curti, C. & Rodrigues, T. (2006). Effects of flavonoids on mitochondria: An overview on pharmacological and toxicological aspects. In Moreno, A.; Oliveira, P. & Palmeira, C., eds, *Mitochondrial Phamacology and Toxicology*, pp. 147-161, ISBN Transworld Research Network, Kerala, India.

Dorta, D.J.; Pigoso, A.; Mingatto, F. et al. (2005). The interaction of flavonoids with mitochondria: effects on energetic processes. *Chemico-Biological Interactions*, Vol. 152, Issue 2-3, pp. 67-78.

Droge, W. (2002). Free radicals in the physiological control of cell function. *Physiological Reviews*, Vol. 82, Issue 1, pp. 47-95, ISSN 0031-9333.

Duguez, S.; Sabido, O. & Freyssenet, D. (2004). Mitochondrial-dependent regulation of myoblast proliferation. *Experimental Cell Research*, Vol. 299, Issue 1, pp. 27-35, ISSN 0014-4827.

Eid, H.M.; Martineau, L.C.; Saleem, A. et al. (2010). Stimulation of AMP-activated protein kinase and enhancement of basal glucose uptake in muscle cells by quercetin and quercetin glycosides, active principles of the antidiabetic medicinal plant Vaccinium vitis-idaea. *Molecular Nutrition & Food Research*, Vol. 54, Issue 7, pp. 991-1003, ISSN 1613-4125.

Feige, J.N.; Lagouge, M.; Canto, C. et al. (2008). Specific SIRT1 Activation Mimics Low Energy Levels and Protects against Diet-induced Metabolic Disorders by Enhancing Fat Oxidation. *Cell Metabolism*, Vol. 8, Issue 5, pp. 347-358, ISSN 1550-4131.

Fiorani, M.; Guidarelli, A.; Blasa, M. et al. (2010). Mitochondria accumulate large amounts of quercetin: prevention of mitochondrial damage and release upon oxidation of the extramitochondrial fraction of the flavonoid. *The Journal of Nutritional Biochemistry*, Vol. 21, Issue 5, pp. 397-404.

Fujisawa, K.; Nishikawa, T.; Kukidome, D. et al. (2009). TZDs reduce mitochondrial ROS production and enhance mitochondrial biogenesis. *Biochemical and Biophysical Research Communications*, Vol. 379, Issue 1, pp. 43-48.

Gledhill, J.R.; Montgomery, M.G.; Leslie, A.G.W. et al. (2007). Mechanism of inhibition of bovine F1-ATPase by resveratrol and related polyphenols. *Proceedings of the National Academy of Sciences*, Vol. 104, Issue 34, pp. 13632-13637.

Goldberg, D.A.; Yan, J. & Soleas, G.J. (2003). Absorption of three wine-related polyphenols in three different matrices by healthy subjects. *Clinical Biochemistry*, Vol. 36, Issue 1, pp. 79-87.

Gomez-Cabrera, M.C.; Domenech, E.; Ji, L.L. et al. (2006). Exercise as an antioxidant: it up-regulates important enzymes for cell adaptations to exercise. *Science & Sports*, Vol. 21, Issue 2, pp. 85-89, ISSN 0765-1597.

Gomez-Cabrera, M.C.; Domenech, E. & Vina, J. (2008). Moderate exercise is an antioxidant: Upregulation of antioxidant genes by training. *Free Radical Biology and Medicine*, Vol. 44, Issue 2, pp. 126-131.

Grubisha, O.; Smith, B.C. & Denu, J.M. (2005). Small molecule regulation of Sir2 protein deacetylases. *Febs Journal*, Vol. 272, Issue 18, pp. 4607-4616, ISSN 1742-464X.

Guarente, L. (2008). Mitochondria - A nexus for aging, calorie restriction, and sirtuins? *Cell*, Vol. 132, Issue 2, pp. 171-176, ISSN 0092-8674.

Hao, J.; Shen, W.; Yu, G. et al. (2010). Hydroxytyrosol promotes mitochondrial biogenesis and mitochondrial function in 3T3-L1 adipocytes. *The Journal of Nutritional Biochemistry*, Vol. 21, Issue 7, pp. 634-644, ISSN 0955-2863.

Harman, D. (1956). Aging: a theory based on free radical and radiation chemistry. *J Gerontol*, Vol. 11, Issue 3, pp. 298-300, ISSN 0022-1422.

Hawley, J.A. & Holloszy, J.O. (2009). Exercise: it's the real thing! *Nutrition Reviews*, Vol. 67, Issue 3, pp. 172-178, ISSN 0029-6643.

Higuchi, M.; Cartier, L.J.; Chen, M. et al. (1985). SUPEROXIDE-DISMUTASE AND CATALASE IN SKELETAL-MUSCLE - ADAPTIVE RESPONSE TO EXERCISE. *Journals of Gerontology*, Vol. 40, Issue 3, pp. 281-286, ISSN 0022-1422.

Hodnick, W.F.; Bohmont, C.W.; Capps, C. et al. (1987). Inhibition of the mitochondrial NADH-oxidase (NADH-Coenzyme Q oxido-reductase) enzyme system by flavonoids: a structure-activity study. *Biochemical Pharmacology*, Vol. 36, Issue 17, pp. 2873-2874.

Hodnick, W.F.; Kung, F.S.; Roettger, W.J. et al. (1986). Inhibition of mitochondrial respiration and production of toxic oxygen radicals by flavonoids: A structure-activity study. *Biochemical Pharmacology*, Vol. 35, Issue 14, pp. 2345-2357.

Holloszy, J.O. & Coyle, E.F. (1984). Adaptations of skeletal muscle to endurance exercise and their metabolic consequences. *J Appl Physiol*, Vol. 56, Issue 4, pp. 831-838.

Hood, D.A.; Irrcher, I.; Ljubicic, V. et al. (2006). Coordination of metabolic plasticity in skeletal muscle. *Journal of Experimental Biology*, Vol. 209, Issue 12, pp. 2265-2275, ISSN 0022-0949.

Hoppeler, H.; Lüthi, P.; Claassen, H. et al. (1973). The ultrastructure of the normal human skeletal muscle. *Pflügers Archiv European Journal of Physiology*, Vol. 344, Issue 3, pp. 217-232.

Howitz, K.T.; Bitterman, K.J.; Cohen, H.Y. et al. (2003). Small molecule activators of sirtuins extend Saccharomyces cerevisiae lifespan. *Nature*, Vol. 425, Issue 6954, pp. 191-196, ISSN 0028-0836.

Hsun-Wei Huang, T.; Prasad, B.; Valentina Razmovski, K. et al. (2005). Herbal or Natural Medicines as Modulators of Peroxisome Proliferator-Activated Receptors and Related Nuclear Receptors for Therapy of Metabolic Syndrome. *Basic & Clinical Pharmacology & Toxicology*, Vol. 96, Issue 1, pp. 3-14, ISSN 1742-7843.

Hu, D.; Cao, P.; Thiels, E. et al. (2007). Hippocampal long-term potentiation, memory, and longevity in mice that overexpress mitochondrial superoxide dismutase. *Neurobiology of Learning and Memory*, Vol. 87, Issue 3, pp. 372-384.

Huang, J.H. & Hood, D.A. (2009). Age-associated Mitochondrial Dysfunction in Skeletal Muscle: Contributing Factors and Suggestions for Long-term Interventions. *Iubmb Life*, Vol. 61, Issue 3, pp. 201-214, ISSN 1521-6543.

Institute of Medicine (1998). Panel on dietary antioxidants and related compounds report: Dietary Reference Intakes. Proposed definition and plan for review of dietary antioxidants and related compounds. In Standing comittee on the scientific evaluation of dietary reference intakes, F.a.N.B., Institute of Medicine, ed. National Academy Press, Washington DC.

Iwasaki, R.; Ito, K.; Ishida, T. et al. (2009). Catechin, green tea component, causes caspase-independent necrosis-like cell death in chronic myelogenous leukemia. *Cancer Science*, Vol. 100, Issue 2, pp. 349-356, ISSN 1347-9032.

Jackson, M.J. (2008). Free radicals generated contracting muscle: By-products of metabolism or key regulators of muscle function? *Free Radical Biology and Medicine*, Vol. 44, Issue 2, pp. 132-141.

Ji, L.L.; Radak, Z. & Goto, S. (2008). Hormesis and Exercise: How the Cell Copes with Oxidative Stress. *American Journal of Pharmacology and Toxicology*, Vol. 3, Issue 1, pp. 44-58.

Joseph, J.A.; Fisher, D.R.; Cheng, V. et al. (2008). Cellular and Behavioral Effects of Stilbene Resveratrol Analogues: Implications for Reducing the Deleterious Effects of Aging. *Journal of Agricultural and Food Chemistry*, Vol. 56, Issue 22, pp. 10544-10551, ISSN 0021-8561.

Juan, M.E.; Wenzel, U.; Daniel, H. et al. (2008). Resveratrol induces apoptosis through ROS-dependent mitochondria pathway in HT-29 human colorectal carcinoma cells. *Journal of Agricultural and Food Chemistry*, Vol. 56, Issue 12, pp. 4813-4818, ISSN 0021-8561.

Kaeberlein, M.; McDonagh, T.; Heltweg, B. et al. (2005). Substrate-specific activation of sirtuins by resveratrol. *Journal of Biological Chemistry*, Vol. 280, Issue 17, pp. 17038-17045, ISSN 0021-9258.

Kalt, W.; Blumberg, J.B.; McDonald, J.E. et al. (2008). Identification of anthocyanins in the liver, eye, and brain of blueberry-fed pigs. *Journal of Agricultural and Food Chemistry*, Vol. 56, 705-712, ISSN 0021-8561.

Kalt, W.; Foote, K.; Fillmore, S.A.E. et al. (2007). Effect of blueberry feeding on plasma lipids in pigs. *British Journal of Nutrition*, Vol. 100, Issue 01, pp. 70-78, ISSN 0007-1145.

Knez, W.; Jenkins, D. & Coombes, J. (2007). Does antioxidant supplementation prevent favorable adaptations to exercise training? - Response. *Medicine and Science in Sports and Exercise*, Vol. 39, Issue 10, pp. 1888-1888.

Koren, E.; Kohen, R. & Ginsburg, I. (2010). Polyphenols enhance total oxidant-scavenging capacities of human blood by binding to red blood cells. *Experimental Biology and Medicine*, Vol. 235, Issue 6, pp. 689-699, ISSN 1535-3702.

Kushnareva, Y.; Murphy, A.N. & Andreyev, A. (2002). Complex I-mediated reactive oxygen species generation: modulation by cytochrome c and NAD(P)(+) oxidation-reduction state. *Biochemical Journal*, Vol. 368, 545-553, ISSN 0264-6021.

Lagouge, M.; Argmann, C.; Gerhart-Hines, Z. et al. (2006). Resveratrol improves mitochondrial function and protects against metabolic disease by activating SIRT1 and PGC-1 alpha. *Cell*, Vol. 127, Issue 6, pp. 1109-1122, ISSN 0092-8674.

Li, W.; Nie, S.; Yu, Q. et al. (2009). Epigallocatechin-3-gallate Induces Apoptosis of Human Hepatoma Cells by Mitochondrial Pathways Related to Reactive Oxygen Species. *Journal of Agricultural and Food Chemistry*, Vol. 57, Issue 15, pp. 6685-6691.

Li, Y.; Huang, T.-T.; Carlson, E.J. et al. (1995). Dilated cardiomyopathy and neonatal lethality in mutant mice lacking manganese superoxide dismutase. *Nat Genet*, Vol. 11, Issue 4, pp. 376-381.

Lopez-Lluch, G.; Hunt, N.; Jones, B. et al. (2006). Calorie restriction induces mitochondrial biogenesis and bioenergetic efficiency. *Proceedings of the National Academy of Sciences of the United States of America*, Vol. 103, Issue 6, pp. 1768-1773, ISSN 0027-8424.

Lu, Z.; Zhongbo, L.; Zhihui, F. et al. (2010). Hydroxytyrosol protects against oxidative damage by simultaneous activation of mitochondrial biogenesis and phase II detoxifying enzyme systems in retinal pigment epithelial cells. *Journal of Nutritional Biochemistry*, Vol. 21, Issue 11, pp. 1089-1098, ISSN 0955-2863.

Marfe, G.; Tafani, M.; Indelicato, M. et al. (2009). Kaempferol Induces Apoptosis in Two Different Cell Lines Via Akt Inactivation, Bax and SIRT3 Activation, and Mitochondrial Dysfunction. *Journal of Cellular Biochemistry*, Vol. 106, Issue 4, pp. 643-650, ISSN 0730-2312.

Murase, T.; Haramizu, S.; Ota, N. et al. (2009). Suppression of the aging-associated decline in physical performance by a combination of resveratrol intake and habitual exercise in senescence-accelerated mice. *Biogerontology*, Vol. 10, Issue 4, pp. 423-434, ISSN 1389-5729.

Nieman, D.C.; Henson, D.A.; Maxwell, K.R. et al. (2009). Effects of Quercetin and EGCG on Mitochondrial Biogenesis and Immunity. *Medicine and Science in Sports and Exercise*, Vol. 41, Issue 7, pp. 1467-1475, ISSN 0195-9131.

Nieman, D.C.; Williams, A.S.; Shanely, R.A. et al. (2010). Quercetin's Influence on Exercise Performance and Muscle Mitochondrial Biogenesis. *Medicine and Science in Sports and Exercise*, Vol. 42, Issue 2, pp. 338-345, ISSN 0195-9131.

Nunn, A.V.W.; Bell, J.D. & Guy, G.W. (2009). Lifestyle-induced metabolic inflexibility and accelerated ageing syndrome: insulin resistance, friend or foe? *Nutrition & Metabolism*, Vol. 6, ISSN 1743-7075.

Nunn, A.V.W.; Guy, G.W. & Bell, J.D. (2010). Endocannabinoids, FOXO and the metabolic syndrome: Redox, function and tipping point - The view from two systems. *Immunobiology*, Vol. 215, Issue 8, pp. 617-628, ISSN 0171-2985.

Ortega, R. & Garcia, N. (2009). The flavonoid quercetin induces changes in mitochondrial permeability by inhibiting adenine nucleotide translocase. *Journal of Bioenergetics and Biomembranes*, Vol. 41, Issue 1, pp. 41-47, ISSN 0145-479X.

Pan, M.H.; Chang, Y.H.; Badmaev, V. et al. (2007). Pterostilbene induces apoptosis and cell cycle arrest in human gastric carcinoma cells. *Journal of Agricultural and Food Chemistry*, Vol. 55, Issue 19, pp. 7777-7785, ISSN 0021-8561.

Poderoso, J.J.; Boveris, A. & Cadenas, E. (2000). Mitochondrial oxidative stress: A self-propagating process with implications for signaling cascades. *BioFactors*, Vol. 11, Issue 1-2, pp. 43-45, ISSN 0951-6433.

Powers, S.K. & Jackson, M.J. (2008). Exercise-induced oxidative stress: Cellular mechanisms and impact on muscle force production. *Physiological Reviews*, Vol. 88, Issue 4, pp. 1243-1276, ISSN 0031-9333.

Radak, Z.; Chung, H.Y. & Goto, S. (2008). Systemic adaptation to oxidative challenge induced by regular exercise. *Free Radical Biology and Medicine*, Vol. 44, Issue 2, pp. 153-159.

Ristow, M. & Zarse, K. (2010). How increased oxidative stress promotes longevity and metabolic health: The concept of mitochondrial hormesis (mitohormesis). *Experimental Gerontology*, Vol. 45, Issue 6, pp. 410-418, ISSN 0531-5565.

Ristow, M.; Zarse, K.; Oberbach, A. et al. (2009). Antioxidants prevent health-promoting effects of physical exercise in humans. *Proceedings of the National Academy of Sciences*, Vol. 106, Issue 21, pp. 8665-8670.

Robb, E.L.; Winkelmolen, L.; Visanji, N. et al. (2008). Resveratrol Affects Mitochondrial Reactive Oxygen Species Metabolism. *Free Radical Biology and Medicine*, Vol. 45, S90-S90, ISSN 0891-5849.

Roy, P.; Kalra, N.; Prasad, S. et al. (2009). Chemopreventive Potential of Resveratrol in Mouse Skin Tumors Through Regulation of Mitochondrial and PI3K/AKT Signaling Pathways. *Pharmaceutical Research (Dordrecht)*, Vol. 26, Issue 1, pp. 211-217, ISSN 0724-8741.

Santos, A.C.; Uyemura, S.A.; Lopes, J.L.C. et al. (1998). Effect of naturally occurring flavonoids on lipid peroxidation and membrane permeability transition in mitochondria. *Free Radical Biology and Medicine*, Vol. 24, Issue 9, pp. 1455-1461, ISSN 0891-5849.

Scheffler, I.E. (2008). Mitochondria. In, Ed Second. Wiley, Hoboken, p 462pp.

Schroeder, E.K.; Kelsey, N.A.; Doyle, J. et al. (2009). Green Tea Epigallocatechin 3-Gallate Accumulates in Mitochondria and Displays a Selective Antiapoptotic Effect Against Inducers of Mitochondrial Oxidative Stress in Neurons. *Antioxidants & Redox Signaling*, Vol. 11, Issue 3, pp. 469-480, ISSN 1523-0864.

Shakibaei, M.; Harikumar, K.B. & Aggarwal, B.B. (2009). Resveratrol addiction: To die or not to die. *Molecular Nutrition & Food Research*, Vol. 53, Issue 1, pp. 115-128, ISSN 1613-4125.

Stevenson, D. & Lowe, T. (2009). Plant-derived compounds as antioxidants for health – are they all really antioxidants? *Functional Plant Science and Biotechnology*, Vol. 3(S1), 1-12.

Stevenson, D.E.; Scheepens, A. & Hurst, R.D. (2009). Bioavailability and metabolism of dietary flavonoids - much known - much more to discover. In Keller, R.B., ed, Flavonoids: biosynthesis, biological effects and dietary sources, Nova Science Publishers Inc.

Stevenson, D.E.; Cooney, J.M.; Jensen, D.J. et al. (2008). Comparison of enzymically glucuronidated flavonoids with flavonoid aglycones in an in vitro cellular model of oxidative stress protection. *In Vitro Cellular & Developmental Biology-Animal*, Vol. 44, Issue 3-4, pp. 73-80.

Stevenson, D.E. & Hurst, R.D. (2007). Polyphenolic phytochemicals - just antioxidants or much more? *Cellular and Molecular Life Sciences*, Vol. 64, 2900-2916.

Tan, L.; Yu, J.T. & Guan, H.S. (2008). Resveratrol exerts pharmacological preconditioning by activating PGC-1 alpha. *Medical Hypotheses*, Vol. 71, Issue 5, pp. 664-667, ISSN 0306-9877.

Tapia, P.C. (2006). Sublethal mitochondrial stress with an attendant stoichiometric augmentation of reactive oxygen species may precipitate many of the beneficial alterations in cellular physiology produced by caloric restriction, intermittent fasting, exercise and dietary phytonutrients: "Mitohormesis" for health and vitality. *Medical Hypotheses*, Vol. 66, Issue 4, pp. 832-843.

Theodorou, A.A.; Nikolaidis, M.G.; Paschalis, V. et al. (2011). No effect of antioxidant supplementation on muscle performance and blood redox status adaptations to eccentric training. *The American Journal of Clinical Nutrition*, Vol. 93, Issue 6, pp. 1373-1383.

Uchida, K.; Shiraishi, M.; Naito, Y. et al. (1999). Activation of stress signaling pathways by the end product of lipid peroxidation - 4-hydroxy-2-nonenal is a potential inducer of intracellular peroxide production. *Journal of Biological Chemistry*, Vol. 274, Issue 4, pp. 2234-2242, ISSN 0021-9258.

van Ommen, B.; Keijer, J.; Heil, S.G. et al. (2009). Challenging homeostasis to define biomarkers for nutrition related health. *Molecular Nutrition and Food Research*, Vol. 53, Issue 7, pp. 53 (57) 795-804, ISSN 1613-4125.

Vincent, H.K.; Bourguignon, C.M.; Vincent, K.R. et al. (2006). Antioxidant supplementation lowers exercise-induced oxidative stress in young overweight adults. *Obesity*, Vol. 14, Issue 12, pp. 2224-2235.

Wilson, L.; Yang, Q.; Szustakowski, J.D. et al. (2007). Pyruvate induces mitochondrial biogenesis by a PGC-1alpha-independent mechanism. *American Journal of Physiology-Cell Physiology*, Vol. 292, Issue 5, pp. C1599-C1605, ISSN 0363-6143.

Yang, H.Y.; Baur, J.A.; Chen, A. et al. (2007). Design and synthesis of compounds that extend yeast replicative lifespan. *Aging Cell*, Vol. 6, Issue 1, pp. 35-43, ISSN 1474-9718.

Zoechling, A.; Liebner, F. & Jungbauer, A. (2011). Red wine: A source of potent ligands for peroxisome proliferator-activated receptor [gamma]. *Food & Function*, Vol. 2, Issue 1, pp. 28-38, ISSN 2042-6496.

9

Erythrina, a Potential Source of Chemicals from the Neotropics

R. Marcos Soto-Hernández, Rosario García-Mateos,
Rubén San Miguel-Chávez, Geoffrey Kite,
Mariano Martínez-Vázquez and Ana C. Ramos-Valdivia
[1]Colegio de Postgraduados, Campus Montecillo Mexico, Universidad Autónoma Chapingo, Preparatoria Agrícola, Mexico,
[2]Royal Botanic Gardens, Kew Richmond,
[3]Universidad Nacional Autónoma de México, Instituto de Química Mexico,
[4]Centro de Investigación y Estudios Avanzados del Instituto Politécnico Nacional, Unidad Zacatenco,
[1,3,4]México
[2]UK

1. Introduction

The history of *Erythrina* research begins at the end of the nineteen century. During the last two decades of that time extracts from species of *Erythrina* have been found to exhibit curare-like neuro muscular blocking activities which are caused by alkaloids occurring there in (Rey, 1883; Altamirano, 1888; Greshoff, 1890; Folkers & Unna, 1938).

It was Altamirano (1888), who obtained a silky shining, crystalline compound as well as Greshoff (1890) who already isolated several basic unspecified compounds. Because of their remarkable biological activity he suggested a systematic phytochemical examination of the genus *Erythrina*. But it still has taken at most half a century before this has been realized for the first time by Folkers. He has shown that more than fifty Erythrina species e.g. *Erythrina americana* (Fig. 1) are containing the typical alkaloids exhibiting the same curare-like activity reported before (Folkers & Unna, 1939; Folkers & Major, 1937). Moreover, his group succeeded in isolation the first erythrinane alkaloid named erythroidine (**14**, Fig. 3) (Folkers & Koniouszy, 1939). Soon after numerous alkaloids have been isolated, e.g. erythramine (**8**) (Folkers & Koniouszy, 1940a), erythraline (**3**) (Folkers & Koniouszy, 1940b), erythratine (**9**) (Folkers & Koniouszy, 1940c), erysodine (**6**), erysopine (**4**) and erysovine (**5**) (Carmag, et al. 1951).

Another decade later the fundamentals investigations of Prelog (Kenner, et al., 1951; Tsuda & Sano, 1996) and Boekelheide (Boekelheide, et al. 1953) have finally led to the correct structural framework of the erythrinane alkaloids (Parent compounds 1, Fig. 2)

Due to the increasing attraction and rapid extension in this field the *Erythrina* alkaloids have been regularly reviewed concerning occurrence, structure, analytical, spectral properties,

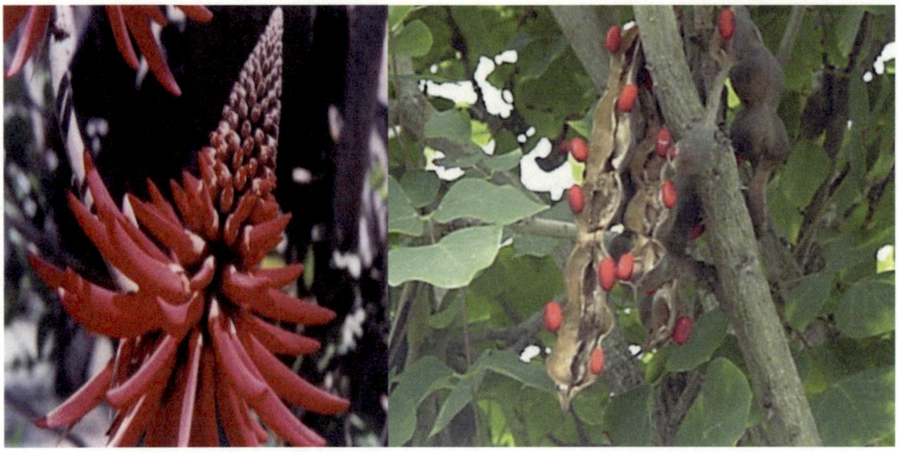

Fig. 1. *Erythrina americana Mill* (Colorin)

biosynthesis, total synthesis and biological activities covering the literature up to date. Besides compounds as flavonoids, isoflavonoids, lectins, saponins have received special attention mainly by their biological activity or toxicity.

This review has the aim to show the evolution in the knowledge of these ubiquitous compounds that remark the *Erythrina* genus and emphasize their importance and interest in different areas.

2. Structural classification of *Erythrina* alkaloids

The alkaloids of *Erythrina* type are characterized by their unique skeleton of a tetracyclic spiroamine. They are classified in two main groups: alkaloids possesses a skeleton of a 6,5,6,6 indoloisoquinoline called erythrinanes and those with a skeleton of 6,5,7-6 indolobenzazepine called schelhammerans or homoerythrinane alkaloids (Fig. 2).

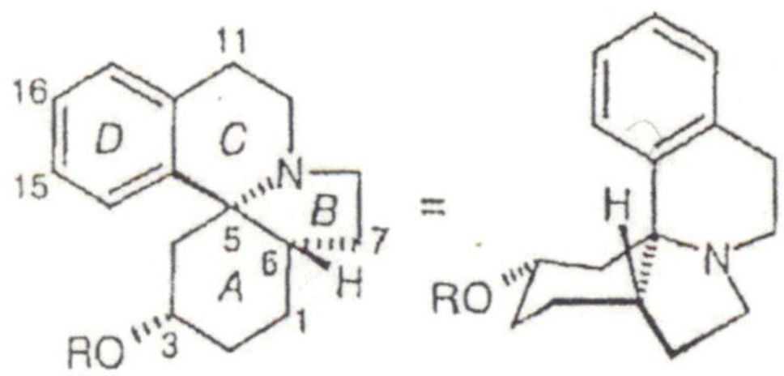

(3R,5S,6S/3S,5R,6R)-Erythrinane (1)

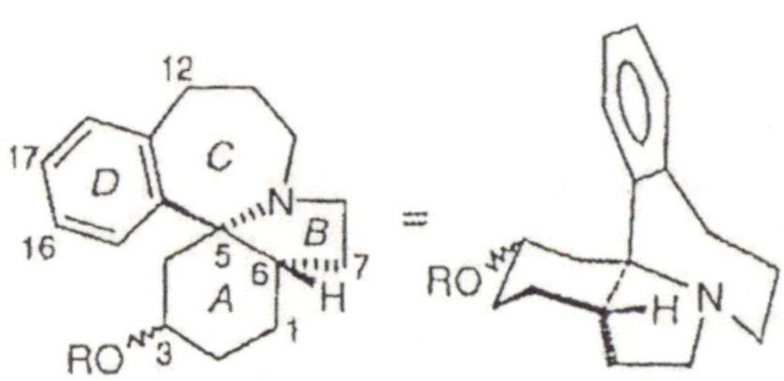

(5S,6S / 5R,6R)-Schelhammerane (2)
(homoerytrinane alkaloids)

Depending of the nature of D ring both groups can be subdivide in aromatic and non aromatic. In this last group that include in the D ring oxa compounds, are those called lactonic alkaloids. Besides, in both series have been isolated alkaloids with a pyridinium group instead of a phenyl group, for example the erymelanthine (**11**) and the holidine (**12**).

Dienoid Type: Alkenoid Type:

Aromatics

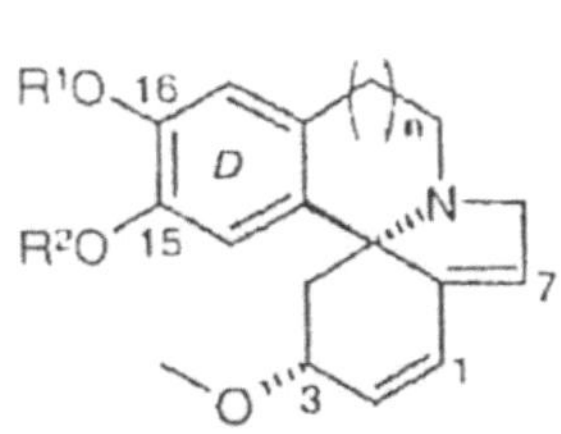

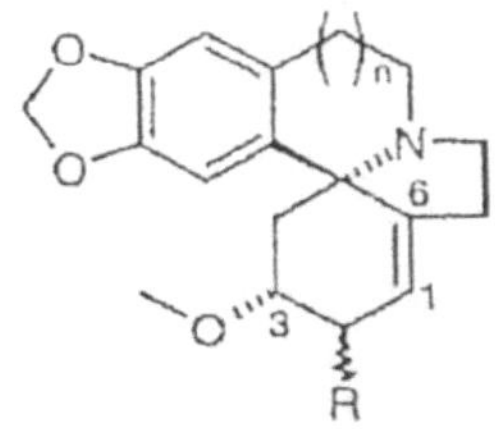

R^1-R^2=CH_2;n=1: Erythraline (**3**)

R^1=H;R^2=H;n=1 Erysopine (**4**)

R^1= CH_3;R^2=H;n=1 Erysovine (**5**)

R^1=H;R^2=CH_3;n=1 Erysodine (**6**)

R^1-R^2=CH_2;n=2: Schelhammeridine (**7**)

R=H; n=1: Erythramine (**8**)

R= β-OH;n=1 Erythratine (**9**)

R=H;n=2:Schelhammericine (**10**)

Heteroaromatics

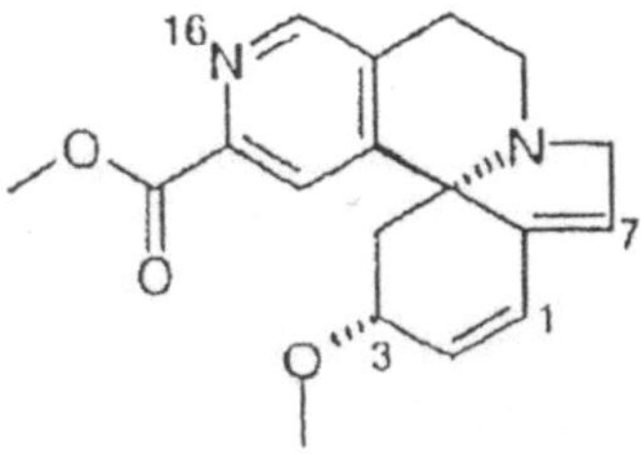

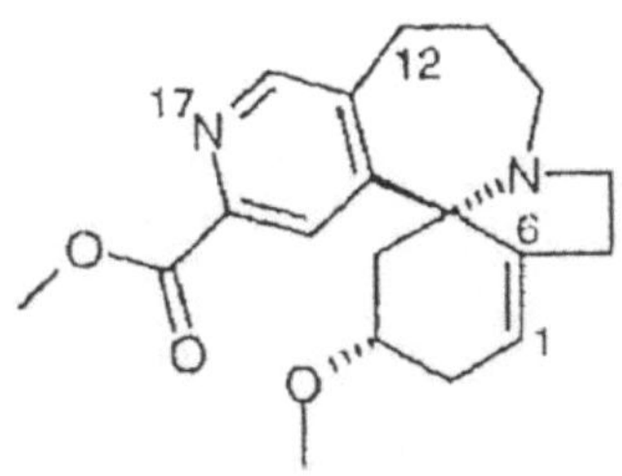

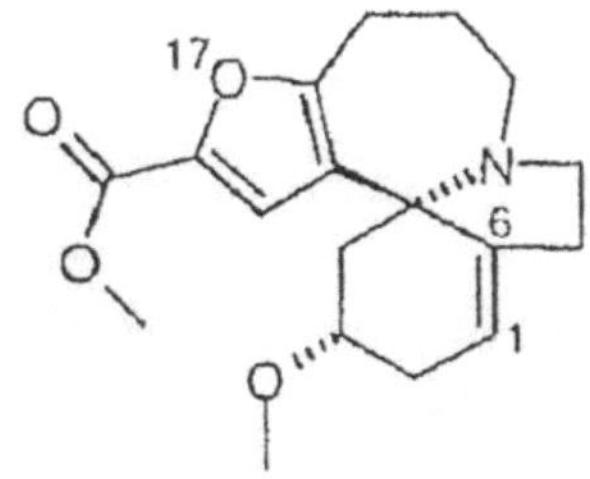

Erymelanthine (**11**) Holıdine (**12**) Selaginoidine (**13**)

Non-aromatics
(lactonic)

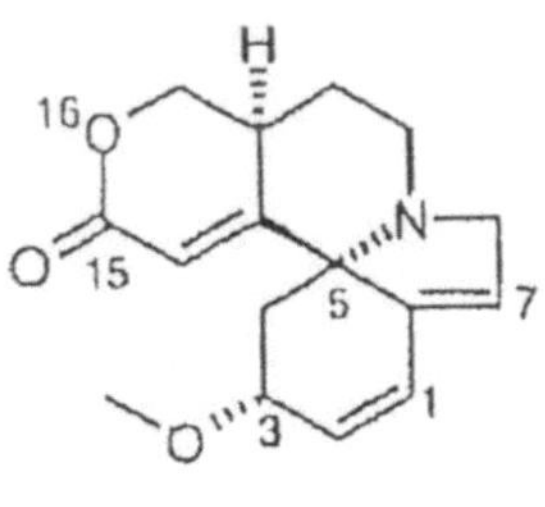

Erythroidine (**14**)

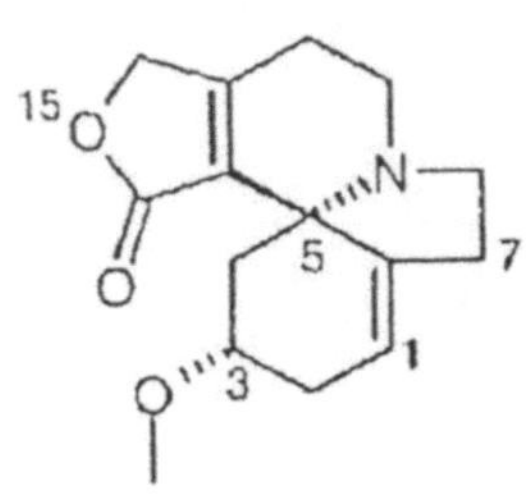

Cocculolidine (**15**)

Fig. 2. General classification of *Erythrina* alkaloids: Dienoid and alkenoid type alkaloids and D ring modifications.

Besides, the specific position and number of double bonds in the A and B rings have taken to another alkaloid sub division: dienoid and alkenoid in both series. The first ones are characterized by a conjugated diene in the 1,2,6 and 7 carbons whereas the last ones possesses only one a double bond in the position 1,6 (**8,9**).

As aromatic erythrinane alkaloids and homoerythrinanes as well show a substitution characteristics pattern, e.g. present oxygenated substituents in the 3,15 and 16 carbons mainly and besides there is a group of alkaloids deoxygenated in C-16,the saturated compounds in both series of alkaloids have cis configuration in the fussion A/B independently that had obtained by transformation of natural alkaloids or by synthesis (Mondon, et al., 1970; Reiman & Ettmayr, 2004).

Generally these alkaloids are dextrorotatory and their absolute configuration in the carbon 5 is (S) to respect to basic skeleton (Amer, et al., 1991), although is observed some exceptions as the wilsonine (**49**) has configuration (R) in the carbon 5.

The carbon 3 of the erythrinanes always have the configuration R.

3. Biosynthesis of the erythrinane alkaloids

A series of experiment *in vivo* and *in vitro* done by Barton and coworkers (Barton & Cohen, 1957; Barton et al.,1970) demonstrated that a derivative of an isoquinoline, the (**5**)-norprotosinomenine (Bencyl-tetrahydroisoquinoline (**34**) is the main precursor to which is cyclized through a phenolic coupling *p-p* to a derivative of a neoproaphorfine (**35**).

In this is effected a rearrangement to form a dibenzazonine (**36**). Its hydrogenation product (**37**) is oxydized to the corresponding diphenoquinone **38**. To the end occurs an intramolecular addition type Michael to form the erysodienone (**39**) which already has the skeleton of an erythrinane (Barton & Cohen, 1957; Barton, et al., 1970; Barton, et al., 1974). Both precursors **34** and **37** are compounds of natural origin (Scheme 1). Later on this route was reinvestigated by Maier & coworkers (Maier & Zenk 1997; Maier, et al., 1999) because was observed only occurred a small rate of relative incorporation of non protosinomenine (**34**) in the erythraline (**3**) (0.1 - 0.25%) someone not usual to the group of alkaloids with isoquinoline skeleton derivated of (**S**) reticuline (**40**: NCH_3 instead of NH) e.g. aporphines, protoberberine, bisbencylisoquinolines, morphinones, pavines and benzophenanthridines.

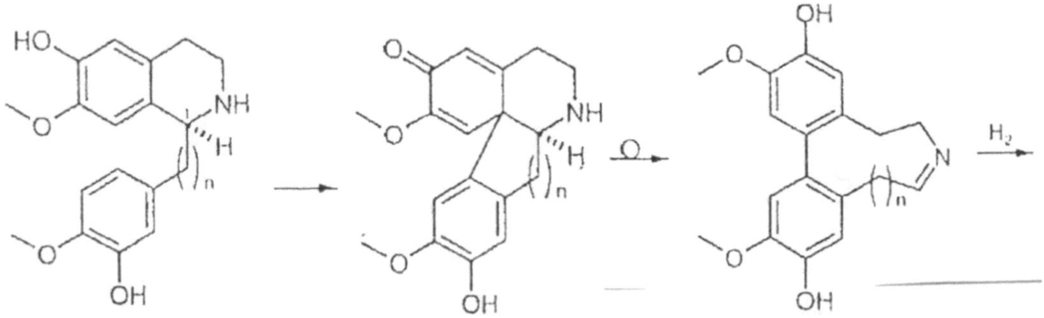

S-Norprotosinomenine (**34**) Neoproaporphine (**35**) (**36**)

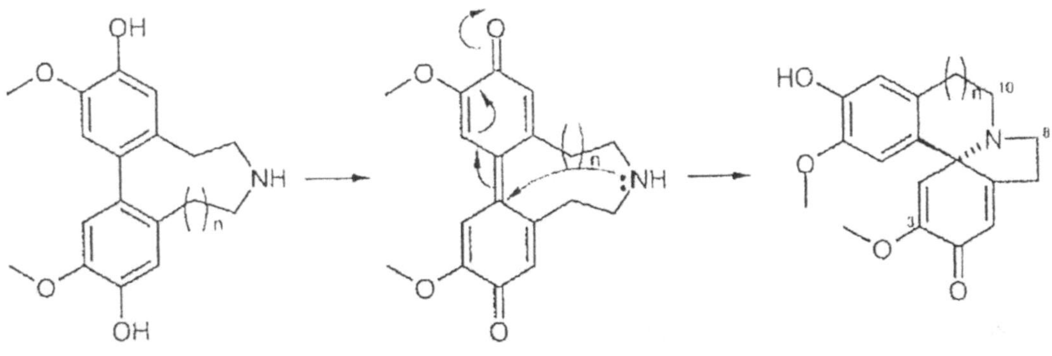

Dibenzazonine (**37**) Dibenzazonine dione (**38**) Erysodienone (**39**)

Scheme 1.

It was observed by this way that the (S)- non reticuline (40) is the biosynthetic precursor more important to the erythrinane alkaloids and that the rate of incorporation surpassed by for that of (**S**) norprotosinomenine(34) previously found (7.9%) against 0.25% in the case of erythraline and this last one did not transform in another alkaloids. This can suggest a new route and mechanism to the biosynthesis of the alkaloids (Scheme 2)

In this model, the *p-p* coupling of the (S) nor reticuline should take to the derivative of the morphinanedienone, the norisosalutanidine (**41)** and not to the neoproaporphine derivative (**35**).

The last one, after formation the function benzo [1,3]dioxol forms the noramurine (**42**), which can rearrange via the ion neoespirinic (**43)** to the unsymmetrical dibenzazonine oxidation of the free phenolic residue proceeds through a SET mechanism to form diallylic cation **(45),** the last one is supposed that reacts with the nitrogen atom to get Δ^3erythratinone (**46**).

The subsequent steps leading to erythraline (**3**) are similar to those already established (Maier, et al., 1999).

4. Syntheses of *Erythrina* alkaloids and compounds type Erythrine

Since some time ago had interest in the total synthesis of the *Erythrina* alkaloids because their unique structure and biological activity. In this way has been developed to date numerous synthetic approaches to the tetracyclic skeleton. Considering that three of the rings A,B and C can be joint in a final step,have been developed two synthetic strategies to this type of compounds: the formation of one of the mentioned rings (route A, B, or C) or the simultaneous or sequential formation of more than one cycle for example A/B, A/C, B/C or A/B/C in one step (called routes A/B, B/C, etc. schemes 3,4).

Various subtypes of the synthesis result depending of the bond formed (Schemes 3,4): for example the formation of the C ring can be attain through the method (a) or (b) = route C (a) or C (b).

According to this can be generate two different subdivisions to the simultaneous construction of the B and C rings (= route B/C (a) or B/C (b) (Kawasaki, 2001)

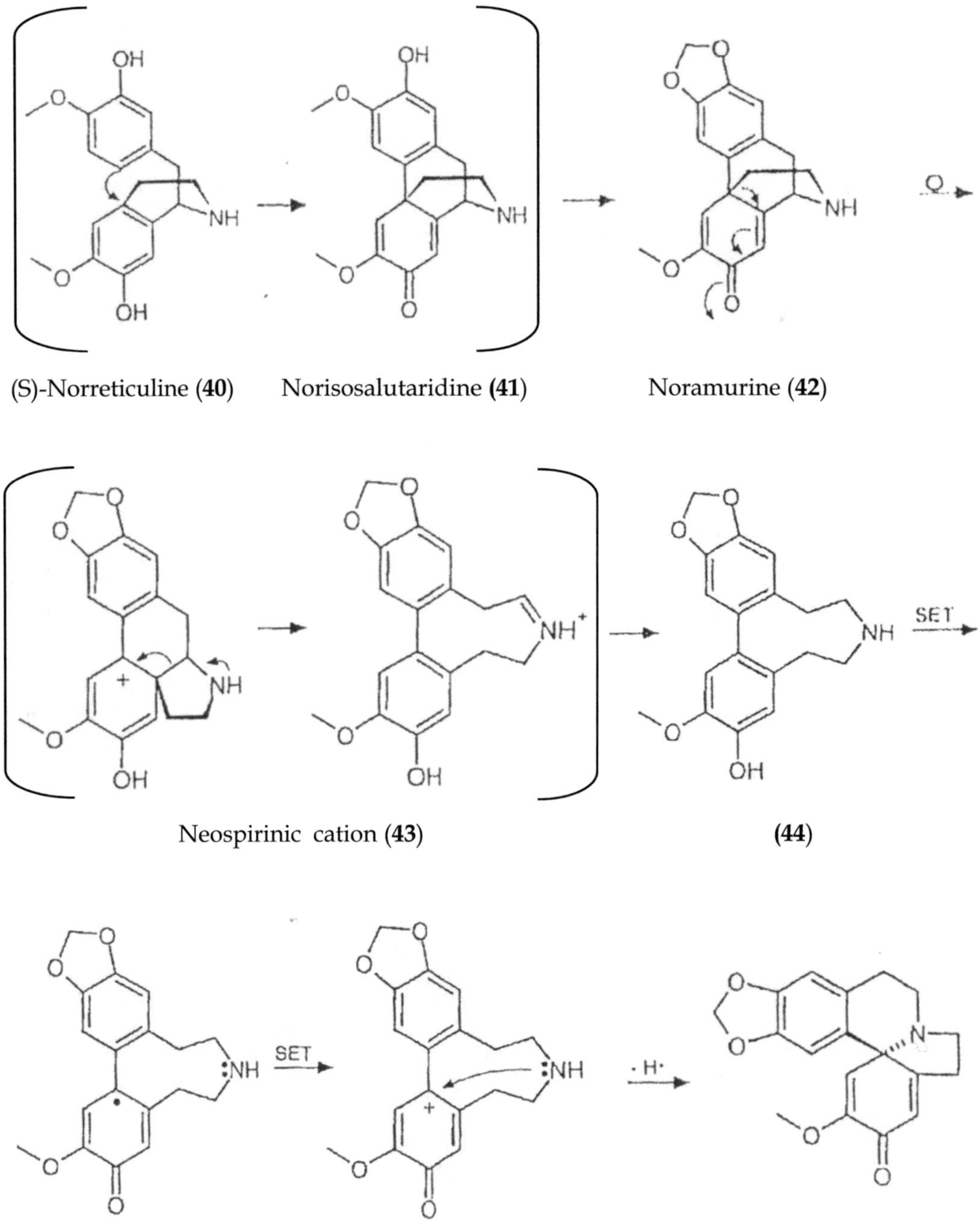

(S)-Norreticuline (**40**) Norisosalutaridine (**41**) Noramurine (**42**)

Neospirinic cation (**43**) (**44**)

(**45**) Δ^3-Erythratinone (**46**)

Scheme 2. Biosynthetic pathway of *Erythrina* alkaloids suggested by Maier, et al. (1999)

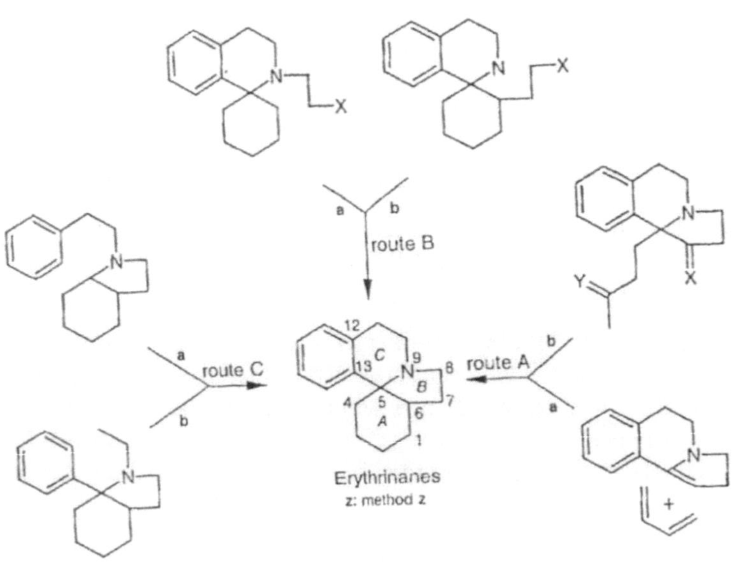

Scheme 3. Synthetic strategies to the aromatic erythrinane alkaloids. Generation of an alicyclic ring in the final step

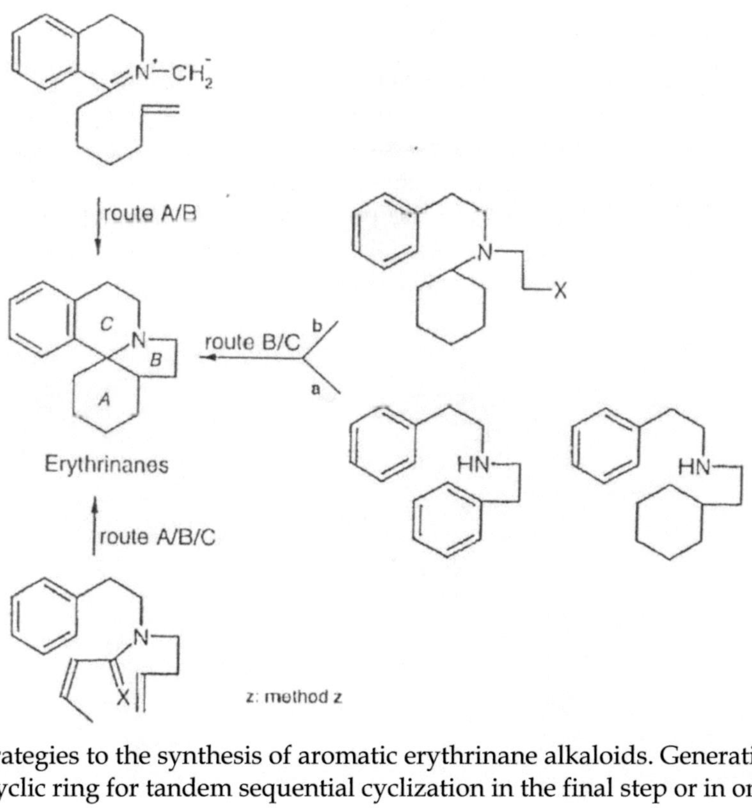

Scheme 4. Strategies to the synthesis of aromatic erythrinane alkaloids. Generation of more than one alicyclic ring for tandem sequential cyclization in the final step or in one step.

In the case of the non aromatic *Erythrine* alkaloids, only has described one total synthesis so far. Thus the synthesis of the (±) coculolidine (15) has been completed in 0.42% total yield through 21 steps (Kawasaki, et al., 2001). Also has been described several synthetic approaches to the D ring of the oxaerythrinane skeleton (Studa & Sano, 1996).

5. Spectroscopic characteristics of the *Erythrina* alkaloids

In the structural determination of these alkaloids have been used widely the common spectroscopic techniques e.g. UV, IR, and ^{1}H NMR ^{13}CNMR, besides of mass spectrometry and X ray crystallography.

The aromatic alkaloids show IR absorption to 1610 cm^{-1} and in the UV in the range of 285-290 nm (aromatic deoxygenated ring) and 235-240 nm (of the diene residue). The alkenoid alkaloids absorb in the UV about of 225 nm, whereas the enone residue shows absorption to 230 nm and in IR between 1675-1698 cm^{-1}. The lactonic alkaloids absorb in the IR to 1720 cm^{-1} (carbonyl of the lactone) whereas in the UV its absorption is about 224 and 238 nm.

The ^{1}H- NMR easily distinguish to the dienoid alkaloids by the presence of a ABX system comes from the three olefinic protons pattern does not presented the alkenoid alkaloids or the lactonic alkaloids.

The ^{13}C spectra of various erythrinane alkaloids has been assigned by comparison with series of related compounds or well through the case of model compounds, the spirocenter at C-5 usually absorb at δ 63-68. The tertiary aromatic carbons of those of C-14 present a chemical shift to high field (δ 108-112) whereas that at C-17 is observed about δ 111-117.

The mass spectrometry had an important role in the structural identification of these alkaloids particularly when is combined with gas chromatography or liquid chromatography. An analysis of a mass spectrum to those alkaloids shows in the case of those aromatic or lactonic that occurs a main fragmentation of the methyl or methoxy group in C-3 (Fig. 3) In the series of the alkenoid alkaloids also is observed this type of fragmentation, but is observed another peak at M^{+}-58 which corresponds to a retro Diels-Alder fragmentation. Loss of C-3, C-4 and methoxy group at C-3 also is observed in this series (Fig. 4).

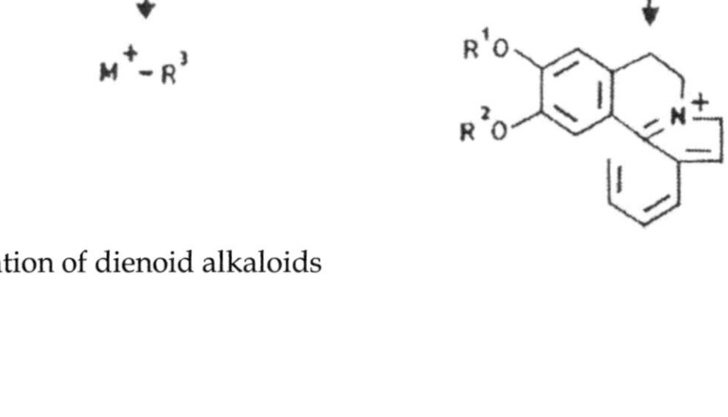

Fig. 3. Fragmentation of dienoid alkaloids

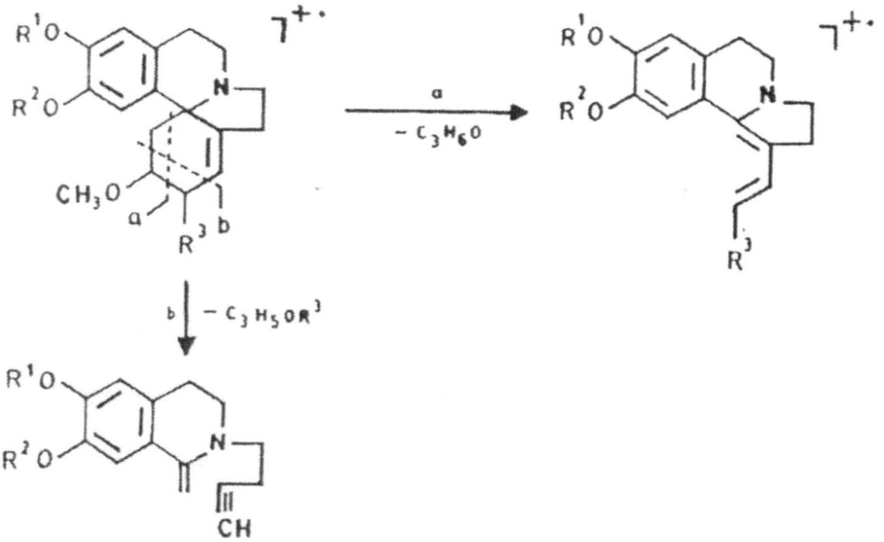

Fig. 4. Fragmentation of the alkenoid alkaloids

Following MS/MS analysis in an ion trap analyser, *Erythrina* alkaloids methoxylated at C3 show the neutral loss of methanol from the protonated molecule but few other abundant fragments. Thus MS3 analysis of the $[(M+H)-CH_3OH]^+$ is necessary to obtain a greater array of fragments, which is necessary to confirm identities against standards of for library spectra (Fig. 5). Several product ions generated from the $[(M+H)-CH_3OH]^+$ fragment appear to be produced by radical losses of methyl or hydroxyl groups. Glycosylated forms of *Erythrina* alkaloids are also evident in some species when crude extracts are analysed by LC-MS, and they may be the most abundant types present. Fragmentation of the glycosides proceeds via neutral loss of the glycosyl unit to yield a protonated aglycone ion that fragments in the same manner at the free protonated alkaloid. Undoubtedly, systematic surveys of native Erythrinane alkaloids in *Erythrina* species by LC-MS will reveal a greater variety of glycosilated or other conjugated forms than have presently been isolated.

In this sense all parts of *Erythrina* plants have been screened to describe new compounds, for instance Wanjala & Majinda (2000) described the structures of two novel alkaloids from *E. latissima* seeds; from the wood of *E. poeppigiana* Tanaka et al, (2001) isolated a new erythrina alkaloid, 8-oxo-α-erythroidine. From the flowers of *E. speciosa* two alkaloids were isolated, erysotrine and erythartine and the leaves furnished one alkaloid, nororientaline, Faria, et al (2007.) Three new alkaloids, 10,11-dioxo-erythrartine, 10,11-dioxoepierythratidine and 10,11-dioxo erythratidinone and a new pterocarpan 1-methoxyerythrabissin were isolated from the bark of *E. subumbrans* (Rukachaisirikul, et al., 2008). A new *Erythrina* alkaloid, 10-hydroxy-11-oxo-erysotrine has been isolated from the flowers of *E. herbacea* (Tanaka & Hattori, 2008). From the bark of *E. crista-galli* two new alkaloids, cristanines A and B were isolated (Ozawa, et al., 2010) and from the seeds of *E. velutina* were isolated four new alkaloids, three of them were found to be novel sulfated erythrinane alkaloids (Ozawa, et al., 2011).

It is interesting to note that in the 2000 decade the literature described not only the isolation of new structures but also related them with biological activity, for instance Juma & Majinda (2004) described the isolation of fourteen different *Erythrina* alkaloids from the flowers and pods of *E. lysistemon* and tested their DPPH radical scavenging properties against stable 2,2-diphenyl-1-picrylhydrazyl (DPPH) radical. The antifeedant activities of the *Erythrina* alkaloids from the seeds, seed pods and flowers of *E. latissima* were investigated in laboratory dual-choice bioassays using third –instar *Spodoptera littoralis* (Boisduval) larvae (Wanjala, et al., 2009) and they found a dependant activity at concentrations between 100-500 ppm. The seed pods of *E. latissima* were studied by Wanjala & coworkers (Wanjala, et al., 2002), they found in this tissue the known alkaloids, erysotrine and erysodine and a new alkaloid, 10,11-dioxoerysotrine, which was lethal to brine shrimp and a 2-(5′-hydroxy-3′-methoxy phenyl)-6-hydroxy-5-methoxybenzofuran, which showed strong antimicrobial activity against the yeast spores, Gram-positive and Gram-negative bacteria.

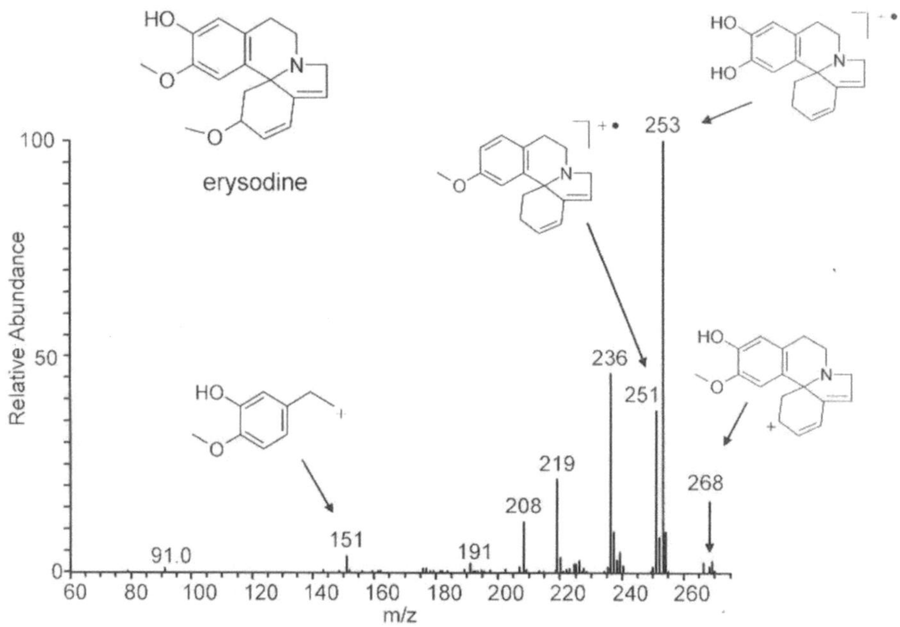

Fig. 5. MS (*m/z* 313 $[MH]^+ \rightarrow 268$) spectrum of erysodine recorded on a Thermo-Scientific I.CQ Classic quadrupole ion trap mass spectrometer.

6. Analysis of *Erythrina* alkaloids by liquid chromatography

These alkaloids has been analyzed traditionally by gas chromatography coupled to mass spectrometry (GC-MS). Although is possible analyze some of these alkaloids directly by this technique (Mantle, 1995) the method is improved with chemical derivatization, for example with trimethyl silylation the volatility of the compounds in increased (Jackson, et al., 1982). The glycosylated compounds are hydrolyzed to release the aglycone and facilitate the analysis. By this way the technique has been valuable in the analysis of several species of *Erythrina* (Soto-Hernandez & Jackson, 1994) also to compare hydrolyzed form with non hydrolyzed the levels of conjugated alkaloids can be deducted.

Besides, the high resolution of the hyphenated technique helps in the distinction of isomers, but the derivatization could complicate the analysis to form artifacts or could be incomplete and the method is consuming time.These observation made to look another technique with lesser inconveniences e.g. the coupling of HPLC with mass spectrometry referred as HPLC-MS. As these alkaloids easily accept protons, are ionized efficiently in positive mode with ionic sources as electrospray (ESI) or chemical ionization at atmospheric pressure (APCL). This last ionization mode is obtained higher sensitivity to the aglucones. Being basic compounds is low probable that their ionization is depleted in positive mode by other compounds, allowing that is detected easily by direct injection of a crude extract of alkaloids. However when is presented isomeric forms should be separated them before their analysis by mass spectrometry.

In one first step, the analysis of these alkaloids by HPLC with UV detection has been done with a normal phase column (Soto-Hernandez & Jackson, 1994). Later on was used the columns in reverse phase C-18 which at the beginning had low resolution and presented adverse effects to occur interactions between the charged alkaloids and negative residue charge from the stationary phase of the column. Also these compounds have been analyzed in the ionic pair mode. To diminish the positive charge of them, this mode (Fabre, et al. 2000) took to propose a method of analysis with the combination HPLC-MS, but the use of the present C-18 columns can remove the participation of the ionic volatile reagent (Verpoorte & Niesse, 1994).With them are managed in basic pH to increase the retention of the alkaloids and suppress the ionization of the OH groups in the stationary phase, this criteria helped in the analysis of the alkaloids of *Erythrina herbacea* that allowed a good separation and detection of the alkaloids, starting from a crude extract of the plant in which was used a programmed gradient of 0.1% ammonium acetate (at pH 7.4) and methanol (Garin-Aguilar, et al., 2005). However, with the recent incorporation of C-18 column with phenyl group linked to ethers, designed specifically to retain polar aromatic compounds, results suitable to the analysis of these alkaloids using simply a gradient of aqueous methanol and the method is still acceptable in acidic methanol (Fig. 5) by this way the acidic mobile phase promote the protonation of the alkaloids and improve their sensitivity.

7. Pharmacology

The biological activity of extracts of *Erythrina* species is known since long time ago. Thus, the natives of South America used concentrated extracts of these species as arrow poisons as antidote against strychnine or as an hypnotic and antiepileptic (Folkers & Unna, 1938). Also was observed that when is applied to dogs at different doses an alcoholic extract of seeds of *E. americana* provoked a similar activity to that of tubocurarine, this action was confirmed later on (Lozoya & Lozoya, 1982)

The first crystalline alkaloid pharmacologically active was isolated from *E. americana* (Folkers & Major, 1937) called erythroidine. Altamirano used this name but he related it as a unknown constituent of the plant. The subsequent analysis showed that this material was a mixture of isomeric alkaloids to which were called α- and β- erythroidines(**47, 48**)

Between 1940 and 1950 the systematic review of more than 50 species of *Erythrina* showed that all the isolated alkaloids produced similar effects to those of the curare alkaloids (Pick & Unna, 1945) used before as adjuvants in surgical anaesthesia, this stimulated the systematic investigation of the *Erythrina* species related to the biological properties of their extracts.

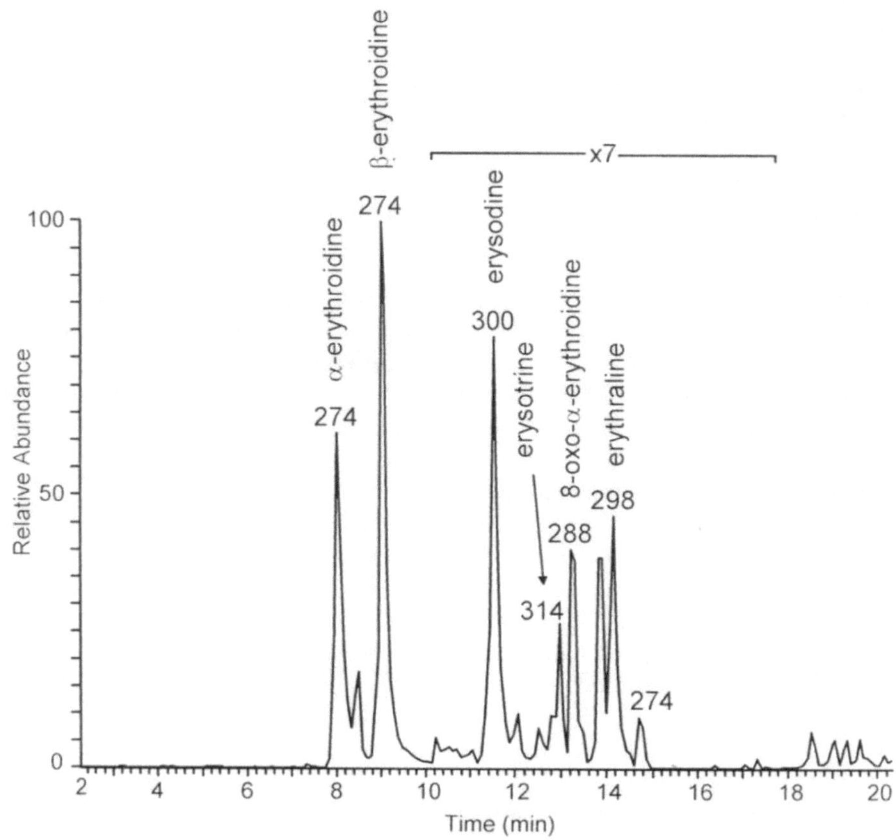

Fig. 6. Chromatogram of a LC-MS analysis of a methanol crude extract of *E. americana* seeds. The analysis was done in a phenomenex RP polar column of 150 x 46 mm, using a gradient of 0-10% methanol in the mobile phase (acidified with 1% acetic acid). Detection with APCI. The figures near to the peaks are the values of [M+H].

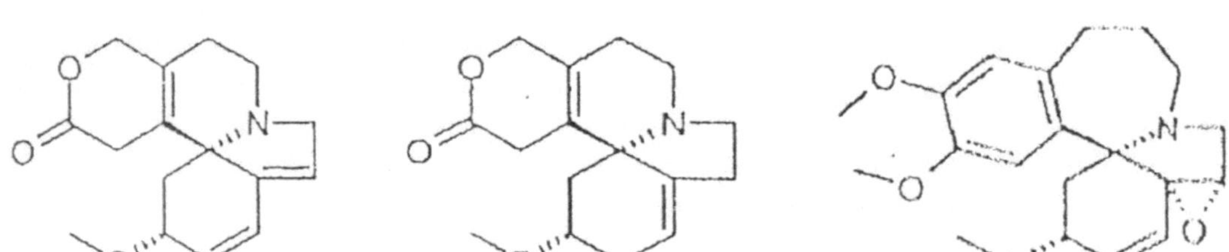

β-erythroidine (**47**) Dihydro-β-erythroidine (**48**) Wilsonine (**49**)

Fig. 7. Structure of various *Erythrina* alkaloids with special pharmacological properties.

Several species have been used in the indigenous medicine as eyewashes or wounds, for pain relief of arthritis or as calm and relaxants agents (Garin-Aguilar, et al., 2000). Interesting also has been described the hypoglycemic activity of *E. variegata* leaf in streptozotocin-induced diabetic rats (Kumar, et al., 2011) and the authors conclude that leaf of this plant has promising hypoglycemic action in STZ-induced diabetic rats substantiating in this way the ethnomedical use. The study of the antidiarrhoeal effects of ethanolic leaf extract of *E. indica* L. in experimental animals done by Sonia and coworkers (Sonia, et al., 2011) showed that this extract elicit potential antidiarrhoeal effects and thus substantiated its traditional claim as an antidiarrohoeal agent, also their findings suggest that the main constituents of the extracts were alkaloids

Also they have been related with antiasthmatic, diuretic or hypnotics properties. The alkaloidal extracts of *E. variegata* besides of its smooth properties as muscular relaxant has found depressed activity of the CNS and anticonvulsant, also increase the hypnosis provoked by pentobarbital and inhibit the acetyl choline induced spasm. Extracts of *E. velutina* and *E.suberosa* have spasmolytic and antineoplastic activity (Ghosal, et al., 1972; Craig, 1955). In recent researches crude extracts of *E. americana* as well their pure constituents: β-erythroidine and dihydro-β-erythroidine (Fig. 7) diminished the aggressive behavior in rats when is used diazepam as control. These effects are attributed to an interaction between the cholinergic and GABAergic receptors. Besides was determined the LD_{50} of the extracts as well to the pure alkaloids. From all the pure alkaloids tested the α- and β-erythroidine showed the highest activity (Garin-Aguilar, et al., 2000). It is considered that they are responsible of the hypnotic activity of the extracts of the flowers of *E. americana* (Tsuda & Sano, 1996). The β-erythroidine and its more potent derivative (2,7-dihydro) (**48**) have been used as muscular relaxants in numerous clinical applications (Lozoya & Lozoya, 1982). This activity is attributed to a antagonistic action of the dihydro β-erythroidine with the nicotinic receptors of acetyl choline (Tsuda & Sano, 1996; Cheeta, et al., 2001; Schoffelmer, et al., 2002).

Subsequently the group of Iturriaga-Vasquez and coworkers (Iturriaga-Vasquez, et al., 2010) studied the molecular determinants for competitive inhibition of α4β2 nicotinic acetylcholine receptors provoked by the dihydro-β-erythroidine (DHβE). They addressed this issue by examining the effects of DHβE and a range of aromatic *Erythrina* alkaloids on $[^3H]$ cytisine binding and receptor function in conjunction with homology models of the α4β2 nAChR, mutagenesis and functional assays. They found that the lactone group of DHβE and a hydroxyl group at position C-16 in aromatic *Erythrina* alkaloids were identified as major determinants of potency, which was decreased when the conserved residue Tyr 126 in loop A of the α4 subunit was substituted by alanine.

Erysodine (**6**) has found as competitive reversible antagonist of nicotine and the induced release of dopamine. It is equipotent with the dihydro-β-erythroidine (**48**) and can be used as tool to characterize neuronal nicotinic receptors of acetyl choline.

The anxiolytic effects of the *E. velutina* aqueous alcoholic crude extract and the purified alkaloids of the flowers of this plant were evaluated using the elevated T-maze test, and the light dark transition model(Flausino, et al., 2007a; Flausino, et al., 2007b). They observed a moderate activity but explain the use of the plant as calm agitation and other disorders of the nervous system. Subsequently, Carvalho, et al., (2009) showed an evidence of the mechanism of action of the leaves aqueous extract of this plant and they found that this extract provokes a $GABA_A$ receptor activation, acetylcholine release, muscarinic receptor activation, augmentation of Ca^{2+} entry though L-type calcium channels, and calcium release from the intracellular stores and they mention that their findings provide further support for *E. velutina* traditional uses.

However the study of Silva and coworkers (Silva et al., 2011) put in attention the use of this plant because through genotoxicity and cytotoxicity experiments on the root meristem cells of *Allium cepa* showed that the decoction of the leaves can have genotoxic effects at some doses and they recommend caution when using this plant for the preparation of teas and other medicinal products.

The group of Atsarno & coworkers (Atsarno, et al., 2011) evaluated the potential toxicity of the decoction of the stem bark of *E. senegalensis* which is used traditionally in Cameroon against liver disorders. Their results demonstrated that there is a wide margin of safety for the therapeutic use of this decoction and further corroborated the traditional use of this extract as hepatoprotective agent.

The analgesic properties of extracts and fractions from *E. crista-galli* leaves were tested by Fischer, et al., (2007) and they found that one of the fractions was the most active, being about 7-fold more active than the reference drugs(acetyl salicylic acid and acetaminophen)

It is important to mention that the curare alkaloids as quaternary salts and by their potent solubility in water are administered parentally. In contrast the *Erythrina* alkaloids are tertiary amines and they are able to develop their pharmacologic effects by oral via.

8. Chemotaxonomy

The alkaloids has been proposed as possible taxonomic markers is several species of angiosperms and this has helped to the resolution of some taxonomic problems, their limited distribution make that they can not be employed in the higher level of taxonomic classification only in those orders and classes where they are represented.

In this way the chemotaxonomy of alkaloids is found well documented but only to certain families of angiosperms (Hegnauer, 1963). In the case of *Erythrina* plants has been studied the alkaloid content in approximately half of the known species and the relationship of them is reflected in the presence of a series of alkaloids with isoquinoline skeleton.

Although the pattern of alkaloids of this genus is characteristic, their concentration varies. Hargreaves & coworkers mentioned that in the American species the proportion of alkaloids differs widely. The results indicate that in the genus, the dienoid alkaloids erysodine, erysovine and erysopine are the most abundant and widely distributed. In the American species the alkaloids generally do not contain oxygenated functions in C-11 may be by the enzymatic lack to hydroxylate this position (Hargreaves, et al., 1974). Aguilar & coworkers pointed out that in *E. americana* is typical to find lactonic alkaloids as main compounds (Aguilar, et al., 1981).

In *E. folkersii* has been found alkaloids of the type 1,6-diene and in *E. salviflora* those of alkenoid type. Ghosal & coworkers mentioned that erysotrine is the most abundant alkaloid in bark of *E. variegata* var. *orientalis* but also has been identified the erysodine in a lesser amounts (Ghosal, et al., 1972), whereas Dyke & Quessy mentioned that only is found erysodine in the bark of the same species (Dyke & Quessy, 1981). In some species is frequent to find alkaloids to contain oxygenated functions in the C-8 and C-11 position of the erythrinane skeleton, still exist doubts respect if one species is synonym to other. As the case of *E. americana* which some authors mention is synonym of *E. coralloides*. To prove that they are different species San Miguel-Chavez & coworkers found that the plantlets of one month age of *E. americana* synthetize erysosalvine, erythraline, N-oxide, erythratine and 8-oxo-α-erythroidine, whereas those of *E. coralloides* presented only erythraline and erysopine. These observations together with those of the morphology of the plantlets gives the idea of both species are different (San Miguel-Chavez et al., 2006).

9. Biotechnology in the production of Erythrinane alkaloids

Is well known that most of the drugs using in medicine are synthetic but some of them are of natural origin. Their demand is so high that some of plants are cultivated to this aim and to get enough biomass for the extraction of the drugs.

To satisfy the demand and protect the natural resources, has been developed alternative methods as Biotechnology plant cell tissue culture or the chemical synthesis and has been observed better results comparing with the traditional methods (Bougard, et al., 2001; Murphy, 2011).

Except to cultivated plants (e.g. *Papaver somniferum*) most of secondary metabolites are accumulated after certain age or maturity of the plant e.g. trees or shrubs (*Cinchona, Rauwolfia, Campotheca, Ochrosia, etc*)

The plants obtain their maturity before accumulate the active principles in higher amounts and is difficult increase the plantation to particular species. To avoid all of these limitations is required alternative methods to get a constant material all the year. To collect the plants in their natural environment is difficult but also put in risk of extinction some of them. When the plant material is not obtained during the year in enough amount to industrial scale and the chemical synthesis is not possible particularly in the case of complex molecules, the biotechnological methods give an excellent alternative. However to get this option should be consider cost/benefit of the product and then justify its its production (Bourgard, et al., 2001; Murphy, 2011).

E. americana had a wide distribution in México but recently its natural populations have started down because to the disappearance of its habitats.

This species also have interest because by the production of alkaloids with pharmacological and antimicrobial properties. Also has been explored the possibility of the *in vitro* tissue culture. In a first approach was obtained calluses from cotyledons of germinated seeds and maintained in a MS medium. These calluses were analyzed in the production of alkaloids and were observed that erythraline and the erythtroidines are the major alkaloids (Garcia-Mateos, et al., 1999; San Miguel-Chávez, et al., 2003.)

Subsequently cell suspension culture were induced from calluses what showed an efficient production of alkaloids in MS medium plus sucrose. The alkaloids obtained in these tissue culture were erythraline, 8-oxo-erythraline erysodine, α-and β-erythroidine, erysotramidine, and 8-oxo-α-erythroidine, but with levels below of those of the calluses (San Miguel-Chávez, et al., 2003). Trying to increase the alkaloid production in cell suspension culture, the concentration and type of plant growth regulation has been managed, and kinetin, indol acetic acid, naphthalene acetic acid and 2,4-phenoxyacetic acid have been tested and the treatment with MS medium plus 2,4-D+ kinetin (2 mg l^{-1}each one) gave the best results (San Miguel-Chávez, et.al., 2003).

In another step it has been elicited the cell suspension culture with jasmonic acid and only erysodine increased its production (San Miguel-Chávez, et al., 2007).

10. Compounds of non alkaloid composition

Besides of the presence of alkaloids in the *Erythrina* plants, has been detected the presence of diverse metabolites, for example glucoproteins or lectins with the characteristic to agglutinate cells (Ortega, et al. 1990). Stojanovic & coworkers , characterized a lectin isolated from *E. velutina* which is a good agglutinant agent of erytrocites A, B and O in human beings (Stojanovic, et al., 1994).

The saponins sigmoidin C and D were isolated from the steam bark of *E. sigmoidea* Hua and have been used in Cameroon as antimicrobial agents (Mbafor, et al., 1997). Also from this species have been recently isolated a new antibacterial triterpenoid saponin called Sigmoiside E (Kouam, et al., 2007). In *E. crista-galli* were isolated 3 new pterocapans: cristacarpin, erystagallin and phaseollidin with phytoalexin properties and possessing antimicrobial activity against Gram- positive bacteria (Tanaka, et al., 1997). The erystagallin-A also isolated from the stem bark of *E. variegata* L. showed significant anti-cancer activity against breast cancer T47D cell-lines *in vitro* using the Sulforhodamine B(SRB) assay and anti-malarial activity against *Plasmodium falciparum* *in vitro* using the lactate dehydrogenase (LDH) assay (Tati, et al., 2011). It is interesting to note that the pterocarpene, erycristagallin isolated from root bark of *E. mildbraedii* (Njamen, et al., 2003) showed anti-inflammatory properties through its capacity to inhibit the arachidonic acid metabolism via the 5-lipooxygenase pathway.

Fomum and coworkers (1986) found in the bark of *E.sigmoidea* three new phenyl flavanones: sigmoidine A, B and C with a notorious activity against, Gram- positive bacteria (Fomum, et al., 1986).

In the seeds of *Erythrina* also have been detected protease inhibitors, for instance Joubet & coworkers found this kind of compounds against tripsine, which acts as activator of the plasminogen tissue (Joubet, et al. 1987). In this way, continue an intense research with diverse species of *Erythrina* with the aim to characterize other compounds with notorious antibiotic activity and anticancer for example Cui & coworkers described four new chalcones 1 to 4 called abyssinones A-D isolated from *E. abyssinica*. They showed a moderate cytotoxic against Caco2 cell line of human colorectal cancer with IC_{50} 13.3, 15.1 and 11.1 μM respectively(Cui, et al. 2008).

Previously in this species Yenesew & coworkers (2004) found in the ethyl acetate extract of the bark, anti plasmodial activity against the chloroquine sensible (D6) and chloroquine-resistant (W-2) strains in *Plasmodium falciparum* with values of IC_{30} of 7.9 ± 1.1 and 5.3 I 0.7 mg ml respectively (Yenesew, et al. 2003, 2004).

Also several flavonoids (Chacha, et al. 2005; Chukwujekwu, et al., 2011; Doughari, 2011), isoflavonoids (Sato, et al., 2006; Kamdem Waffo, et al., 2006; Redko, et al., 2007) and pterocarpanes (Rukachaisirikul, et al., 2007a; 2007b) have been mentioned as antimicotic and antibacterial agents. For instance, an arylbenzofuran, erypoegin F and four isoflavonoids, erypoegins G-J were isolated from the roots of *E. poeppigiana* and their structure were elucidated by spectroscopic evidence (Tanaka, et al., 2003).

Also is important to mention the study done by Tanaka & coworkers (Tanaka, et al. 2010) in which they isolated two new compounds from the roots of *E. herbaceae*, erybacin A and erybacin B, as a 1-hydroxy-1,3-diphenylpropan-2-one derivatives. These compounds were evaluated for their antibacterial activities against 13 strains of methicillin resistant *Staphylococcus aureus* (MRSA), the erybacy B showed a potent bactericidal activity against MRSA.

The stem bark of *E. senegalensis* studied by its hepatoprotective properties have been recently studied by the presence of prenyl isoflavonoids as novel HIV-1 protease inhibitors (Lee, et al., 2009). These authors found that the prenyl isoflavonoids had a dose-dependant inhibitory activities on HIV-1 PR with IC50 values from 0.5 to 30 µM and mention that the isoflavonoid with prenyl groups at 6 and 8 positions of the ring A and one hydroxyl group in the 4´ position of B ring was the most potent HIV-1 PR inhibitor.

11. Conclusions

This review represents the work done in the last seventy five years in the knowledge of the *Erythrina* genus, a group of 120 species of the Leguminosae, with seventy of them in the Neotropics, 50 species are in Mexico, Central America and Caribbean where is used as ornamental (coral or lucky bean tree) , shade tree, timber (construction, implements), living fences and enclosures, green manure, livestock, fodder, medicine and seeds are used for necklaces.

These features have contributed to a deep research of their chemical constituents as alkaloids, flavonoids, isoflavonoids, saponins and lectins. The review remarked the potential which each type of compounds have now days.

Alkaloids for instance with their unique structure have attracted attention for their synthesis and structural elucidation or their pharmacological potential given by the relaxant properties.

The flavonoids and isoflavonoids represent other of the potentials of the genus because in recent years the literature has described not only novel structures but also notorious biological activity mainly related with antimicrobial agents.

Their impact is large in developing countries due to a relative unvailability of medicines and the emergence of widespread drug resistance. Therefore researchers are increasingly diverting their attention to folk medicine, looking for new leads to develop better drugs against microbial infections

It is hoped that this review can stimulate the development of new strategies in the manage of these kind of compounds and possibly to find new active agents from this beautiful genus of plants.

12. References

Aguilar, M.I.; Giral, F. & Espejo, O. (1981) Alkaloids from the flowers of *Erythrina americana. Phytochem* 20: 2061-2062.

Altamirano, F. (1888) Nuevos Apuntes para el estudio del Colorin, *Erythrina coralloides. Gaceta Médica de Mexico* 23: 369

Amer, M.E.; Shamma, M. & Freyer, A.J. (1991) The Tetracyclic *Erythrina* Alkaloids, *J Nat Prod* 54:329-363

Atsarno, AD.; Nguelefack, T.B.; Datte, J.Y. & Kamanyi, A. (2011) Acute and subchronic oral assessment of the aqueous extract from the stem bark of *Erythrina senegalensis* DC(Fabaceae) in rodents, *J. Ethnopharmacol.* 134 (3): 697-702.

Barton, D.H.R. & Cohen, T. (1957) Some Biogenetic Aspects of Phenol Oxidation. In Festschrift Professor Dr. Artur Stoll. Basel: Birkhäuser

Barton, D.H.R.; Boar, R.B. & Widdowson, D.A. (1970) Phenol Oxidation and Biosynthesis Part XXI. The Biosynthesis of the *Erythrina* Alkaloids, *J Chem Soc C* 1213.

Barton, D.H.R.; Potter, C.J. & Widdowson, D.A. (1974) Phenol Oxidation and Biosynthesis Part XXIII. On the benzyltetrahydroisoquinoline Origins of the *Erytrina* Alkaloids. *J Chem Soc Perkin Trans* 1 346

Barton, D.H.R.; James, R.; Kirby, G.W.; Turner, D.W. & Widdowson, D.A. (1968) Phenol Oxidation and Biosynthesis. Part XVIII.The Structure and Biosynthesis of *Erythrina* Alkaloids. *J Chem Soc C* 1529

Boekelheide, V. ;Weinstock, J.; Grundon, M.F.; Sauvage, G.L. & Agnello, E.J. (1953) The structure of β-Erythoidine and its derivatives. *J. Amer. Chem. Soc.* 75:2550

Bourgard, F.; Gravot, A.; Milesi, S. & Gontier, E. (2001) Production of plant secondary metabolites: a historical perspective, *Plant Science* 161, 839-851.

Carvalho, A.C.C.S.; Almeida, D.S.; Melo, M.G.D.; Cavalcanti, S.C.H. & Marçal, R.M. (2009) Evidence of the mechanism of action of *Erythrina velutina* Wild (Fabaceae) leaves aqueous extract, *J.Ethnopharmacol.* 122: 374-378.

Carmack, M., MacKusick, B.C. & Prelog, V. (1951) *Erythrina*-Alkaloide,2. Mitt Über das Apo-erysodin und das Apo-erythralin. *Helv Chim Acta* 34:1601

Chacha, M.; Bojase-Moleta, G. & Majinda, R.R.T. (2005) Antimicrobial and radical scavenging flavonoids from the stem wood of *Erythrina latissima, Phytochemistry.* 66 (1): 99-104.

Cheeta, S.; Tucci, S. & File, S.E. (2001) Antagonism of the Anxiolytic Effect of Nicotine in the dorsal raphé nucleus by dihydro-β-erythroidine, *Pharmacol. Biochem Behavior* 70:491-496

Chukwujekwu, J.C.; Van Heerden, F.R. & Van Staden, J. (2011) Antibacterial Activity of Flavonoids from the Stem Bark of *Erythrina caffra* Thumb., *Phytother. Res.* 25: 46-48.

Craig, L.E. (1955) Curare-like Effects In: The alkaloids, Chemistry and Physiology Vol.5-Pharmacology. Manske, R.H.F. (Ed.) p. 265-290, Academic Press, New York.

Cui, L. ; Thuong,P.T.; Lee, H.S; Njamen, D.; Mbafor, J.T.; Fomum, Z T , Lee, J.; Kim Y.H. & Oh, W.K. (2008) Four new chalcones from *Erythrina abyssinica, Planta Medica,* 74 (4): 422-426.

Decker, M.W.; Anderson, D.J.; Brioni, J.D.; Donelly-Roberts, D.L.; Kang, C.H.; O´Neill, A.B.: Piattoni-Kaplan, M.; Swanson, S. & Sullivan, J.P. (1995) Erysodine, a competitive antagonist at neuronal nicotinic acetylcholine receptors, *Eur J. Pharmacol* 280: 79.

Dominguez, M. & Altamirano, F. (1877) Del Colorín, *Gaceta Médica de México* 12:77.

Doughari, J.H. (2010) Evaluation of antimicrobial potential of stem bark extracts of *Erythrina senegalensis* DC , *Afr. J. Microbiol. Res.* 4(7): 1836-1841.

Dyke, S.F. & Quessy S.N. (1981). *Erythrina* and related alkaloids, In: The Alkaloids. Vol. 18. Manske R F H (ed.),1-98 Academic Press. New York.

Fabre, N.; Claparols, C.; Richelme, S.; Angelin, M.L.; Fourasté, I. & Moulis, C. (2000) Direct characterization of isoquinoline alkaloids in a crude plant extract by ion-pair liquid chromatography-electrospray ionization tandem mass spectrometry: example of *Eschscholziacalifornica, J. Chromatogr. A.* 904, 35-46

Faria, T.D.J. , Cafèu, M.C.; Akiyoshi, G.; Ferreira, D.T.; Galao, O.F., Andrei, C.C.; Pinge Filho, P.; Paiva, M.R.C.; Barbosa, A.D.M. & Braz-Filho, R. (2007) Alkaloids from flowers and leaves of *Erythrina speciosa* Andrews, *Quimica Nova* 30 (3): 525-527.

Fischer, L.G..O.; Leitao, R.; Etcheverry, S.R.; De Campos-Buzzi, F.; Vazquez, A.A.; Heinzen, H.A. & Filho, C.(2007) Analgesic properties of extracts and fractions from *Erythrina crista-galli* (Fabaceae) leaves, *Nat. Prod. Res.* 21(8): 759-766.

Flausino, O. Jr.; de Avila Santos, L.; Verli, H.; Pereira, AM., da Silva Bolzani, V. & Nunez-de-Souza R.L. (2007a) Anxiolytic Effects of Erythrinan Alkaloids from *Erythrina mulungu*, *J. Nat. Prod.* 70: 48-53.

Flaustino, O.P. Jr.; Pereira, A.M., da Silva Bolzani, V & Nunez-de-Souza R.L. (2007b) Effects of Erythrinan Alkaloids isolated from *Erythrina mulungu* (Papilionaceae) in Mice Submitted to Animal Model of Anxiety, *Biol. Pharm. Bull.* 30(2): 375-378.

Folkers, K. & Major, R.T. (1937) Isolation of Erythroidine, an Alkaloid of Curare Action from *Erythrina americana* Mill. *J. Am Chem Soc* 59:1580

Folkers, K. & Koniuszy, F. (1939) *Erythrina* alkaloids, III. Isolation and Characterization of a new alkaloid, *Erythramine, J. Am Chem Soc* 31:1232

Folkers, K. & Koniuszy, F. (1940a) *Erythrina* Alkaloids. VII. Isolation and Characterization of the New Alkaloids, *Erythraline* and *Erythratine, J. Am Chem Soc* 62:436

Folkers, K. & Unna K. (1938) Erythrina alkaloids, II. A review, and New Data on the Alkaloids of Species of the Genus *Erythrina. J. Am Pharm Assoc* 27:693

Folkers, K. & Unna, K. (1939) *Erythrina* alkaloids V. Comparative Curare-like Potencies of Species of the Genus *Erythrina. J. Pharm Assoc* 28:1019.

Folkers, K.& Koniuszy, F. (1940b) *Erythrina* alkaloids VIII. Studies on the Constitution of *Erythramine* and *Erythraline, J Am Chem Soc* 62:1673

Folkers, K.& Koniuszy, F. (1940c) *Erythrina* Alkaloids. IX. Isolation and Characterization of *Erysodine, Erysopine, Erysocine* and *Erysovine, J Am Chem Soc* 62: 1677

Fomum, Z.T.; Ayafor, J.F.; Mbafor, J.T. & Mbi, Ch.M. (1986) Erythrina studies. Part 2. Structures of three novel prenylated antibacterial flavanones, sigmoidins A-C, from *Erythrina sigmoidea* Hua, *J Chem Soc Perkin* Trans I: 33-37.

García-Mateos, R.; Garín-Aguilar, M.E.; Soto-Hernández, M &. Martínez-Vazquez, M. (2000) Effect of β-Erythroidine and β-Dihydroerythroidine from *Erythrina americana* on rats Aggressive Behavior, *Pharm Pharmacol Lett* 10:34

García-Mateos, R.; Soto-Hernández, M.; Martínez-Vázquez, M. & Villegas- Monter A. (1999) Isolation of alkaloids of *Erythrina* from tissue culture, *Phytochemical analysis.* 10: 12-16.

Garín-Aguilar, M.E.; Ramírez- Luna, J.E.; Soto-Hernández, M.; Valencia del Toro, G. & Martínez- Vazquez, M. (2000) Effect of crude Extracts of *Erythrina americana* Mill. on aggressive behaviour in Rats, *J. Ethnopharmacol* 69:189

Garín-Aguilar, M.E.; Valencia del Toro, G., Soto-Hernández, M. & Kite, G. (2005) High-performance liquid chromatography-mass spectrometric analysis of alkaloids extracted from seeds of *Erythrina herbacea, Phytochemical Analysis* 16: 302-306

Ghosal, S.; Dutta, S. & Bhattacharya, S.K. (1972) *Erythrina* - Chemical and Pharmacological Evaluation II: Alkaloids of *Erythrina variegata 1, J. Pharm Sci* 61:1274

Greshoff, M (1890) Mitteilungen aus dem chemisch-pharmakologisehen Laboratorium de Botanischen Gartens zu Buitenzorg (Java), *ChemBer* 23: 3537.

Hargreaves, R.T., Johnson, R.D.; Millington, D.S.; Mondal, M.H.; Beavers, W.; Becker, L.; Young, C., & Rinehart, K.L. Jr (1974) Alkaloids of American Species of *Erythrina*, *Lloydia* 37:569-580

Hegnauer, R. (1963). Chemotaxonomy, past and present. *Lloydia* 28: 267-278.

Iturriaga-Vasquez, P.; Carbone, A.L.; García-Beltrán, O.; Livingstone, P.D; Biggin, P.C.; Cassels, B.K.; Wonnacott, S.; Zapata-Torres, G. & Bemudez, I. (2010) Molecular Determinants for Competitive Inhibition of α4β2 Nicotinic Acetylcholine Receptors, *Molec Pharmacol*. 78(3): 366-375.

Jackson, A.H.; Ludgate, P.; Mavraganis, V. & Redha, F.M. (1982). Studies of *Erythrina* alkaloids, part V.GC/MS investigation of alkaloids in the seeds of *E. subumbrans, E. lanata, E. rubinervia, E. acanthocarpa, E. variegate* and *E. melanacantha, Allertonia* 3: 47-51

Joubet, J.J.; Merrifiel, E.H. & Dowdle, E.B.D. (1987). The reactives sites of proteinase inhibitors from *Erythrina* seeds, *International Journal of Biochemistry* 19: 601-606.

Juma, B. & Majinda, R.R.T. (2004) Erythrinaline alkaloids from the flowers and pods of *Erythrina lysistemon* and their DPPH radical scanvenging properties, *Phytochem*. 65: 1397-1404.

Kamdem Waffo, A.F.; Coombes, P.H.; Mulholland, D.A.; Nkengfack, A.E. & Fomum Z.T. (2006) Flavones and isoflavones from the west African Fabaceae *Erythrina vogelii*, *Phytochem* 67: 459-463

Kawasaki, T.; Onoda, N.; Watanabe, H. & Kitara, T. (2001) Total Synthesis of (±) Cocculolidine. *Tetrahedron Lett* 42: 8003

Kenner, G.W., Khorana, H.G. & Prelog, V. (1951) *Erythrina*-Alkaloide, 3. Mitt. Über den *Hoffman*´schenAbbau des Tetrahydro-erysotrins und des Tetrahydro-erythralins. *Helv Chim Acta* 34:1969

Kouam, J. ; Noundou, X.Siewe Noundou, X.; Kouitcheu Mebeku, L.B.; Meli Lannang, A.; Choudhary, M.I. & Fomum, Z.T.(2007) Sigmoiside E: A New Antibacterial Triterpenoid Saponin from *Erythrina sigmoidea* HUA, *Bull. Chem. Soc Ethiop* 21(3): 373-378.

Kumar, A; Lingadurai, S.; Shirivastava, T.P.; Bhattacharya, S. & Haddar, P.K. (2011) Hypoglycemic activity of *Erythrina variegata* leaf in streptozotocin-induced diabetic rats, *Pharm. Biol*. 49(6): 577-582.

Lee, J.S.; Oh, W.K.; Ahn, J.S.; Kim, Y.H.;Mbafor, J.T.; Wandji, J. & Fomum, Z.T. (2009) Prenylisoflavonoids from *Erythrina senegalensis* as Novel HIV-1 Protease Inhibitors, *Planta Med*. 75:268-270.

Lehman, A.J. (1936) Curare-Actions of *Erythrina americana, Proc Soc Exp Biol Med* 33: 501

Lehman, A.J. (1937) Action of *Erythrina americana*, a possible Curare Substitute, *J Pharmacol Exp Ther* 60: 69

Lozoya, X. & Lozoya, M. (1982) Flora Medicinal de México. In*: Plantas Indígenas del Seguro Social*, México, D.F. p 174

Maier, U.H. & Zenk, M.H. (1997), (S)-Norrreticuline is the precursor for the biosynthesis of *Erythrina* alkaloids, Chem Commun.2313-2314.

Maier, U.H.; Rödl, W.; Deus-Neumann B. & Zenk, M.H. (1999) Biosynthesis of *Erythrina* Alkaloids in *Erythrina crista-galli* . *Phytochemistry* 52: 373

Mantle, P.G. (1995). Direct analysis of aromatic diene *Erythrina* alkaloids by capillary GC-MS *Phytochemistry* 38: 135-1316

Mbafor, T. J.; Ndom, J.C. & Fomum, T.Z..(1997). Triterpenoids saponins from *E. sigmoidea*, *Phytochemistry* 44 (6): 1151-1155.

Mondon, A.; Hansen, K.F.; Boehme, K.; Faro, H.P.; Nestler, H.J.; Vilhuber, H.G. & Böttcher, K. (1970) SynthetischeArbeiten in der Reidhe der aromatischen *Erythrina*-Alkaloide, XI; Anwendungen der Glyoxylester-Synthese, *Chem Ber* 103:615

Murphy, A.C. (2011) Metabolic engineering is key to sustainable chemical industry, *Nat Prod Rep* 28, 1406-1425.

Nagaraja, T.S., Mahmood, R.; Krishna, V. & Maruthi,E.T. (2011) Evaluation of antimicrobial activity of *Erythrina mysorensis* Gamb. *Int J. Drug Devel. & Res.*, 3 (2):198-202.

Njamen,D.; Talla, E.; Mbafor, J.T.; Fomum, Z.T.; Kamanyi, A.; Mbanya, J.C.; Cerda-Nicolas, M.; Giner, R.M.; Recio, M.C. & Ríos, J.L.(2003) Anti-inflammatory activity of erycristagallin, a pterocarpene from *Erythrina mildbraedii, Eur. J. Pharmacol.* 468:67-74.

Ortega, M.; Sánchez, C.; Chacón, E.; Rendón, L.J.; Estrada, R.; Masso, F. Montaño, F.L. & Zenteno,E. (1990) Purification and characterization of a lectin from *Erythrina americana* by affinity chromatography, *Plant Science* 72: 133-140.

Ozawa, M.; Kawamata, S.; Etoh, T.; Hayashi, M.; Komiyama, K.; Kishida, A.; Kuroda, Ch. & Ohsaki, A. (2010) Structures of new Erythrinan alkaloids and Nitric Oxide Production Inhibitors from *Erythrina crista-galli, Chem Pharm. Bull.* 58(8): 1119-1122

Ozawa, M.; Kishida, A. & Ohsaki, A. (2011) Erythrinan Alkaloids from Seeds of *Erythrina velutina, Chem Pharm. Bull.* 59(5):564-567.

Pick, E.P. & Unna, K. (1945) The effect of Curare and Curare -like substances on the Central Nervous System, *J. Pharmacol. Exp Therap* 83:59

Ramírez, E. & Rivero, M.D. (1935) Pharmacodynamic Action of *Erythrina americana* Mill [family leguminosae]. *Anales Inst. Biol.* (Mex) 6:301 .

Redko, F. ; Clavin, M.L.; Weber, D.; Ranea, F.; Anke, T. & Martino, V. (2007) Antimicrobial isoflavonoids from *Erythrina crista galli* infected with *Phomopsis* sp., Z. Naturforschung. C, 62 (3-4):164-168.

Reiman, E. & Ettmayr, C. (2004) An Improved Stereocontrolled Route to *cis*-Erythrinanes by Combined Intramolecular Strecker and Bruylants Reaction. *Monatsh Chem* 135:1143

Rey, P. (1883) Note sur les proprietés thérapeutiques de l´*Erythrina corallodendron Le Journal de Terapeutique* 10: 843

Rukachaisirikul,T.; Innok, P.; Aroonrerk, N.; Boonamnuaylap, W.; Limrangsun, S.; Boonyon, Ch.; Woonjina, U.;Suksamrarn, A. (2007) Antibacterial pterocarpans from *Erythrina subumbrans, J Ethnopharmacol.* 110 (1): 171-175.

Rukachaisirikul, T.; Saekee, A.; Tharibun, Ch.; Watkoulham, S. & Suksamrarn, A.(2007b) Biological Activities of the Chemical Constituents of *Erythrina stricta* and *Erythrina subumbrans, Arch Pharm Res* 30(11): 1398-1403

Rukachaisirikul, T.; Innok, P. & Suksamrarn, A. (2008) *Erythrina* Alkaloids and a Pterocarpan from the Bark of *Erythrina subumbrans, J. Nat Prod.* 71: 156-158.

San Miguel-Chávez, R.; Soto-Hernández, M.; Ramos-Valdivia A.C. & Kite, G. (2007) Alkaloid production in elicited cell suspension cultures of *Erythrina americana* Miller, *Phytochem Rev.* 6: 167-173.

San Miguel-Chávez, R.; Soto-Hernández, M.; Ramos-Valdivia, A.C.; Kite, G.; Martínez-Vázquez, M.; García-Mateos, R.& Terrazas, T. (2003) Production of alkaloids by *in vitro* culture of *Erythrina americana* Miller, *Biotechnol Lett. 25(13):* 1055-1059.

San Miguel-Chávez, R.; Soto-Hernández, M.; Terrazas, T. & Kite,.G. (2006) Morphology and alkaloidal profile of the seedlings of *Erythrina americana* Mill, and *E. coralloides* A.D, *Feddes Repertorium.* 117 (3-4): 232-239.

Sato, M.; Tanaka, H.; Tani, N.; Nagayama, M. & Yamaguchi, R.(2006). Different antibacterial actions of isoflavones isolated from *Erythrina poeppigiana* against methicillin-resistant *Staphylococcus aureus*, *Letters Applied Microbiology*. 43 (3): 243-248.

Schoffelmer, A.N.M.; De Vries, T.J.; Wardeh, G.; van de Ven, H.W.M. & Venderschuren I. J.M.J. (2002) Psychostimulant-Induced Behavioral Sensitization Depends on Nicotinic Receptor Activation, *J. Neurosci* 22:3269

Silva, D.S.B.S.; Garcia, A.CF.S.; Mata, S.S.; de Oliveira, B.; Estevam, Ch.S.; Scher, R. & Pantaleao, S.M. (2011) Genotoxicity and citotoxicity of *Erythrina velutina* Willd., Fabaceae, on the root meristem cells of *Allium cepa*, *Braz. J. Pharmacog*. 21(1):92-97.

Sonia, J.; Latha, P.G; Gowsalya, P.; Anuja, G.I.; Suja, S.R.; Shine, V.J.; Shymal, S.; Shikha, P.; Krishnakumar, N.M.; Sreejith, G.; Sini, S.& Sekharan, S. (2011) Antidiarrhoeal effects of ethanolic leaf extract of *Erythrina indica* L. in experimental animals, *Med. Plants* 3(1)

Soto-Hernández, M. & Jackson, A.H. (1994) *Erythrina* alkaloids: isolation and characterization of alkaloids from seven *Erythrina* species, *Planta Med* 60: 175-177

Stojanovic, D.; Fernández, M.; Casale, I.; Trujillo, D. & Castes, M.. (1994). Characterization and mitogenicity of a lectin from *Erythrina velutina* seeds, *Phytochem* 37: 1069-1074.

Tanaka, H.; Tanaka, T. & Etoh, H.(1997). Three pterocarpans from *E. crista-galli*, *Phytochem* 45 (4): 835-838.

Tanaka, H.; Etoh, H.; Shimizu, H.; Oh-Uchi, T.; Terada, Y. & Tateishi, Y.(2001) Erythrinan alkaloids and isoflavonoids from *Erythrina poeppigiana*, *Planta Med* 67:871-873.

Tanaka, H.; Oh-Uchi, T.; Etoh, H.; Sako, M.; Sato, M.; Fukai, T. & Tateishi, Y. (2003) An arylbenzofuran and four isoflavonoids from the roots of *Erythrina poeppigiana*, *Phytochem* 63: 597-602.

Tanaka, H.; Hattori, H.; Tanaka, T.; Sakai, E.; Tanaka, N.; Kulkarni, a. & Etoh H.(2008) A new *Erythrina* alkaloid from *Erythrina herbacea*, *J Nat Med* 62:228-231.

Tanaka, H.; Sudo, M.; Kawamura, T.; Sato, M.; Yamaguchi, R.; Fukai, T.; Sakai, E. & Tanaka N. (2010) Antibacterial Constituents from the Roots of *Erythrina herbacea* against Methicillin-resistant *Staphylococcus aureus*, *Planta Med* 76: 916-919.

Tati, H.; Nurlelasari ; Dikdik, K.; Unang, S. and Zalinar, U. (2011) In vitro anticancer and antimalarial Erystagallin-A from *Erythrina variegata* (L) stem bark, *Med Plant* 3(1)

Tsuda, Y. & Sano, T. (1996) *Erythrina* and Related Alkaloids. In: The Alkaloids, vol. 48, G.A Cordell (Ed.), 249-338 Academic Press, Inc., New York.

Verpoorte, R. & Niesse, W.M.A. (1994). Liquid chromatography coupled with mass spectrometry in the analysis of alkaloids. *Phytochem. Anal.* 5. 217-232

Wanjala, C.C.W. & Majinda, R.T. (2000) Two Novel Glucodienoid Alkaloids from *Erythrina latissima* Seeds, *J Nat Prod* 63: 871-873.

Wanjala, C. C.W.; Juma, B.F.; Bojase, G.; Gashe, B.A. & Majinda, R.R.T. (2002) Erythrinaline alkaloids and Antimicrobial Flavonoids from *Erythrina latissima*, *Planta Med* 68:640-642

Wanjala, C.W., Akeng´a, T.; Obiero, G.O. & Lutta, K.P. (2009) Antifeedant Activities of the Erythrinaline Alkaloids from *Erythrina latissima* against *Spodoptera littoralis* (Lepidoptera noctuidae), *Rec. Nat. Prod.* 3(2):96-103

Yenesew, A.; Derese, S.; Irungu, B.; Midiwo, J.O.; Waters, N.C., Liyala, P.; Akala, H.;Heydenreich, M. & Peter, M.G. (2003) Flavonoids and Isoflavonoids with Antiplasmodial Activities from the Root Bark of *Erythrina abyssinica*, *Planta Med* 69:658-661

Yenesew, A.; Induli, M.; Derese, S.; Midiwo, J. O.; Heydenreich, M.; Peter, M.G.; Akala, H.; Wangui, J.; Liyala, P.& Waters, N.C. (2004) Anti-plasmodial flavonoids from the stem bark of *Erythrina abyssinica*, *Phytochem* 65 (22): 3029-3032

10

Zanthoxylum Genus as Potential Source of Bioactive Compounds

L. Oscar Javier Patiño, R. Juliet Angélica Prieto and S. Luis Enrique Cuca
Laboratorio de Productos Naturales Vegetales, Universidad Nacional de Colombia, Colombia

1. Introduction

Natural products have been used for thousands of years for the benefit of mankind, as important sources of food, clothing, cosmetics, building materials, tools, medicines and crop protection agents. They have made enormous contributions to human health through compounds such as quinine, morphine, aspirin (a natural product analog), digitoxin and many others. Researches in this field are becoming more numerous, to the point of getting about half of pharmaceuticals and pesticides from natural sources (Newman & Cragg, 2007). The main reasons because natural products are so important to undertake research are that they can be a source of new compounds because they produce many bioactive secondary metabolites that are used as a chemical defense against predators. Also, in the past, they have provided many new drugs, some of which can't be obtained by other sources and because they can provide the necessary templates to design new products in the future (Colegate and Molyneux, 2008; Kaufman et al., 2006; Cragg et al., 2005).

Dissatisfied therapeutic needs in the treatment of bacterial, parasitic, viral and fungal infections, cancer, Alzheimer's and AIDS, among other diseases, have led to the search of new substances with therapeutic applications. Although for most diseases there is a treatment, many of them have begun to be ineffective due to the development of resistance to medicaments that were initially effective and to the low security that they exhibit for patients. Consequently, the development of effective and safe therapeutic alternatives is essential to ensure the availability of new products that reduce mortality and morbidity due to diseases (Pan et al., 2010; Nwaka & Hudson, 2006; Segal & Elad, 2006; Waldvogel, 2004).

The search for new phytosanitary agents to control plant pests and diseases that affect many plant sources of food and/or industrial use is also of great interest, because the indiscriminate and permanent use of agrochemicals has led to the emergence of resitant pests and phytopathogenic microorganisms, that can cause partial or complete loss of crops (Agrios, 2005; Strand, 2000).

Research in plants represents an invaluable source discovering new substances, considering that each of these can contain hundreds or even thousands of secondary metabolites. From the 250,000 to 300,000 plant species reported, only a small part has been the subject of phytochemical and biological activity studies (Tringali, 2001).

This chapter shows information about the importance of ethnobotany, phytochemistry and biological activities of species of the genus *Zanthoxylum*, information that can be the base for undertaking future research.

2. Overview of *Zanthoxylum* genus

Zanthoxylum genus belongs to the Rutaceae family. It is economically important because of their alimentary, industrial and medicinal applications (Seidemann, 2005; Chase et al., 1999). *Zanthoxylum* comes from the word *Xanthoxylum* wich derives from Greek: "xanthon xylon" that means "yellow wood", hence the use of the terms *Xanthoxylum* or *Zanthoxylum* by some authors. The genus *Zanthoxylum* was created by Linné in 1757 and since its inception has been confused with the genus *Fagara*. In 1896, Engler made the distinction between the two genera by the following characteristics: species of the genus *Zanthoxylum* have a simple perianth, while in species of the genus *Fagara* is twofold. Brizicky in 1962, discovered some species with intermediate perianth, which showed that simple perianth of *Zanthoxylum* drift from the *Fagara* due to failure of some sepals, and concluded that *Fagara* and *Zanthoxylum* genus are the same. Finally, in 1966, Hartley grouped *Zanthoxylum* and *Fagara* under the name of *Zanthoxylum*. However, some authors still use the term *Fagara* (Chaaib, 2004).

Zanthoxylum comprises about 549 species distributed worldwide mainly in tropical and temperate regions (Global Biodiversity Information Facility, 2010). This genus includes trees and shrubs, usually dioecious. The trees have leafy crown, with few branches and reach up to 20 meters. The species of this genus are characterized by the presence of recurved spines on its trunk and branches. The leaves are varied, may be alternate or opposite, simple or composed, imparipanadas or parimpanadas with up to 15 pairs of leaflets. The inflorescences are usually in form of panicles or umbels compound, axillary or terminal of small flowers. The flowers are actinomorphic, hermaphrodite and unisexual, rarely bisexual, usually white or green. The fruits are follicles or esquizocarp, contains from one to five carpels usually aromatic, and the are ordinarily bivalve with a single red or black, shiny seeds (Melo & Zickel, 2004; Silva & Paoli, 2004).

The genus *Zanthoxylum* has great importance due to its ethnobotanics, phytochemistry and biological activity, and it is a promising source of various secondary metabolites including benzophenanthridine alkaloids.

3. Ethnobotanical uses

Species of this genus are of economic importance as sources of edible fruits, oils, wood, raw materials for industries, medicinal plants, ornamentals, culinary applications, and are characterized by a satin wood commonly used in woodworking (Yang, 2008; Da Silva *et al.*, 2006; Adesina, 2005; Seidemann, 2005). For example in Africa is used the wood of *Z. gillettii*, *Z. tessmannii*, *Z. lemairei* and *Z. leprieurii* for houses, buildings, drums and ships construction, and for decorative woodwork, carpentry, and paper industry. In some countries of this continent, root bark and stem of many species of *Zanthoxylum* for used as a vermifuge, febrifuge and piscicides (Adesina, 2005).

Zanthoxylum species are also used in the field of perfumery and food industry because of its essential oils from leaves, fruits and inflorescences. The most used essential oils are obtained from *Z. xanthoxyloides* (Ngassoum et al., 2003), *Z. gillettii* (Jirovetz et al., 1999) and *Z. simulans* (Chyau et al., 1996).

A common feature of almost all species of the genus *Zanthoxylum* is the ability to produce tires, which could be used in the pharmaceutical industry as encapsulants, emulsifying agents or diluents. Some investigations have been conducted on the rubber collected on the bark of *Z. tessmannii* (Adesina, 2005).

Many species of the *Zanthoxylum* genus have been used in different parts of the world especially in Asia, Africa and America to treat a number of diseases in humans and animals (McGaw et al., 2008; Rochfort et al., 2008; Adesina, 2005; Chaaib, 2004; Diéguez et al., 2004; Patiño, 2004). For example, the bark of *Z. integrifolioum* is used in traditional medicine by Ya-Mei and Lanyu indigenous tribes in Taiwan, as a remedy for snakebite, dyspepsia and as an aromatic tonic for fever. The bark of *Z. liebmannianum*, is used in Mexico for the treatment of stomach pains, amebiasis, intestinal parasites and as a local anesthetic agent (Ross et al., 2004). Some species are used for the treatment of malaria, such is the case of *Z. rhoifolium* (Jullian et al., 2006; Bertani et al., 2005), *Z. acutifolium* (Arruda et al., 1992), *Z. chalybeum* (Jullian et al., 2006) and *Z. usambarense* (Kirira et al., 2006). Venezuelan traditional medicine is known to use *Z. monophyllum* in the treatment of runny nose or nasal mucosal inflammation, jaundice, ophthalmia and as an anesthetic (Gomez et al., 2007; Diaz & Ortega, 2006). Another use has been given as a textile dye (De Garcia et al., 1989).

According to reports of ethnobotanical properties of the *Zanthoxylum* genus, in general it is emphasized that the most commonly used extraction methods are infusion and decoction, using mainly water as solvent. In Table 1 are summarized the main ethnobotanical uses of 45 species of the genus *Zanthoxylum*, as well as the plant part used and method of preparation. The major ethnobotanical properties attributed to these plant species are: relief of dental problems, treatment of malaria, gastrointestinal disorders, gonorrhea and lung diseases, antidiarrheal use in animals and humans, emmenagogue action, effective for rheumatism, anthelmintic use in animals and humans, aphrodisiac, analgesic, action against various skin diseases, febrifuge, antihemorrhagic, effective for genitourinary diseases, anticancer, diuretic, stomachic, anti-convulsive, tonic and stimulant. In addition to the medicinal properties, some species are also used as pesticides, building materials and textile dyes.

Some plants have been used as components of natural medicines, because of the important ethnomedical properties of *Zanthoxylum* genus species. *Z. tingoassuiba* has been marketed since 1923 by Flora Medicinal J. Monteiro da Silva Laboratory, as part of herbal medicinal product called Uva do Mato®, which is prescribed for muscle cramps and spasms (Da Silva et al., 2008). *Z. rhoifolium* also has been commercialized in Brazil as a component of herbal tea mixtures sold in drugstores, supermarkets and popular markets (Pereira et al., 2010; Da Silva et al., 2007a).

4. Phytochemistry

Phytochemical studies carried out on species of the genus *Zanthoxylum*, alkaloids of various types, lignans, coumarins amides are commonly secondary metabolites reported and have chemotaxonomic importance to the genre. Also, other metabolites have been isolated such as flavonoids, sterols and terpenes, among others (Adesina, 2005; Patiño, 2004, Waterman & Grundon, 1983).

4.1 Alkaloids

The alkaloids are most important compounds for the genus *Zanthoxylum*, because they are present in most species and have been found in all plant organs, being abundant in the trunk and root bark (Dieguez et al., 2004). The main isolated alkaloids from the genus are of two types: isoquinolines (benzophenanthridine, benzylisoquinoline, aporphine, protoberberine and berberine) and quinolines (Krane et al. 1984; Waterman & Grundon, 1983; Cordell, 1981). Other types of alkaloids have also been found in some species of the genus.

4.1.1 Isoquinoline alkaloids

The **benzophenanthridines** are the most frequently reported type of alkaloid in the genus *Zanthoxylum* and have great interest due to important and varied biological activity that they present, among which highlights the antitumor activity (Maiti & Kumar, 2009; Tillequin, 2007; Maiti & Kumar, 2007; Dvorak et al., 2006; Nyangulu et al., 2005; Eun & Koh, 2004; Tang et al. 2003; Slaninová et al., 2001; Simeon et al., 1989). Representatives of these alkaloids have exhibited antimalarial (Nyangulu et al., 2005; Ross et al., 2004), antileukemic (Dupont et al., 2005), antioxidant (Pérez et al., 2003), nematicide (Matsuhashi et al., 2002), HIV (Chang et al., 2003), antibacterial (Gonzaga et al., 2003), antimicrobial (Nissanka et al., 2001) and antifungal activities (Queiroz et al., 2006), among others. Their distribution is very limited in plants, and only they have been isolated from some genera belonging to the families Papaveraceae, Rutaceae and Fumiraceae mainly, where they are considered chemotaxonomic markers. In Rutaceae family they are present in species of the genera *Phellodendron*, *Fagaropsis*, *Tetradium*, *Toddalia* and *Zanthoxylum* (including *Fagara*), the latter with a majority presence of these alkaloids from the others (Krane et al., 1984; Cordell, 1981). The main representatives of this type of alkaloids are fagaronine **1**, nitidine **2**, chelerythrine **3** and sanguinarine **4**. Compounds with similar chemical structure to iwamide **5** and integriamide **6**, isolated from various species of the genus *Zanthoxylum*, have been classified by different authors within benzophenanthridine alkaloids (Krane et al., 1984).

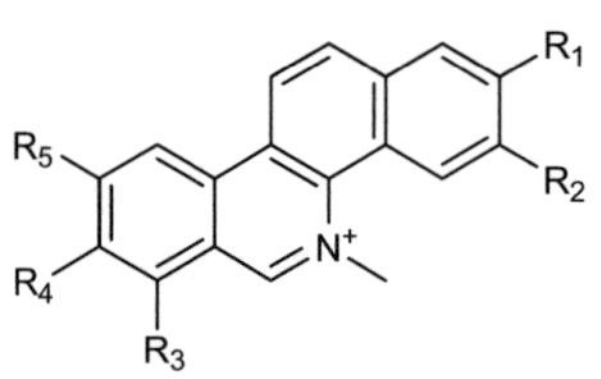

1: R_1 = OH; R_2 = OMe; R_3 = H; $R_4 = R_5$ = OMe
2: $R_1 + R_2 = OCH_2O$; R_3 = H; $R_4 = R_5$ = OMe
3: $R_1 + R_2 = OCH_2O$; $R_3 = R_4$ = OMe; R_5 = H
4: $R_1 + R_2 = R_3 + R_4 = OCH_2O$; R_5 = H

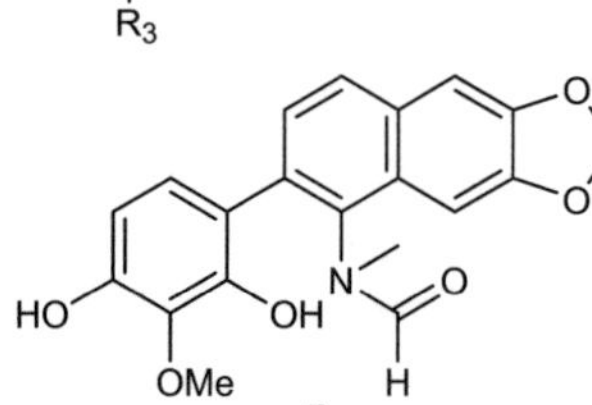

5

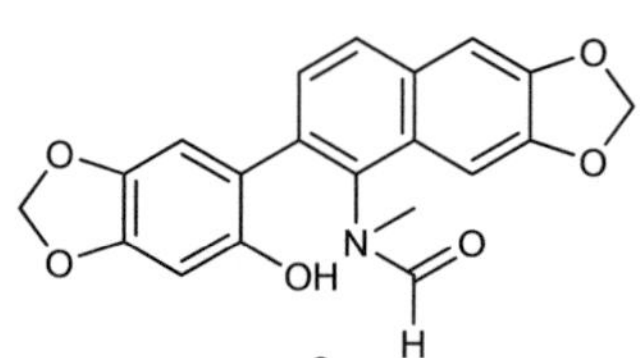

6

PLANT SPECIES	PART USED	POPULAR USES	FORM OF ADMINISTRATION	REFERENCES
Z. acanthopodium DC.	Fruits	As spice. Also has been used to heal stomach ache and toothache.	Oral route (dried fruits, decoction powder).	Suryanto et al., 2004
Z. ailanthoides Siebold.&Zucc.	Bark and fruits Tender leaves Steam	Epigastric pain, vomiting, diarrhea, abdominal pain, colds, snake bites. Substitute for the green onion in Chinese dishes. Myocardium disorder attenuation, cold resistance and bone-injury alleviation.	Local and oral routes (decoction or ointment). Oral route (chopped leaves) Oral route (macerated or decoction powder).	Sheen et al., 1994 Xiong & Shi, 1991 Chou et al., 2011
Z. alatum Roxb.	Fruits, branches and thorns Seeds Bark Fruits	Used as carminative, stomachic and as a remedy for toothache. Spice, aromatic tonic, stomachic and for fever, dyspepsia, cholera. Skin diseases, abdominal pain, anorexia, worm infestation. Mixed with salt for dyspepsia and headache.	Local and oral routes (macerated or decoction). Oral route (powdered seeds, macerated powder). Oral route (macerated or decoction powder). Oral route (dry fruit).	Batool et al., 2010
Z. americanum Mill.	All parts of the plant	To treat rheumatic conditions, toothaches, sore throats and burns, and as a tonic for various ailments.	Local and oral routes (macerated or decoction powder, paste, sticks).	Bafi-Yeboa et al., 2005
Z. armatum DC.	Fruits and seeds Bark, branches	Piscicide, aromatic tonic in fever, dyspepsia, and for expelling roundworms. Carminative, stomachic and	Oral route (Powder and decoction). Oral route (Infusion).	Ranawat et al., 2010 Ramanujam & Ratha, 2008

	and seeds	anthelmintic.		
Z. avicennae (Lam.) DC.	Branches and stems	Stomach tonic, to treat snake bites.	Oral route (Infusion).	Thuy et al., 1999
Z. beecheyanum K. Koch	Leaves	For treat bellyache and skin diseases.	Local and oral routes (macerated or decoction).	Cheng et al., 2004
Z. budrunga Wall.	Leaves Stem bark	Used for treating dyspepsia and some forms of diarrhea. Dysentery, coughs and headache.	Oral route (aqueous extract of the leaves) Oral route (bark juice).	Islam et al., 2001
Z. bungeanum Maxim.	Pericarps	Food condiment and seasoning in China. Treatment of vomiting, toothache, stomach ache and abdominal pain owing to roundworm.	Oral route (dried pericarps, macerated or decoction powder).	Gong et al., 2009
Z. capense (Thunb.) Harv.	Leaves	Treat fever, stomachache, flatulent colic, toothache and epilepsy.	Oral route (infusion)	Amabeoku & Kinyua, 2010
Z. caribeum Lam.	Leaves and stem bark	For asthma, spasm, fever, herpes and skin ulcers.	Oral route (macerated or decoction powder).	Schnee, 1984
Z. chalybeum Engl. *Z. chalybeum* Engl	Leaves Bark Roots	Treating severe colds and pneumonia. Malaria, colds, coughs, and dizziness. Chewed to alleviate toothaches. The Masai and Sonjo use this for small children by adding its juice to milk to give a better appetite. The decoction is given to sick goats, especially those suffering from diarrhea. Malaria, colds, coughs, toothache, sores, wounds and headache.	Local and oral routes (decoction powder, paste, sticks, juice). Local and oral routes (macerated or decoction powder, paste, sticks, juice). Local and oral routes (macerated or	Kamikawa et al., 1996 Matu & Staden, 2003 Nguta et al., 2010

	Fruits	Used in treatment of coughs.	decoction powder, paste, sticks, juice).	
Z. chiloperone var. *angustifolium* Engl.	Root bark	As antimalaric, emmenagogue and antirheumatic properties.	Oral route (decoction).	Ferreira et al., 2007
Z. davyi (I.Verd.) Waterm.	Leaves	To treat snakebite, severe coughs and colds and chest pains.	Local and oral routes (macerated or decoction).	Tarus et al., 2006
	Spines	Used for infected wounds.	Local routes (infusion or decoction material, paste).	
	Stem bark	Treat boils, pleurisy and toothache.		
	Root	Used for mouth ulcers, sore throats and as aphrodisiac.	Local and oral routes (macerated or decoction).	
	Root bark	Tonic both for man and animals and to treat toothache.	Local route (Root-bark decoctions)	
Z. dipetalum H. Mann var. *tomentosum*	Leaves and pericap	Insecticide - ovicidal.	Local route (decoction).	Marr & Tang, 1992
Z. dugandii Standl.	Bark	Diuretic and sudorific.	Oral route (decoction).	Schnee, 1984
Z. ekmanii (URB.) ALAIN.	Leaves and roots	For malaria, in vaginal washes and to relieve toothache.	Local and oral routes (decoction).	Facundo et al., 2005
Z. fagara (L.) Sarg.	Leaves, fruits and seeds	Used as sedative and sudorific.	Oral route (decoction).	Amaro et al., 1988
Z. gillettii (Wild) Waterm.	Leaves	Antihypertensive, analgesic and to treat gonorrhea.	Oral route (infusion).	Addae et al., 1989 Jirovetz et al., 1999 Adesina, 2005
	Wood	Used in house and boat-building, decorative paneling, joinery, construction of talking drums and in the paper and pulp industry.	Wood	
Z. hawaiiense Hbd.	Leaves and pericap	Insecticide - ovicidal.	Local route (decoction).	Marr & Tang, 1992
Z. hyemale A. St. Hil.	Leaves	As painkiller, sudorific, emetic and	Oral route (tea of leaves).	Guy et al., 2001

		to favor the salivation		
Z. integrifoliolum Merr.	Bark	Folk remedy for snake-bite by Ya-Mei aborigines.	Oral route (macerated or decoction powder).	Cheng et al., 2007
*Z. lemairie (*De Wild) Waterm.	Wood	House and boat-building, decorative paneling, joinery, construction of talking drums and in the paper and pulp industry.	Wood.	Adesina, 2005
Z. leprieurii Guill. et Perr.	Leaves	Used for traditional treatment of stomatitis, gingivitis, bilharzia.	Oral route (macerated or decoction powder).	Ngane et al., 2000
	Roots	As antiulcerative, antiseptic, urinary antiseptic, anti-sickler, antibacterial.	Local and oral routes (macerated powder, paste).	
	Stem barks	Used as antimicrobial, digestive aid, antidiarrheic, anticancerous, anti-odontologic and parasticide.	Local and oral routes; rectal injection (macerated or decoction powder, sticks).	Ngoumfo et al., 2010
	Fruits	Used as spices.	Oral route (dried fruits).	
	Wood	Used in house and boat-building, decorative paneling, joinery, construction of talking drums and in the paper and pulp industry.	Wood.	Adesina, 2005
Z. liebmanianum (Engler.) P. Wilson	Bark	Used to treat amebiasis, intestinal parasites, and as a local anesthetic.	Local and oral routes (decoction powder, sticks)	Navarrete, 1996 Arrieta et al., 2001
Z. limonella Alston.	Bark	Used as febrifugal, sudorific and diuretic.	Oral route (infusion, macerated powder).	Somanabandhu et al., 1992
Z. macrophylla Engl.	Bark and seeds	Used for toothache, colds, fever, malaria, stomachache, rheumatism and urogenital affections,	Local and oral routes (macerated or decoction powder, paste, sticks).	Kuete et al., 2011 Tringali et al., 2001

		as well as to prepare poisonous arrows.		
Z. monophyllum (Lam.) P. Wilson	Bark	Used as a colorant and to treat of runny nose, jaundice, ophthalmia and as an anesthetic.	Local and oral routes (macerated or decoction powder, paste, sticks).	Patiño & Cuca, 2011
Z. naranjillo Griseb.	Leaves	Preparations have been used to treat illness associated with inflammatory process.	Oral route (tea of leaves).	Bastos et al., 2001 Guy et al., 2001
Z. nitidum (Roxb.) DC	Fruits Root	Spice and in to treat stomachache, vomiting, diarrhea, cough, colic, and paresis and as an aromatic, stimulant and piscicide.	Oral route (dried fruits, infusion or decoction material). Local and oral routes (infusion or decoction material, paste).	Chen et al., 2011
Z. nitidum (Roxb.) DC	Branches, seeds and stem bark	Used in toothache, stomachache, fever, rheumatism, paresis, boils and as an insecticide and piscicide. Used in fever, diarrhea and cholera.	Oral route (infusion or decoction material).	Bhattacharya et al., 2009
Z. piperitum DC.	Pericarp All parts of the plant	Commonly used as a spice in Japan. Used to heal vomiting, diarrhea, and abdominal pain.	Oral route (ground pericarp) Oral route (macerated or decoction powder).	Lee & Lim, 2008 Yamazaki et al., 2007
Z. rhetsa Roxb.	Spines Seeds	Applied on the breast to give relief from pain and increase lactation in nursing mothers. Used as antiseptic, disinfectant, and for treat asthma, toothache and rheumatism.	Local route (paste prepared by rubbing the hard spines on a rock along with water). Local and oral routes (seeds oil, infusion or decoction material, paste).	Lalitharani et al., 2010 Reddy & Jose, 2011
Z. riedelianum Engl.		Used in different types of inflammations, rheumatism and skin stains.	Oral route (decoction)	Fernandes et al., 2009
Z. rigidum Humb. & Bonpl.	Wood	Used in building houses.	Wood	Moccelini et al., 2009

ex Willd.	Leaves	Used for toothache	Local route (ointment)	Schnee, 1984
Z. rhoifolium Lam.	Root bark	Used as a tonic, a febrifuge, against inflammatory and microbial processes, and in the treatment of malaria.	Oral route (infusion or decoction of roots bark).	Pereira et al., 2010
	Bark	Used to treat toothache and earache, also is used as an anti-venom serum, anti-tumor and in the treatment of hemorrhoids.	Oral route (decoction bark)	da Silva et al., 2007a
Z. schinifolium Sieb. & Zucc.	Leaves and ripe pericarp	Used as culinary applications and drugs for epigastric pain.	Oral route (macerated or decoction powder, crushed material).	Cao et al., 2009 Cui et al., 2009 Chang et al., 1997
Z. simulans Hance.	Roots	Used for snake bites and gastrointestinal disorders	Oral route (macerated powder).	Chen et al., 1994a Chen et al., 1994b
Z. tessmannii Engl.	Stem bark	Used for treat tumors, swellings, inflammation and gonorrhea.	Oral route (macerated or decoction powder).	Mbaze et al., 2007
	Root bark	Used as a toothbrush	Cleaning the teeth.	
	Wood	House and boat-building, joinery, decorative paneling and in the paper and pulp industry.	Wood	Adesina, 2005
Z. tetraspermum Wight and Arn.	Stem bark	Used for the treatment of dyspepsia, rheumatism and some forms of diarrhea.	Oral route (decoction).	Nissanka et al., 2001
Z. tingoassuiba A. St. Hil.	Stem bark	Antispasmodic, muscle relaxant, analgesic, sudorific, antifungal, diuretic, antiplatelet, antiparasitic and antihypertensive.	Oral route (teas or infusions).	Da Silva et al., 2008
Z. usambarense (Engl.) Kokwaro	Bark	Used to treat rheumatism.	Oral route (infusion or decoction powder).	Matu & Staden, 2003
	Young	Used as	Local route (cleaning	

	twigs	toothbrushes.	the teeth with twigs).	Nanyingi et al., 2008
	Seeds	For respiratory tract infections, malaria and catarrhal fevers.	Oral route (Grinding, hot decoction)	
Z. xanthoxyloides Waterm	Seeds	Condiment in Cameroon.	Oral route (crushed seeds)	
	Leaves and bark	Used against cough, fever, colds, toothache and snake bite.	Local and oral routes (infusion material, paste).	Kassim et al., 2009
	Leaves	As scaring and as antiseptic, astringent and laxative.	Local and oral routes (macerated or decoction).	
	Roots	Used as antiseptic, anti-sickler, digestive aid and parasticide. Also are generally used as chewing sticks for teeth cleaning.	Local and oral routes; rectal and vaginal injections (macerated or decoction powder, paste, sticks).	Ngassoum et al., 2003
Z. xanthoxyloides Waterm	Stem bark	Antirheumatic, anti-odontalgic, diurectic, urinary antiseptic, digestive aid and parasticide.	Local and oral routes (macerated or decoction powder, paste, sticks).	Ngane et al., 2000

Table 1. Main ethnobotanical uses of some species of the *Zanthoxylum* genus.

Benzylisoquinoline alkaloids have a restricted distribution in plants similar to that of benzophenanthridines. In the Rutaceae family they are present in a group of five genera named proto-Rutaceae (*Phellodendron, Fagaropsis, Tetradium, Toddalia* and *Zanthoxylum*) (Ling et al., 2009; Waterman, 2007). In the genus *Zanthoxylum* they are not the most common but have been found in some species, such as quaternary alkaloids (*R*)-(+)- isotembetarine **7** and (*S*)-(-)-xylopinidine **8** that have been isolated from the bark of *Z. quinduense* (Patiño & Cuca, 2010).

Berberine and **protoberberine alkaloids** have been reported in several species of the genus *Zanthoxylum*, for example tetrahydroberberines such as *N*-methyltetrahydrocolumbamine **9** and *N*-methyltetrahydropalmatine **10**, have been isolated from the bark of *Z. quinduense* (Patiño & Cuca, 2010). Berberine **11** is characterized by its significant leishmanicidal and antimicrobial activities and is usually the responsible for the yellowing observed in wood and bark of some species of this genus, as in the case of *Z. monophyllum* that is used as a dye (Patiño & Cuca, 2011).

In the genus *Zanthoxylum*, **aporphine alkaloids** there are not the most representative, but they have been isolated from various species and are of great importance because several have antitumoral activity (Adesina, 2005). For example, N,N-dimethyllindicarpine **12**, obtained from the root bark of *Z. zanthoxyloides* (Queiroz et al., 2006).

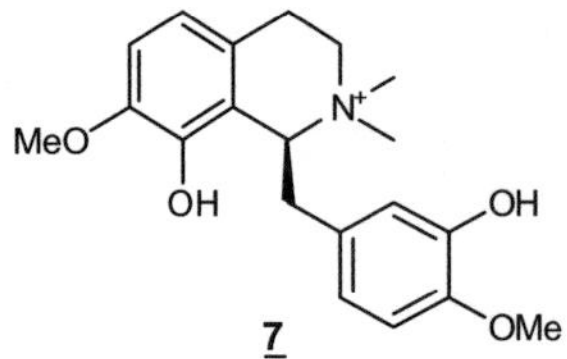

7

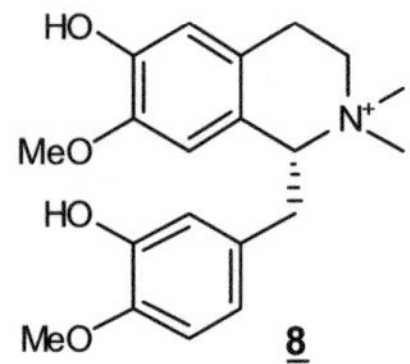

8

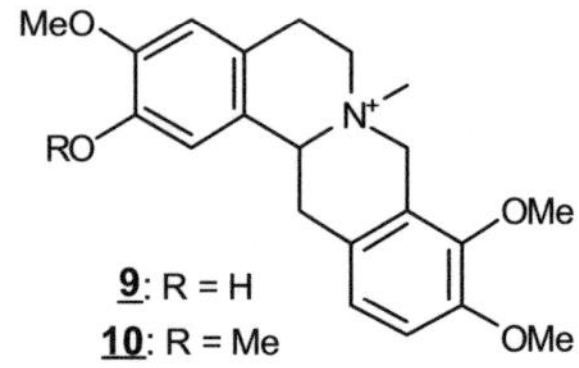

9: R = H
10: R = Me

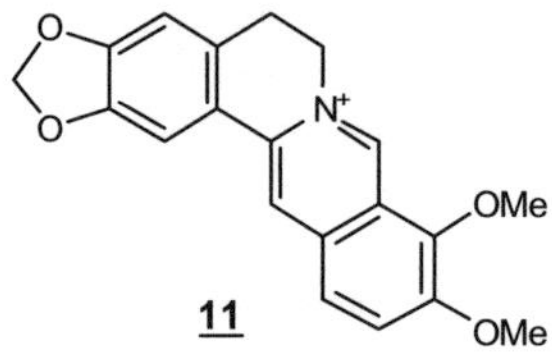

11

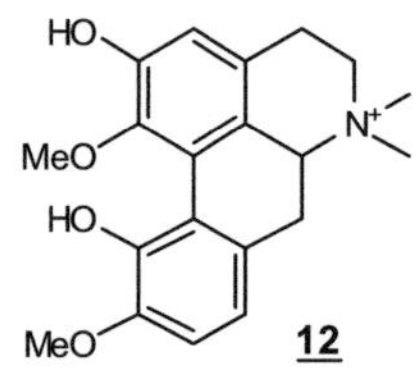

12

4.1.2 Quinoline alkaloids

Quinoline alkaloids are very common in the genus *Zanthoxylum*, usually have been found two types: furoquinolines and pyranoquinolines. Many of them are characterized by contain a carbonyl group in position 2 of the simple quinolinic nucleus and are called 2-quinolones (Waterman & Grundon, 1983). Alkaloids of this type have been isolated from the bark of Z. *budrunga* founding two pyranoquinoline: N-methylflindersine **13** and zanthobungeanine **14**, together with two furoquinolines dictamine **15** and skimmianine **16** (Rahman et al., 2005). From Z. *simulans* also have been isolated pyranoquinoline alkaloids as zhantosimulin **17** and huajiaosimulim **18**, with cytotoxic activity (Chen et al., 1997).

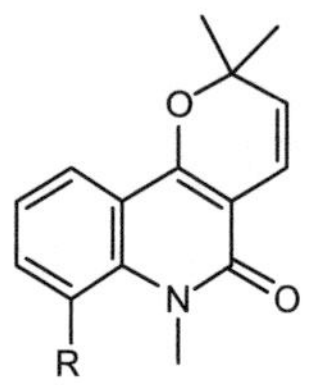

13: R = H
14: R = OMe

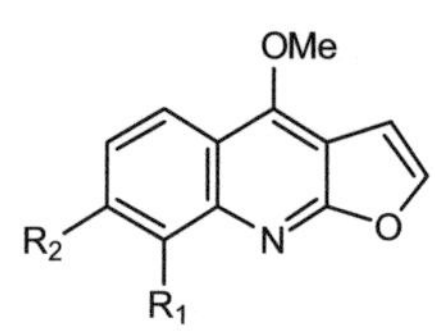

15: $R_1 = R_2 = H$
16: $R_1 = R_2 = OMe$

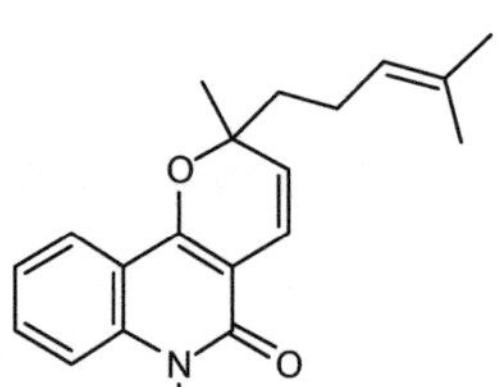

17

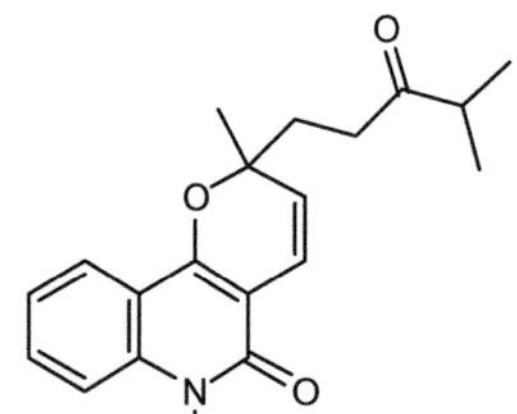

18

4.1.3 Other alkaloids

Bishoderninyl terpene, indolopyridoquinazoline, canthin-6-one, quinazoline and carbazole alkaloids, among others, are not very common in the genus *Zanthoxylum*, they have been found in some particular species. Bishoderninyl terpene alkaloids such as **19** have been isolated from the leaves of Z. *integrifoliolum* (Liu et al., 2000). Indolopyridoquinazoline alkaloids with significant antiplatelet activity as 1-hydroxyrutaecarpine **20**, rutaecarpine **21**, and 1-methoxyrutaecarpine **22** have been obtained from the fruits of Z. *integrifoliolum* (Sheen

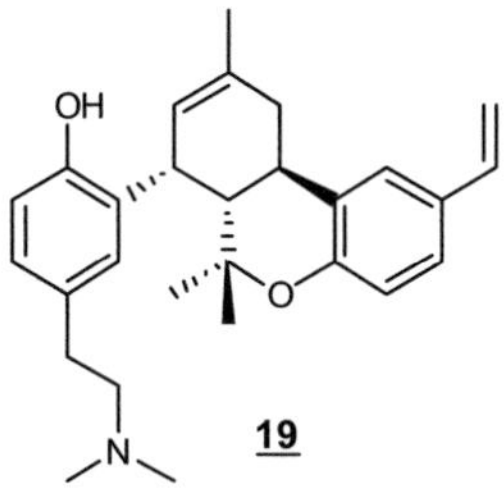

19

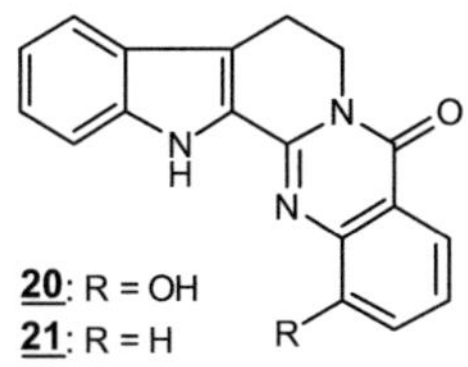

20: R = OH
21: R = H
22: R = OMe

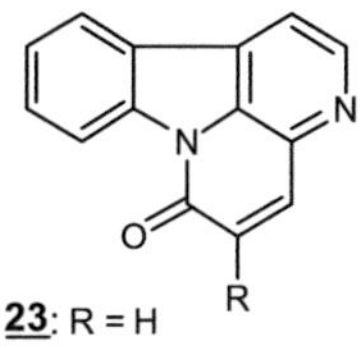

23: R = H
24: R = OMe

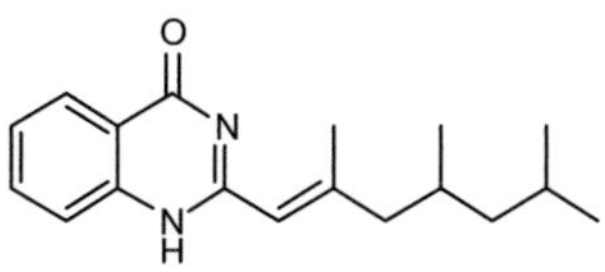

25

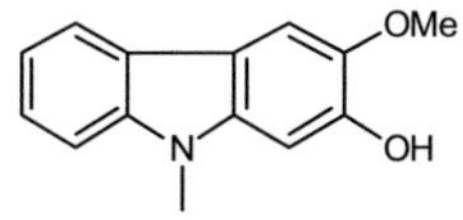

26

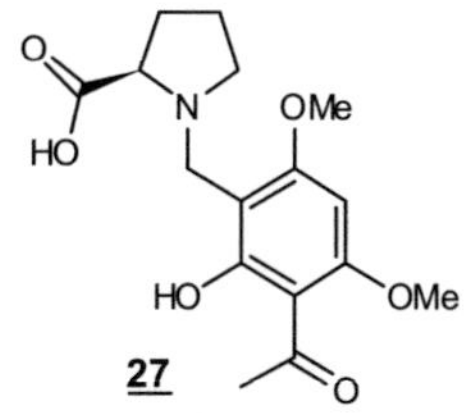

27

et al., 1996). Canthin-6-one alkaloids of importance for its leishmanicidal activity are rare in the family Rutaceae, are found in a few genders including *Zanthoxylum*. For example from *Z. rugosum* (Diehl et al., 2000), *Z. chiloperone* (Ferreira et al., 2002) and *Z. budrunga* (Rahman et al., 2005), have been isolated canthin-6-one **23** and 5-methoxycanthin-6-one **24**. Quinazoline alkaloids have been isolated from *Z. budrunga,* as is the case lunacridina **25** (Ahmad et al., 2003). Carbazole alkaloids such as 3-methoxy-9-methyl-9H-carbazol-2-ol **26** were obtained from the wood of *Z. rhoifolium* (Taborda & Cuca, 2007). Recently, from the bark of *Z. monophyllum* was isolated an alkaloid derived from proline, called monophyllidin **27** with antibacterial activity against *Enterococcus faecalis* (Patiño & Cuca, 2011).

4.2 Lignans

Lignans are also widely distributed in higher plants and have numerous biological activities among which include the antimicrobial, antioxidant, antitumor, antiviral, antihepatotoxic, antituberculous, insecticides and inhibit specifically certain enzymes. At the ecological level, there is the evidence that lignans play a role in plant-fungus, plant-plant and plant-insect interactions. Some lignans are toxic to fungi and insects. They are biogenetically derived by the oxidative dimerization of two C6-C3 units, that is, two characteristic phenylpropanoid units. The degree of oxidation and types of substituents determine the emerging lignan structure. There are also naturally occurring dimers that exhibit peculiar-type linkages. Different types of lignans has been described in a large number of plants from the Rutaceae family, but in the genus *Zanthoxylum* the lignans most reported have been of two types, diarylbutirolactones and 2,6-diaryl-3,7-dioxabicyclo[3.3.0]octanes. Neolignans also have been reported in some species of *Zanthoxylum* (Adesina, 2005; Waterman & Grundon, 1983).

Furofuranic lignans as syringaresinol **28** were obtained from *Z. quinduense* and *Z. monophyllum* (Patiño and Cuca, 2010; 2011). From *Z integrifoliolum* (Chen et al., 1999), *Z. culantrillo* (Cuca et al., 1998) and *Z. naranjillo* (Bastos et al., 1999) ha been isolated (+)-sesamin **29**. Diarylbutirolactonic lignans such as (-)-cubebin **30** with trypanocidal activity has been isolated from *Z. monophyllum* (Cuca et al., 1998) and *Z. naranjillo* (Bastos et al., 1999). A nor-neolignan, ailanthoidol **31**, was isolated from the wood of *Z. ailanthoides,* as tree used in folk medicine in Taiwan for the treatment of snake bite and the common cold (Sheen et al., 1994).

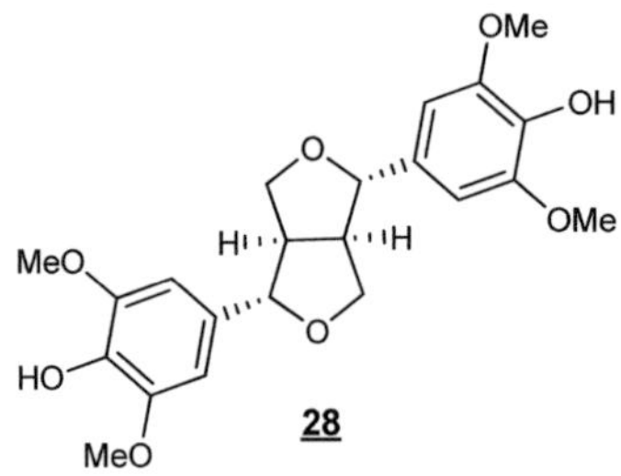

28

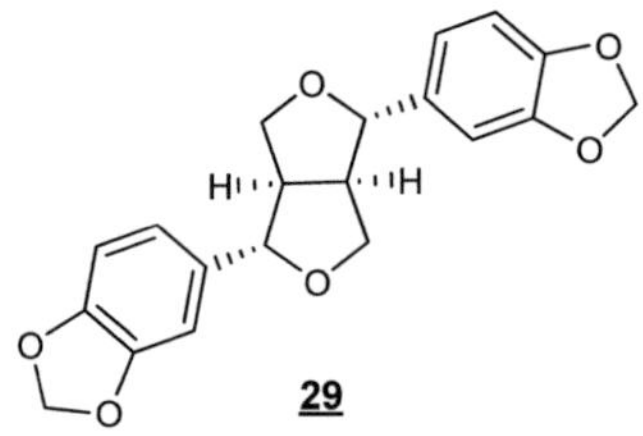

29

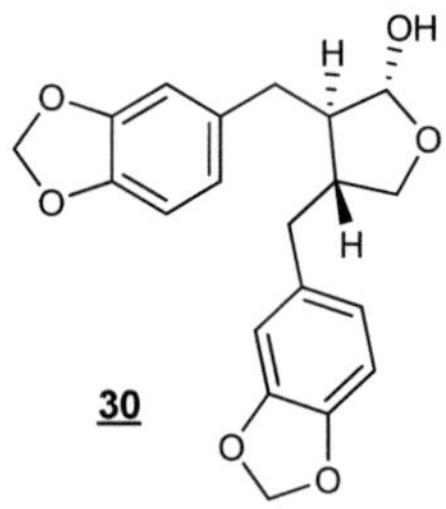

30

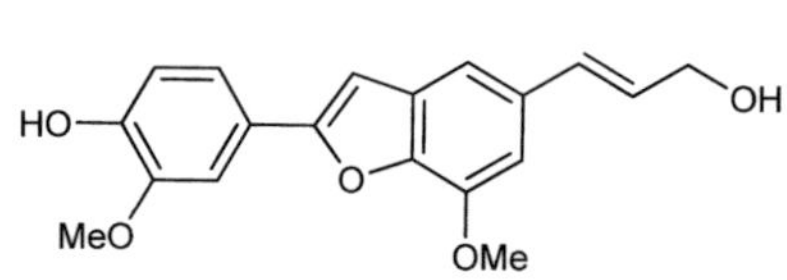

31

4.3 Coumarins

Biologically, coumarins are very useful and many of them have exhibited antibacterial, anti-tumour, vasodilatory (in coronary vessels) and anticoagulant activities. It was long noted that most coumarins are free from toxic side effects and may be given for years without side effects; overdose, however, causes haemorrhages (Murray et al., 1989). Coumarins are widespread in the Angiosperms but they are rather rare in Gymnosperms and lower plants. They are occur in great structural variety especially in the Apiaceae and Rutaceae and are additionally found in many other plants families like the Asteraceae, Poaceae and Rubiaceae (Ribeiro & Kaplan, 2002). The family Rutaceae belongs to the order Rutales characterized by the occurrence of coumarins in all families that comprise it. Coumarins, although are very frequent in the family as a whole, are confined to four sub-families (Aurantioideae, Flindersioideae, Toddalioideae and Rutoideae). In the subfamily Rutoideae is present the genus *Zanthoxylum*, which is characterized by the presence of different types of coumarins (simple, linear, dihydrofurocoumarins, furocoumarins and pyranocoumarins). The linear and angular dihydrofurocoumarins and precursors have been identified in several species of the genus, but angular dihydrofurocoumarins are not common in other species of the family Rutaceae, so it can be chemotaxonomic value for the genus *Zanthoxylum*. The fact that prenyl substitution at C-8 is much less frequent than that at C-6 could explain why angular furanocoumarins are rather rare in the Rutaceae (Murray et al., 1989; Waterman & Grundon, 1983).

From stem of *Z. shinifolium* was isolated larcinatin **32**, a terpenylcoumarin with significant inhibitory activity against the enzyme monoamine oxidase (MAO), which is one of the two isozymes, MAO-B is associated with Parkinson's disease (Jo et al., 2002). In studies done on this species, from the bark of *Z. schinifolium* were isolated auraptene **33** and collinine **34**, terpenylcoumarins with antiplatelet activity and inhibitory activity of DNA replication in hepatitis B virus (Tsai et al., 2000). Furanocoumarins with cytotoxic activity against human tumor cells have been found in berries of *Z. americanum*, for example psoralen **35** (Saquib et al., 1990).

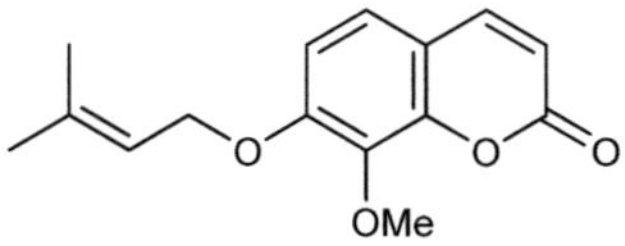

32

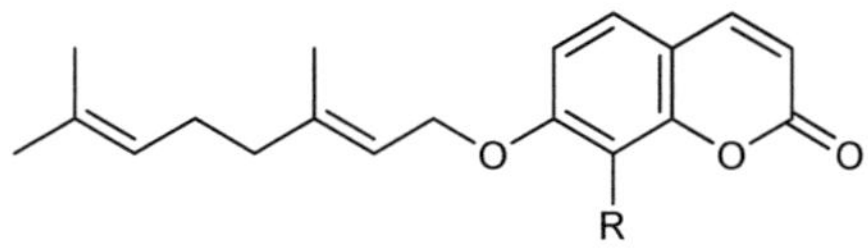

33: R = H
34: R = OMe

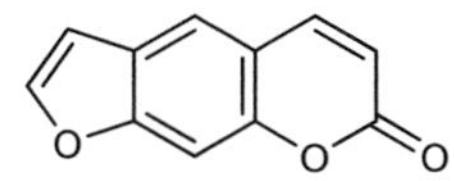

35

4.4 Amides

Amides are compounds that have chemotaxonomic importance for the genus *Zanthoxylum* and have been found mainly in the pericarp of the fruit, stems and roots of these species. The genus *Zanthoxylum* is characterized chemically by the frequent accumulation of olefinic alkamides (unsaturated aliphatic acid amides) and biogenetic capacity derived from the condensation of fatty acids such as linolenic and linoleic acids with isobutyl amines. Biologically, the isobutyl amides have been shown to have strong insecticidal properties. Alkamides have been used medicinally since ancient times as sialogogues, antitussive and analgesic and their presence in the *Zanthoxylum* genus may be of immense benefit to medicine (Adesina, 2005; Chaaib, 2004). An example of such amides is provided by the α-sanshool **36**, isolated from *Z. liebmannianum* and is known for its anthelmintic properties (Navarrete & Hong, 1996).

Other types of amides encountered in the *Zanthoxylum* genus are the aromatic amides described occasionally also as alkaloids or trans-cinnamoylamides. A typical example is the active antiplasmodial syncarpamide **37**, isolated from *Z. syncarpum* (Ross et al., 2004).

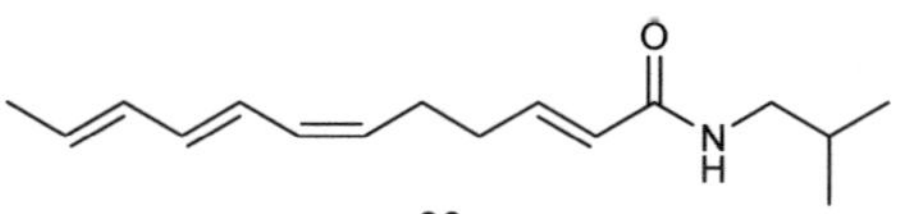

36

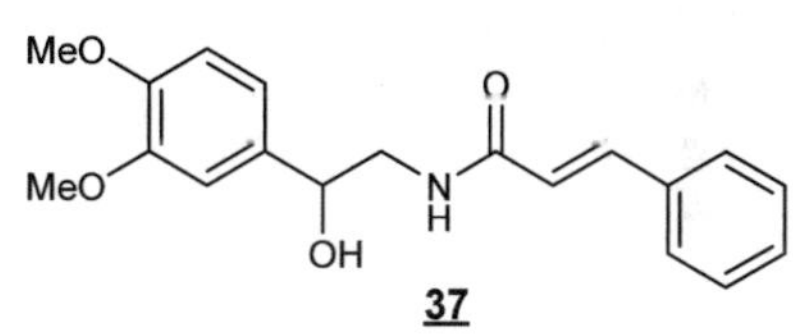

37

4.5 Flavonoids

Flavonoids are phenolic compounds widely available in this genus. They are present in almost all plant organs and play an important role in the antioxidant defense system. These secondary metabolites are known for their diverse biological properties, such as antioxidants, antiinflammatory, antithrombotic, antibacterial, antihepatotoxic, antitumor, antihypertensive, antiviral, antiallergic and estrogenic (Andersson et al. 1996; Harborne & Williams, 2000).

In *Zanthoxylum* genus, flavonoids are mainly represented by glycosides of flavones, flavonols and flavanones. Flavonoids found in the genus *Zanthoxylum*, like those isolated in other genera of the Rutaceae family are characterized to be polymethoxylated (Waterman & Grundon, 1983). Research carried out on fruits of *Z. integrifoliolum* lead to the isolation of 3,5-diacetyltambuline **38**, with significant antiplatelet activity (Chen et al., 1999).

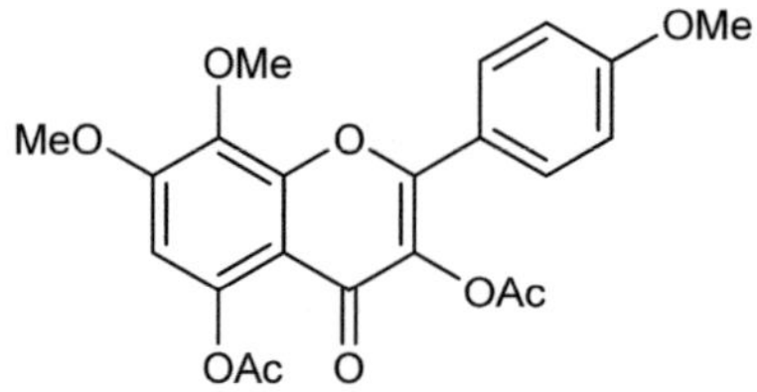

<u>**38**</u>

4.6 Terpenes and sterols

Most species belonging to the family Rutaceae contain glands that secrete volatile substances in different organs of plants such as fruits, leaves, bark, wood, roots, rhizomes and seeds. The essential oils obtained are often complex mixtures of monoterpenes and sesquiterpenes. *Zanthoxylum* genus accumulates volatile oils in leaves, flowers and fruits. Recently was determined the chemical composition of essential oils isolated from fruits of *Z. monophyllum*, *Z. rhoifolium* and *Z. fagara* by steam distillation, as well as were testing their antifungal and insecticidal activities. Gas chromatography-mass spectrometry (GC/MS) analysis allows identified 57 compounds. The main constituents in *Z. rhoifolium* oil were β-myrcene **39** (59.03%), β-phellandrene **40** (21.47%), and germacrene D **41** (9.28%), the major constituents of *Z. monophyllum* oil were sabinene **42** (25.71%), 1,8-cineole **43** (9.19%), and cis-4-thujanol **44** (9.19%), whereas fruit oil of *Z. fagara* mainly contained germacrene D-4-ol **459** (21.1%), elemol **46** (8.35%), and α-cadinol **47** (8.22%). *Z. fagara* showed the highest activity on *Colletotrichum acutatum* (EC$_{50}$ 153.9 μL L-1 air), and *Z. monophyllum* was the most active against *Fusarium oxysporum* f. sp. *lycopersici* (EC5$_0$ 140.1 μL L-1 air). *Z. monophyllum* essential oil showed significant fumigant activity against *Sitophilus oryzae* (Prieto et al., 2011).

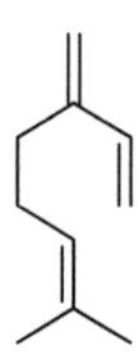

<u>**39**</u>

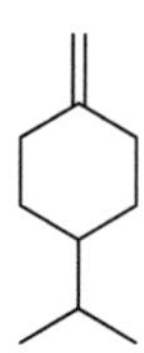

<u>**40**</u>

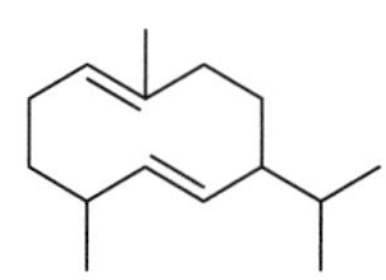

<u>**41**</u>

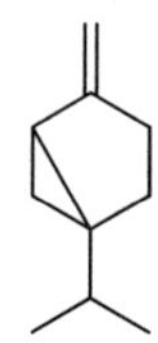

<u>**42**</u>

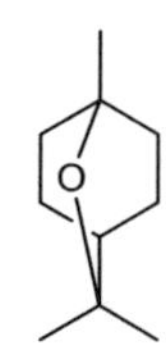

<u>**43**</u>

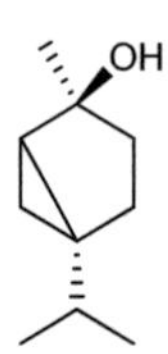

<u>**44**</u>

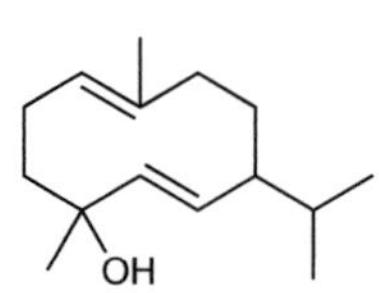

<u>**45**</u>

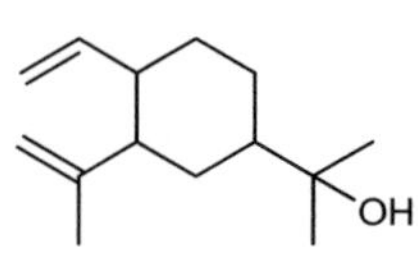

<u>**46**</u>

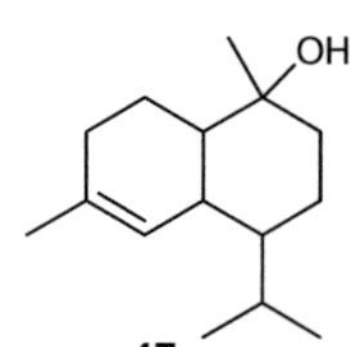

<u>**47**</u>

Sterols are common components of many plants and have been isolated from virtually all plants. Whereas β-sitosterol **48** appears ubiquitous in nature, the triterpene lupeol **49** appears restricted to the *Zanthoxylum* genus. Lupeol, β-sitosterol, usually associated with stigmasterol **50**, campesterol **51** and β-amyrin **52** have been isolated from the various morphological parts of the main species of *Zanthoxylum* studied (Adesina, 2005).

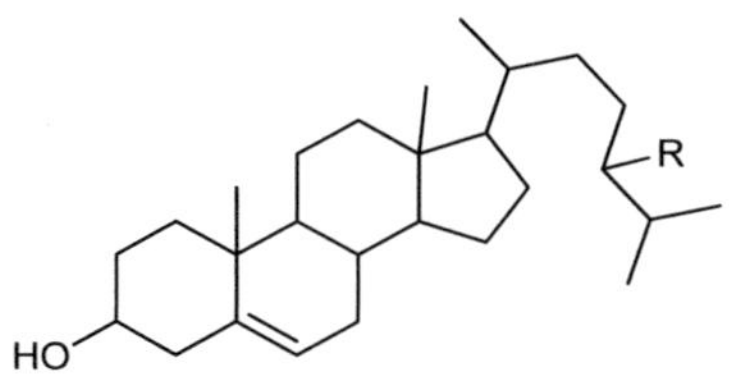

48: R = CH_2CH_3
50: R = CH_3

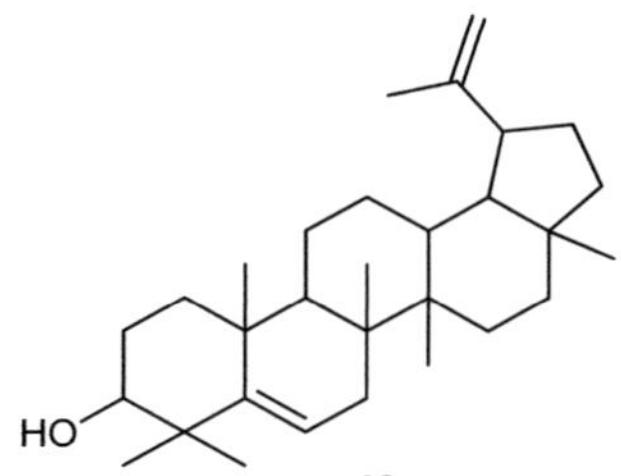

49

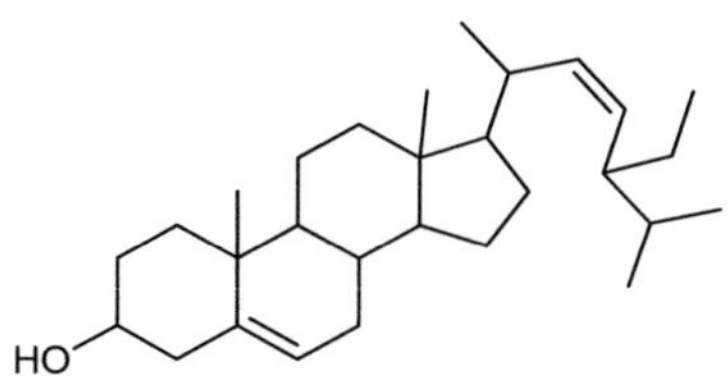

51

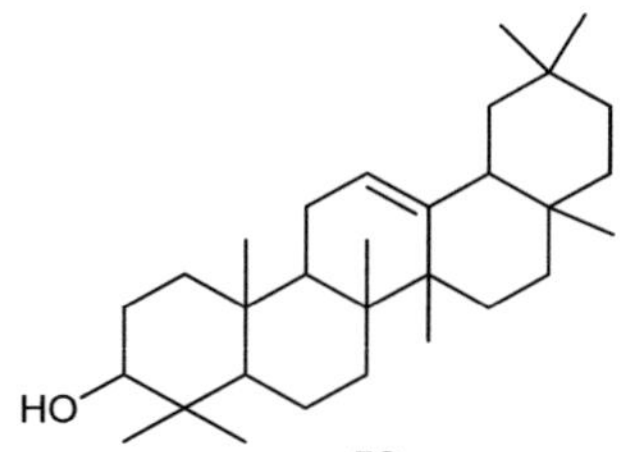

52

5. Biological activity of *Zanthoxylum* genus

As noted in previous sections, *Zanthoxylum* genus is well known for their chemical diversity and ethnobotanical properties, characteristics that have been the basis for developing various biological activity studies, which have helped to find new bioactive extracts and compounds, some of which have good potential for the development of new drugs and different industrial products.

The biological activities for certain species of the genus *Zanthoxylum* are mainly associated with the evaluation of antimicrobial, insecticidal, anti-inflammatory, antioxidant, antiparasitic, antitumor, antihelmitic, antinociceptive and antiviral activities, as well as studies of enzyme inhibition and effects on the central nervous system and cellular components of blood. The information in this section is organized by type biological activity, including the most representative results found for the genus *Zanthoxylum*.

5.1 Allelopathic activity

There are few reports on allelopathic activity of *Zanthoxylum* species. One report shows a bioguided fractionation of the ethyl acetate extract of the *Z. limonella* fruits led to the isolation of xanthoxyline, a substance with allelopathic effects of on Chinese amaranth (*Amaranthus tricolor* L.) and Barnyardgrass (*Echinochloa crus-galli* (L.) Beauv.). At a concentration of 2500 μM, xanthoxyline completely inhibited seed germination and growth of Chinese amaranth, and showed a significantly inhibitory effect on seed germination of Barnyardgrass by 43.59% (Charoenying et al., 2010).

5.2 Analgesic activity

Studies of analgesic activity in the genus *Zanthoxylum* have been focused mainly to validate its traditional uses. An example is the study of analgesic activity made with the aqueous extract of root bark of *Z. xanthozyloides*. This study showed that the extract induced analgesia, probably, by inhibiting prostaglandin production, because some isolated and purified alkaloids of the root bark of Z. *xanthoxyloides* have anti-prostaglandin synthetase activity (Prempeh & Mensah-Attipoe, 2008).

5.3 Anticonvulsant activity

The reports on anticonvulsant activity of *Zanthoxylum* species are few. A recent study of anticonvulsant activity was carried out with the methanol and aqueous extracts from leaves of Z. *capense*. In this report was investigated the effect of both extracts on seizures induced by pentylenetetrazole, bicuculline, picrotoxin, N-methyl-DL-aspartic acid and strychnine in mice. Both extracts showed significant activity in the tests carried out with the five seizures inducing agents, finding that these substances in some cases delay seizures and in some cases act as agonists (Amabeoku & Kinyua, 2010).

5.4 Antihelmitic activity

Antihelmitic activity studies have been advanced mainly in the specie Z. *xanthoxyloides*. Two recent studies reveal that acetone: water (70:30) and ethanol extracts from leaves of Z. *xanthoxyloides* showed promising activity against *Asaris lumbricoides, Haemonchus contortus, Trichostrongylus colubriformis*, three nematodes that of these nematodes provokes production losses, clinical signs and even can lead to deaths in sheep or goats worldwide (Azando et al., 2011; Barnabas et al., 2011).

5.5 Anti-inflamatory activity

The anti-inflammatory effects of the extracts and isolated compounds of some *Zanthoxylum* species have been evaluated employed mainly four methods: 1) paw edema induced by carragenin in rats; 2) ear edema induced by phorbol myristate acetate (PMA), arachidonic acid (AA) and 12-o-tetradecanoyl-phorbol acetate (TPA) in mice; 3) inhibition of superoxide anion generation and 4) elastase release in fMLP/CB-activated human neutrophils in a concentration-dependent manner. In different studies, ethanolic extracts of bark from Z. *elephantiasis*, Z. *fagara*, Z. *martinicense* and Z. *coriaceum*, and hexane, ethyl acetate and ethanolic extracts of leaf from Z. *chiloperone* have presented promising results of anti-inflammatory activity (Villalba et al., 2007; Márquez et al., 2005; Bastos, 2001).

Other studies involving phytochemical and biological activity reported the isolation of various secondary metabolites with anti-inflammatory activity. From the hexane extract of Z. *naranjillo* was isolated a dibenzylbutirolactonic lignan (cubebin) with antiinflammatory properties (Bastos et al., 2001). In the methanol extract of stem wood from Z. *nitidum* were identified benzophenanthridine alkaloids, quinolone alkaloids, lignans and coumarins with promising anti-inflammatory activity (Chen et al., 2011). For the methanol extract of stem wood of Z. *integrifoliolum* and Z. *avicennae* have been reported the presence of phenylpropenoids, lignans, coumarins, quinolone alkaloids and quinoline alkaloids with anti-inflammatory potential (Chen et al., 2008; Chen et al., 2007).

One compound which has gained wide attention of medical professionals, pharmaceutical marketers and researchers all around the world is a dietary triterpene knows as lupeol. This compound is found in most species of the genus presented *Zanyhoxylum*, and has been extensively studied for its inhibitory effects on inflammation under in vitro and in animal models of inflammation (Saleem, 2009).

5.6 Antimicrobial activity

Most reports of biological activity of the *Zanthoxylum* genus are related to the evaluation of antimicrobial activity. This activity has been evaluated mainly using human pathogenic strains, with few cases in which phytopathogenic strains are used. Most studies of antimicrobial activity have been made using disk diffusion method. Here are some examples of antimicrobial activity studies performed with species of the genus *Zanthoxylum*.

The antifungal and antibacterial activities of some compounds isolated from *Z. tessmannii* were determined against *Bacillus subtilis, Escherichia coli, Staphylococcus aureus, Streptomyces viridochromogenes, Mucor miehei, Candida albicans, Chlorella vulgaris, Chlorella sorokiniana and Scenedesmus subspicatus*. 2,6-dimethoxy-1,4-benzoquinone showed activities against seven of the nine strains employed, while *3β*-acetoxy-*16β*-hydroxybetulinic acid showed weak activities against *Bacillus subtilis* and *Escherichia coli*, and *3β, 16β*-hydroxybetulinic acid showed weak activities against *Bacillus subtilis* and *Candida albicans* (Mbaze et al., 2007).

The fruits extract of *Z. armatum* has been tested for their antibacterial activity against *S. aureus, E. coli, Pseudomonas aeruginosa* and *Shigella boydii*. This ethanolic extract was inactive against *P. aeruginosa,* while showed positive activity on the other three strains. These results indicate that the ethanolic extract from fruits of *Z. armatum* may have broad spectrum antibacterial activity because it shows activity against *Gram*-positive and *Gram*-negative bacteria (Panthi & Chaudhary, 2006).

The essential oils of *Z. xanthoxyloides* and *Z. leprieurii*, two Cameroonian plants used as spices in local food, showed antibacterial and antifungal activity against *E. coli, S. aureus, Klebsiella pneumoniae, Enterococcus faecalis, Corynebacterium glutamicum, B. cereus, B. subtilis* and *Aspergillus flavus* (Tatsadjieu et al., 2003).

Aqueous, hexane and methanol extracts of leaves, roots and stem bark obtained from *Z. chalybeum* and *Z. usambarense* were screened for in-vitro antibacterial activity using *Gram*-positive bacteria (*B. subtilis, Micrococcus luteus* and *S. aureus*). The root and stem-bark extracts of the two *Zanthoxylum* species showed high antibacterial activity (Matu & Staden, 2003).

Aqueous, hexane and methanol extracts of leaves, roots and stem bark obtained from *Z. chalybeum* and *Z. usambarense* were screened for in vitro antibacterial activity using *Gram*-positive bacteria (*B. subtilis, Micrococcus luteus* and *S. aureus*). The root and stem-bark extracts of the two *Zanthoxylum* species showed high antibacterial activity (Matu & Staden, 2003).

Ethanolic extracts of bark of *Z.fagara, Z. elephantiasis* and *Z.martinicense* were evaluated against *C. albicans, Saccharomyces cerevisiae, Aspergillus niger, A. flavus, Microsporum canis* and *Trichophyton mentagrophytes* to determined their antifungal activity. All of the extracts assayed showed activity against common dermatophytes of domestic animals, the one being most significant is that exhibited by the ethanolic extract of the bark of *Z. fagara* (Diéguez-Hurtado et al, 2003).

Leaf, fruit, stem, bark and root extracts of *Z. americanum* were investigated for antifungal activity with 11 strains of fungi. All extracts demonstrated a broad spectrum of antifungal activity and inhibited at least eight fungal species, being the fruit and leaf extracts the most active in general. The results provide a basis for the very widespread use of *Z. americanum* in indigenous North American ethnomedical tradition for conditions that may be related to fungal infections (Bafi-Yeboa et al., 2005).

Chelerythrine, N-methyltetrahydrocolumbamine, N-methyltetrahydropalmatine and berberine, four alkaloids isolated from *Z. quinduense*, have exhibited promising antibacterial activity against different *Gram*-positive and *Gram*-negative bacteria, being chelerythrine the most active compound, showing an antibacterial activity comparable to that of the antibiotics kanamycine, tetracycline and anthracycline (Patiño et al., 2011).

5.7 Antinociceptive activity

In order to contribute towards the pharmacological knowledge about *Zanthoxylum* genus, as well as demonstrate the popular uses of some species as a painkiller, have been advanced antinociceptive activity studies with extracts of hexane, ethyl acetate and ethanol obtained from leaves of *Z. chilipirone* and with stem bark ethanolic extract (EtOH), its fractions of partition (hexane, ethyl acetate, aqueous) and lupeol obtained of *Z. rhoifolium*, employing animal models of chemically induced acute pain. The study carried out with *Z. chilipirone* shows that with doses of 100 and 200 mg/kg of each extract is possible to detect significantly inhibition in the paw lick, results that suggest that the extracts from *Z. chiloperone* possess constituents with antinociceptive activity (Villalba et al., 2007). Moreover, the study with extracts of *Z. rhoifolium* sought to confirm its popular use, and shows for the first time that ethanol extract of *Z. rhoifolium* stem bark, its fractions and one of the major constituents (lupeol) have antinociceptive activity when administered orally in different models of chemical nociception in mice (Pereira et al., 2010).

5.8 Antioxidant activity

To determine the antioxidant activity of substances isolated from species of *Zanthoxylum* genus have been used more than ten methods, most based on the determination of free radical scavenging activity. The most common methods are: 1) Total phenolic content; 2) DPPH radical scavenging assay; 3) ABTS radical scavenging activity and 4) superoxide anion scavenging assay.

Studies of antioxidant activity of *Zanthoxylum* species have been advanced mainly extracts from fruits and seeds. For example, the essential oil of seeds of *Z. bungeanum* (Xia et al., 2011), the ethanol extract of fruits of *Z. alatum* (Batool et al., 2010); extracts of hexane, ethyl ether, ethyl acetate and methanol obtained from fruits of *Z. piperitum* (Lee & Lim, 2008; Hisatomi et al., 2000), as well as extracts of hexane, acetone and ethanol from fruits of *Z. achanthopodium* (Suryanto et al., 2004), have demonstrated an interesting antioxidant power.

In a study made by Yamazaki and co-workers shows the isolation of two glycosylated flavonoids (hyperoside and quercitrin) of methanol extract from fruits of *Z. piperitum*, these substances scavenged DPPH radical strongly with IC_{50} values of 16 and 18 μM, respectively (Yamazaki et al., 2007).

5.9 Antiparasitary activity

In the frame of the search for new leads against the most neglegted parasitic diseases, it is of particular interest to evaluate the antimalarial, trypanocidal and antileishmanial potencial of some of the most frequently traditional drugs used.

The information on the frequently utilized antimalarial plant species is an important lead to the species that can be targeted for pharmacological, toxicological and phytochemical tests. The most important antimalarial properties have been observed in alkaloids, sesquiterpene lactones, coumarins, triterpenoids and limonoids. *Z. chalybeum*, *Z. syncarpum*, *Z. zanthoxyloides*, *Z. gilletii*, *Z. limonella*, *Z. rhoifolium* and *Z. usambarense*, among others, are some of the species of *Zanthoxylum* genus that have showed interesting antimalarial properties.

Zanthoxylum chalybeum root bark (IC_{50} of 4.2μg/ml) and some quinoline alkaloids isolated from this species have been exhibited strong antiplasmodial activity on chloroquine resistant *Plasmodioum falciparum* strain (Nguta et al., 2010). Syncarpamide and decarine, two compounds isolated from *Z. syncarpum* have showed strong in vitro antiplasmodial activity against D6 (chloroquine sensitive clone) and W2 (chloroquine resistant clone) *P. falciparum* strains, having IC_{50} values lower than 6.1 μM (Kaur *et al.*, 2009; Ross et al., 2005; Ross et al., 2004). The crude alkaloid extract obtained from the bark of *Z. zanthoxyloides* and fagaronine, a benzophenanthridine alkaloid derived from the root extract of *Z. zanthoxyloides*; inhibited *P. falciparum* growth in vitro at low IC_{50} (Adebayo & Krettli, 2011; Gansane et al., 2010). Also have been reported positive results of antimalarial activity for the ethanolic extract from stem bark of *Z. guilletti* (Zirihi et al, 2009) and for the chloroform crude extract from fruits of *Z. limonella* (Charoenying et al., 2008).

Anti-plasmodial activity of stem bark extracts from *Z. usambarense* was performed against *P. knowlesi* and *P. berghei*. The aqueous extract was remarkably active against the two parasites, while all organic solvents extracts being inactive. These results suggest that the antiplasmodial activity of *Z. usambarense* is due mainly to polar substances (Were et al., 2010).

A study of antimalarial properties of *Z. rhoifolium* bark carried out in order to validate its use and confirm the previously detected in vivo activity, lead to the isolation of antimalarial compounds. The antiplasmodial activity of *Z. rhoifolium* bark was concentrated in the alkaloid fractions showed approximately 44% inhibition of *P. falciparum* growth at 10μg/mL, using LDH micromethod. Three of the seven isolated compounds from alkaloidal fraction displayed antiplasmodial activity, ranging from good (nitidine, the most potent compound) to moderate (avicine and fagaridine) (Jullian et al., 2006). In other research of the antiplasmodial activity of *Z. rhoifolium* was determined that the water infusion from bark inhibited more than 50% the *P. falciparum* development with doses higher than 500 mg/kg (Bertani et al, 2005).

Recently, has been reported the trypanocidal effect of ethanolic extracts of leaves, fruits, stem bark and root bark, canthin-6-one alkaloids and some of its analogs obtained from *Z. chiloperone*, using *in vitro* methods and the mouse model of acute or chronic infection to evaluate the trypanocidal activity. These results demonstrate the anti-*Trypanozoma* activity of canthinones. Additionally, considering the low toxicity of canthin-6-one, is possible to propose this natural product as a possible advantageous phytotherapeutic compared to the current chemotherapy of Chagas disease (Ferreira et al., 2011; Ferreira et al., 2007). In a study carried out with the hexane extract from leaves of *Z. naranjillo* seven lignans were isolated and evaluated as trypanocidals. Four of the seven lignans showed trypanocidal activity in an *in vitro* assay, being (-)-methylpluviatolide the most active compound (Bastos et al., 1999).

Canthin-6-one alkaloids have exhibited interesting antileishmanial activity. For example, in a study carried out with the alkaloidal extract of *Z. chiloperone* stem bark reported that this extract inhibited the growth of *Leishmania braziliensis, L. amazonensis* and *L. donovani* at 100 μg/mL and mentioned that the compounds canthin-6-one and 5-methoxy-canthin-6-one were the two major active constituents (Ferreira et al., 2002). Also has been reported that meglumine antimonate isolated from *Z. chiloperone* showed activity against *L. amazonensis* at dose of 28 mg/kg (Sen & Chatterjee, 2011).

5.10 Antiplatelet activity

The methanolic extract of the stem of *Z. beecheyanum* showed strong antiplatelet activity in vitro using the turbidimetric method. In washed rabbit platelets, thrombin (0.1 U/mL), arachidonic acid (AA 100 M), collagen (100 g/mL), and PAF (2 ng/mL) all caused about 90-95% aggregation.

5.11 Antiviral activity

Zanthoxylum species were used in experiments to test their influence on inhibition of multiplication of porcine epidemic diarrhea virus (PEDV). The extracts of *Z. coreanum* root, *Z. planispinum* leaf and stem, *Z. schinifolium* leaf exhibited antiviral activity with the IC_{50} of 1.0, 6.4, 7.5 and 3.7 μg/mL against PEDV, respectively.

In an anti-HIV screening program, three *Zanthoxylum* species, including the root bark of *Z. ailanthoides*, the root wood of *Z. integrifoliolum*, and the stem bark of *Z. scandens* showed anti-HIV activity. The anti-HIV principles of *Z. ailanthoides* have already been proved to be two alkaloids (decarine and fagarine) and an aromatic amide ((+)-tembamide). Thus, the former two constituents, decarine and fagarine, also isolated of *Z. integrifoliolum*, can be considered as the anti-HIV constituents of the root wood of this species.

5.12 Citotoxic activity

Cancer is the leading cause of death worldwide. Finding a cure for this disease is always an important objective for human endeavor. Natural products have long been considered as potential drug candidates for cancer prevention and treatment (Chou et al., 2011). *Zanthoxylum* species are potential sources for find new antitumor agents, because diverse substances obtained from some of this species have showed strong citotoxic activity against different tumor cell lines. Following are some examples of reports about citotoxic activity of some species of *Zanthoxylum* genus.

The anti-tumor properties of the volatile oil from *Z. rhoifolium* leaves and some terpenes (α-humulene, β-caryophyllene, α-pinene and β-pinene) were investigated in vitro and in vivo using the Ehrlich ascites tumor model. Volatile oil and β-caryophyllene exhibited little direct activity against Ehrlich tumor cells in vitro, while α-humulene, α-pinene and β-pinene did not such activity. Additionally, volatile oil exhibits anti-tumor efficacy and significative immunomodulatory action *in vivo*, which may be related to β- caryophyllene associated to the synergism of other natural compounds presented in volatile oil from *Z. rhoifolium* leaves (Da Silva et al., 2007a). Other study about the citotoxic activity of essential oil from leaves of

Z. rhoifolium permitted to confirm that the essential oil is cytotoxic against tumoral cells (CD_{50} = 82.3, 90.7 and 113.6 µg/ml for A-549 (human lung carcinoma), HeLa (human cervical carcinoma) and HT-29 (human colon adenocarcinoma) cell lines, respectively), while it did not show cytotoxicity against non-tumoral cells (Vero and mice macrophages). Thus, the essential oil from *Z. rhoifolium* leaves seems to present a possible therapeuthic role due to its selective cytotoxic activity against tumoral cell lines (Da Silva et al., 2007b).

The chloroform-soluble fraction of the crude extract of leaves from *Z. ailanthoides* showed cytotoxic activity against human promyelocytic leukemia (HL-60) and myelomonocytic leukemia (WEHI-3) cells with IC_{50} values of 73.06 and 42.22 µg/mL, respectively. From this fraction were obtained four pheophorbide derivatives, where three of these compounds showed cytotoxic activities against both leukemia cells with IC_{50} value in the range of 46.76–79.43 nM (Chou et al., 2011).

The chemical investigation carried out with roots and fruits of *Z. leprieurii* led to the isolation of four acridone derivatives alkaloids were found to be moderately active against lung carcinoma cells (A549), colorectal adenocarcinoma cells (DLD-1) and normal cells (WS1) with IC50 values ranging from 27 to 77 µM (Kuete et al., 2011; Ngoumfo et al., 2010).

A chemical and citotoxic studies of the root bark of *Z. simulans* led the isolation of two citotoxic pyranoquinoline alkaloids (zanthosimuline and huajiaosimulin). These compounds were evaluated against thirteen cultured human cancer cell lines, where zanthosimuline was active against all cell lines employed, while huajiaosimulin only was active against six of the thirteen cell lines (Chen et al., 1994b).

Benzophenanthridine alkaloids are secondary metabolites commonly isolated from species of *Zanthoxylum* genus and are characterized by their potent antitumor activity, being fagaronine and nitidine the most active substances (Tillequin, 2007). Hexahydrobenzophenanthridine alkaloids are also of interest for its cytotoxic activity. Currently the alkaloid chelidonin is used in experimental oncology as the main component of Ukrain ®, an anti-cancer medicament (McManus, et al., 2007).

Berberine, an alkaloid isolated from the bark of *Z. monophyllum* showed activity against HT-29 (colorectal cancer), MCF-7 (breast cancer), HEp-2 (larynx cancer) and MKN-45 (gastric cancer) cell lines (Cordero et al., 2004). Nitidine chloride and 6-methoxy-5,6-dihydronitidine, two benzophenanthridine alkaloids isolated from *Z. macrophylla* seeds also have exhibited antitumor activity against different human cell lines (Kuete et al., 2011).

6. Conclusions

Zanthoxylum genus has proven to be a very valuable genus to the discovery and utilization of medicinal and agrochemical natural products. The collected information provides a means to understand the latest developments in the biological activity and phytochemistry of the genus. The potential for development of leads from *Zanthoxylum* continues to grow, particularly in the development of new antiparasitary, antitumor and antimicrobial agents. The information summarized here is intended to serve as a reference tool to people in all fields of ethnobothany, pharmacology and natural products chemistry.

7. References

Addae-Mensah, I., Munenge, R., Guantai, A. N. (1989). Comparative Examination of two *Zanthoxylum* Benzophenanthridine Alkaloids for Cardiovascular Effects in Rabbits. *Phytotherapy Research*, 3, 165-169. ISSN: 1099-1573.

Adebayo, J. O., Krettli, A. U. (2011). Potential antimalarials fron Nigerian Plants: A review. *Journal of Ethnopharmacology*, 133, 289-302. ISSN: 0378-8741.

Adesina, S. K. (2005). The Nigerian *Zanthoxylum*: Chemical and Biological Values. *African Journal of Traditional, Complementary and Alternative medicines*, 2, 282-301. ISSN: 0189-6016.

Agrios, G. (2005). *Plant Pathology* (5th Edition). Elsevier Academic Press. ISBN: 978-0-12-044565-3, USA. pp. 4-5.

Ahmad, M. U., Rahman, M. A., Hug, E., Chowdhury, R. (2003). Alkaloids of *Zanthoxylum budrunga*. *Fitoterapia*, 74, 191-193. ISSN: 0367-326X.

Amabeoku, G. J., Kinyua, C. G. (2010). Evaluation of the Anticonvulsant of *Zanthoxylum capense* (Thunb.) Harv. (Rutaceae) in Mice. *International Journal of Pharmacology*, 6 (6), 844-853. ISSN: 1811-7775.

Amaro-Luis, J. M., Fronczek, F. R., Massanet, G. M., Pando, E., Rodriguez-Luis, F., Watkins, S. F., Zubia, E. (1988). Meridinol, a Lignan from *Zanthoxylum fagara*. *Phytochemistry*, 27, 3933-3935. ISSN: 0031-9422.

Andersson, C. M., Halberg, A., Hogberg, T. (1996). Advances in the Development of Pharmaceutical Antioxidants. *Advances in Drug Research*, 28, 65-180. ISBN: 0-12-013326-1.

Arrieta, J., Reyes, B., Calzada, F., Cedillo-Rivera, R., Navarrete, A. (2001). Amoebicidal and Giardicidal Compounds from the Leaves of *Zanthoxylum liebmannianum*. *Fitoterapia*, 72, 295-297. ISSN: 0367-326X.

Azando, E. V. B., Hounzangbé-Adoté, M. S., Oloundadé, P. A., Brunet, S., Fabre, N., Valentin, A., Hoste, H. (2011). Involvement of tannins and flavonoids in the *in vitro* effects of *Newbouldia laevis* and *Zanthoxylum zanthoxyloïdes* extracts on the exsheathment of third-stage infective larvae of gastrointestinal nematodes. *Veterinary Parasitology*, 180, 292-297. ISSN: 0304-4017.

Bafi-Yeboa, N. F. A., Arnason, J. T., Baker, J., Smith, M.L. (2005). Antifungal constituents of Northern prickly ash, *Zanthoxylum americanum* Mill. *Phytomedicine*, 28, 370-377. ISSN: 0944-7113.

Barnabas, B. B., Man, A., Ogunrinola, T. S., Anyanwu, P. E. (2011). Screening for Anthelminthic Activities from Extracts of *Zanthoxylum Zanthoxyloides*, *Neocarya Macrophylla* and *Celosia Laxa* Against Ascaris Infection in Rabbits. *International Journal of Applied Research in Natural Products*, 3 (4), 1-4. ISSN : 19406223.

Bastos, J. K., Carvalho, J. C. T., de Souza, G. H. B., Pedrazzi, A. H. P., Sarti, S. J. (2001). Anti-inflammatory activity of cubebin, a lignan from the leaves of *Zanthoxylum naranjillo* Griseb. *Journal of Ethnopharmacology*, 75, 279-282. ISSN: 0378-8741.

Bastos, J. K., Albuquerque, S., Silva, M. L. A. (1999). Evaluation of the Tripanocidal Activity of lignans Isolated from the Leaves of *Zanthoxylum naranjillo*. *Planta Medica*, 65, 541-544. ISSN: 0032-0943.

Batool, F., Mubashir, S., Rocha, J. B. T., Hussain, A., Saied, Z., Dilnawaz, S. (2010). Evualuation of Antioxidant and Free Radical Scavenging Activities of Fruit Extract from *Zanthoxylum alatum*: A Commonly Used Spice from Pakistan. *Pakistan Journal of Botany*, 42 (6), 4299-4311. ISSN: 2070-3368.

Bertani, S., Bourdy, G., Landau, I., Robinson, J. C., Esterre, Ph. Deharo, E. (2005). Evaluation of French Guiana traditional antimalarial remedies. *Journal of Ethnopharmacology*, 98, 45-54. ISSN: 0378-8741.

Bhattacharya, S., Zaman, K.., Ghosh, A. K. (2009). Histological and Physico-chemical Evaluation of *Zanthoxylum nitidum* Stem Bark. *Ethnobotanical Leaflets*, 13, 540-547. ISSN: 1948-3570.

Cao, L. H., Lee, Y. J., Kang, D. G., Kim, J. S., Lee, H. S. Effect of *Zanthoxylum schinifolium* on TNF-α-induced vascular inflammation in human umbilical vein endothelial cells. *Vascular Pharmacology*, 50, 200-207. ISSN: 1537-1891.

Chaaib, K. F. (2004). Investigation Phytochimique d'une Brosse à Dents Africaine *Zanthoxylum zanthoxyloides* (Lam.) Zepernick et Timler (Syn. *Fagara zanthoxyloides* L.) (Rutaceae). Thèse de doctorat. Faculté des Sciences de l'Université de Lausanne. pp. 11-44.

Chang, Y.-C., Hsieh, P.-W., Chang, F. R., Wu, R.-R., Liaw, C.-C., Lee, K.-H., Wu, Y.-C. (2003). Two New Protopine Argemexicaines A and B and the Anti-HIV Alkaloid 6-Acetonyldihydrochelerythrine from Formosan *Argemone mexicana*. *Planta Medica*, 69, 148-152. ISSN: 0032-0943.

Chang, C-T., Doong, S-L., Tsai, I-L., Chen, I-S. (1997). Coumarins and Anti-HBV Constituents from *Zanthoxylum schinifolium*. *Phytochemistry*, 45 (7), 1419-1422. ISSN: 0031-9422.

Charoenying, P., Teerarak, M., Laosinwattana, C. (2010). An allelopathic sibstance isolated from *Zanthoxylum limonella* Alston fruit. *Scientia Horticulturae*, 125, 411-416. ISSN: 0304-4238.

Charoenying, P., Laosinwattana, C., Phuwiwat, W., Lomratsiri, J. (2008). Biological Activities of *Zanthoxylum limonella* Alston Fruit Extracts. *KMITL Science Journal*, 8 (1), 12-15.

Chase, M. W., Morton, C. M., Kallunki, J. A. (1999). Phylogenetic Relationships of Rutaceae: a Cladistic Analysis of the Subfamilies Using Evidence from *rbcL* and *atpB* Sequence Variation. *American Journal of Botany*, 86, 1191-1199. ISSN: 1537-2197.

Chen, J-J., Lin, Y-H., Day, S-H., Hwang, T-L., Chen, I-S. (2011). New benzenoids and anti-inflammatory constituents from *Zanthoxylum nitidum*. *Food Chemistry*, 125, 282-287. ISSN: 0308-8146.

Chen, J-J., Wang, T-Y., Hwang, T-L. (2008). Neolignans, a Coumarinolignan, Lignan Derivatives, and a Chromene: Anti-inflammatory Constituents from *Zanthoxylum avicennae*. *Journal of Natural Products*, 71, 212-217. ISSN: 0163-3864.

Chen, J-J., Chen, P-H., Liao, C-H., Huang, S-Y., Chen, I-S. (2007). New Phenylpropenoids, Bis(1-phenylethyl)phenols, Bisquinolinone Alkaloid, and Anti-inflammatory Constituents from *Zanthoxylum integrifoliolum*. *Journal of Natural Products*, 70, 1444-1448. ISSN: 0163-3864.

Chen, I.-S., Chen, T. L., Chang, Y.-L., Teng, C.-M., Lin, W.-Y. (1999). Chemical Constituents and Biological Activities of the Fruit of *Zanthoxylum integrifoliolum*. *Journal of Natural Products*, 62, 833 -837. ISSN: 0163-3864.

Chen, I. S., Tsai, I.-W., Teng, C.-M., Chen, J.-J., Chang, Y.-L., Ko, F.-N., Lu, M. C., Pezzuto, J. M. (1997). Piranoquinolines Alkaloids from *Zanthoxylum simulans*. *Phytochemistry.*, 46, 525-529. ISSN: 0031-9422.

Chen, I.-S., Wu, S.-J., Lin, Y.-C., Tsai, I.-L., Seki, H., Ko, F.-N., Teng, C.-M. (1994a) Dimeric 2-Quinolone Alkaloids and Antiplatelet Aggregation Constituents of *Zanthoxylum simulans*. *Phytochemistry*, 36, 237-239. ISSN: 0031-9422.

Chen, I-S., Wu, S-J., Tsai, I-L., Wu, T-S., Pezzuto, J. M., Lu, M. C., Chai, H., Shu, N., Teng, C-M. (1994b). Chemical and bioactive constituents from *Zanthoxylum simulans*. *Phytochemistry*, 57 (9), 1206-1211. ISSN: 0031-9422.

Cheng, M-J., Lin, C-F., Wang, C-J., Tsai, I-L., Chen, I-S. (2007). Chemical Constituents from the Root Wood of *Zanthoxylum integrifoliolum*. *Journal of the Chinese Chemical Society*, *54*, 779-783. ISSN: 0009-4536.

Cheng, M-J., Wu, C-C., Tsai, I-L., Chen I-S. (2004). Chemical and Antiplatelet Constituents from the Stem of *Zanthoxylum beecheyanum*. *Journal of the Chinese Chemical Society*, 51, 1065-1072. ISSN: 0009-4536.

Chou, Z-T., Chan, H-H., Peng, H-Y., Liou, M-J., Wu, T-S. (2011). Isolation of substances with antiproliferative and apoptosis-inducing activities against leukemia cells from the leaves of *Zanthoxylum ailanthoides* Sieb. & Zucc. *Phytomedicine*, 18, 344-348. ISSN: 0944-7113.

Colegate, S. M., Molyneux, R. J. (2008). An Introduction and Overview. In: *Bioactive Natural Products: Detection, Isolation, and Structural Determination* (2nd Edition). S. M. Colegate, R. J. Molyneux. pp. 1-3. CRC Press. ISBN: 0849343720, New York.

Cordell, A. G. (1981). *Introduction to Alkaloids -A Biogenetic Approach.* John Wiley & Sons. ISBN: 0471034789, New York. pp. 509-517.

Cordero, C. P., Gómez-González, S., León-Acosta, C. J., Morantes-Medina, S. J., Aristizabal, F. A. (2004). Cytotoxic activity of five compounds from Colombian plants. *Fitoterapia*, 75, 225-227. ISSN: 0367-326X.

Cragg, G. M., Kingston, D. G. I., Newman, D. J. (2005). *Anticancer Agents from Natural Products*. Taylor & Francis Group, ISBN: 0849318637, New York. pp. 1-3.

Cuca, L. E., Martinez, J. C., Monache, F. D.(1998). Constituyentes Químicos de *Zanthoxylum monophyllum*. *Revista Colombiana de Química*, 27, 17-27. ISSN: 0120-2804.

Cui, H. Z., Choi, H. R., Choi, D. H., Cho, K. W., Kang, D. G., Lee, H. S. (2009). Aqueous extract of *Zanthoxylum schinifolium* elicts contractile and secretory responses via β_1-adrenoceptor activation in beating rabbit atria. *Journal of Ethnopharmacology*, 126, 300-307. ISSN: 0378-8741.

Da Silva, C. V., Detoni, C. B., da Silva, E., da Silva, M. L. (2008). Alcalóides e Outros Metabólitos do Caule e Frutos de *Zanthoxylum tingoassuiba* A. ST. HIL. *Quimica Nova*, 31 (8), 2052-2055. ISSN 0100-4042.

Da Silva, S. L., Figueredo, P. M. S., Yano, T. (2007a). Chemotherapeutic potential of the volatile oils from *Zanthoxylum rhoifolium* Lam leaves. *European Journal of Pharmacology*, 576, 180-188. ISSN: 0014- 2999.

Da Silva, S. L., Figueredo, P. M., Yano, T. (2007b). Cytotoxic evaluation of essential oil from *Zanthoxylum rhoifolium* Lam. leaves. *Acta Amazonica*, 37 (2), 281-286. ISSN: 0044-5967.

Da Silva, S. L., Figueredo, P. M. S., Yano, T. (2006). Antibacterial and Antifungal Activities of Volatile Oils from *Zanthoxylum rhoifolium* Lam. Leaves. *Pharmaceutical Biology*, 44, 657-659. ISSN: 1744-5116.

Diéguez, R., Garrido, G., Prieto, S., Iznaga, Y., González, L., Molina, J., Curini, M., Epifano, F., Marcotullio, M. C. (2003). Antifungal activity of some Cuban *Zanthoxylum* species. *Fitoterapia*, 74, 384-386. ISSN: 0367-326X.

Diehl, E. E., Poser, G. L., Henriques, A. T. (2000). Constituents of *Zanthoxylum rugosum* St.-Hil & Tul. *Biochemical Systematic and Ecology*, 28, 275-277. ISSN: 0305-1978.

Dupont, C., Couillerot, E., Gillet, R., Caron, C., Zeches-Hanrot, M., Riou J.-F., Trentesaux, C. (2005). The Benzophenanthridine Alkaloid Fagaronine Induces Erytroleukemic Cell Differentation by Gene Activation. *Planta Medica*, 71, 489- 494. ISSN: 0032-0943.

Dvořák Z., Kubáň V., Klejdus B., Hlaváč J., Vičar J., Ulrichová J., Šimánek V. (2006). Quaternary Benzo[*c*]phenanthridines Sanguinarine and Chelerythrine: A Review of Investigations from Chemical and Biological Studies. *Heterocycles*, 68, 2403-2422. ISSN: 0385-5414.

Eun, J.-P., Koh, G. Y. (2004). Suppression of Angiogenesis by the Plant Alkaloid, Sanguinarine. *Biochemical and Biophysics Research Communications*, 317, 618-624. ISSN: 0006-291X.

Facundo, V. A., Pinto, A. S., Filho, R. B., Pinto, A. C., Rezende, C. M. (2005). Constituintes Químicos de *Zanthoxylum ekmanii* (URB.) ALAIN. *Quimica Nova*, 28 (2), 224-225. ISSN 0100-4042.

Fernandes, C. C., Vieira, P. C., da Silva, V. C., Dall'Oglio, E. L., da Silva, L. E., de Sousa, P. T. (2009). 6-Acetonyl-N-methyl-dihydrodecarine, a New Alkaloid from *Zanthoxylum riedelianum*. *Journal of Brazilian Chemical Society*, 20 (2), 379-382. ISSN: 0103-5053.

Ferreira, M. E., Cebrián-Torrejón, G., Corrales, A. S., Vera, N., Rolón, M., Vega, C., Leblanc, K., Yaluf, G., Schinini, A., Torres, S., Serna, E., Rojas, A., Poupon, E., Fournet, A. (2011). *Zanthoxylum chiloperone* leaves extract: First sustainable Chagas disease treatment. *Journal of Ethnopharmacology*, 133, 986-993. ISSN: 0378-8741.

Ferreira, M. H., Nakayama, H., Rojas, A., Schinini, A., Vera, N., Serna, E., Lagoutte, D., Soriano-Agatón, F., Poupon, E., Hocquemiller, R., Fournet, A. (2007). Effects of canthin-6-one alkaloids from *Zanthoxylum chiloperone* on *Trypanosoma cruzi*-infected mice. *Journal of Ethnopharmacology*, 109, 258-263. ISSN: 0378-8741.

Ferreira, M. E., Rojas, A., Torres, S., Inchausti, A., Nakayama, H., Thouvenel, C., Hocquemiller, R., Fournet, A. (2002). Leishmanicidal Activity of Two Canthin-6-one Alkaloids, Two Major Constituents of *Zanthoxylum chiloperone* var. *angustifolium*". *Journal of Ethnopharmacology*, 80, 199-202. ISSN: 0378-8741.

Gansane, A., Sanon, S., Ouattara, P. L., Hutter, S., Ollivier, E., Azas, N., Traore, A., Traore, A. S., Guissou, I. P., Nebie, I., Sirima, B. S. (2010). Antiplasmodial Activity and Citotoxicity of Semi Purified Fractions from *Zanthoxylum zanthoxyloides* Lam. Bark of Trunk. *International Journal of Pharmacology*, 6 (6), 921-925. ISSN: 1811-7775.

Gong, Y., Huang, Y., Zhou, L., Shi, X., Guo, Z., Wang, M., Jiang, W. (2009). Chemical Composition and Antifungal Activity of the Fruit Oil of *Zanthoxylum bungeanum* Maxim.(Rutaceae) from China. *Journal of Essential Oil Research*, 21, 174-178. ISSN: 1041-2905.

Gonzaga, W. A., Weber, A. D., Giacomelli, S. R., Dalcol, I. I., Hoelzel, S. C. S., Morel, A. F. (2003). Antibacterial alkaloids from *Zanthoxylum rhoifolium*. *Planta Medica*, 69, 371-374. ISSN: 0032-0943.

Global Biodiversity Information Facility: Biodiversity occurrence data, In: *GBIF Data Portal*. March 20, 2010, Available from: http://data.gbif.org/species/.

Guy, I., Charles, B., Guinaudeau, H. (2001). Essential Oils from Leaves of Two Paraguayan Rutaceae: *Zanthoxylum hyemale* A. St. Hil. And *Z. naranjillo* Griseb. *Journal of Essential Oil Research*, 13, 200-201. ISSN: 1041-2905.

Harbone, J. B., Williams, C. A. (2000). Advances in Flavonoid Research since 1992. *Phytochemistry*, 55, 481-504. ISSN: 0031-9422.

Hisatomi, E., Matsui, M., Kobayashi, A., Kubota, K. (2000), Antioxidative Activity in the Pericaprp and Seed of Japanese Pepper (*Xanthoxylum piperitum* DC). *Journal of Agricultural and Food Chemistry*, 48, 4924-4928. ISSN: 0021-8561.

Islam, A., Sayeed, A., Bhuiyan, M.S.A., Mosaddik, M.A., Islam, M. A. U., Astaq Mondal Khan, G. R. M. (2001). Antimicrobial activity and citotoxicity of *Zanthoxylum budrunga*. *Fitoterapia*, 72, 428-430. ISSN: 0367-326X.

Jirovetz, L., Buchabauer, G., Fleischhacker, W., Ngassoum, M. B. (1999). Analysis of Leaf Volatiles of *Zanthoxylum gillettii* Used in Folk Medicine of Cameroon. *Planta Medica*, 65, 181-183. ISSN: 0032-0943.

Jo, Y. S, Huong, D. T. L., Bae, K., Lee, M. K., Kim, Y. H. (2002). "Monoamine Oxidase Inhibitory Coumarin from *Zanthoxylum schinifolium*". *Planta Medica*. 68, 84-85. ISSN: 0032-0943.

Jullian, V., Bourdy, G., Georges, S., Maurel, S., Sauvain, M. (2006). Validation of use of a traditional remedy from French Guiana, *Zanthoxylum rhoifolium* Lam. *Journal of Ethnopharmacology*, 106, 348-352. ISSN: 0378-8741.

Kamikawa, T., Hanaoka, Y., Fujie, S., Saito, K. Yamagiwa, Y., Fukuhara, K., Kubo, I. (1996). SRS-A Antagonist Pyranoquinolone Alkaloids from East African *Fagara* Plants and their Synthesis. *Bioorganic & Medicinal Chemistry*, 4 (8), 1317-1320. ISSN: 09680896.

Kassim, O. O., Loyevsky. M., Amonoo, H., Lashley, L., Ako-Naic, K. A., Gordeuk, V. R. (2009). Inhibition of in-vitro growth of *Plasmodium falciparum* by *Pseudocedrela kotschyi* extract alone and in combination with *Fagara zanthoxyloides* extract. *Transactions of the Royal Society of Tropical Medicine and Hygiene*, 103, 698-702. ISSN: 0035-9203.

Kaufman, P. B., Kirakosyan, A., McKenzie, M., Dayanandan, P., Hoyt, J. E., Li , C. (2006). The Uses of Plant Natural Products by Humans and Risks Associated with Their Use. In *Natural Products from Plants*. L. Cseke, A. Kirakosyan, P. Kaufman, S. Warber, J. Duke, H. Brielmann. pp. 442–468. CRC Taylor & Francis, ISBN: 0849329760, New York..

Kaur, K., Jain, M., Kaur, T., Jain, R. (2009). Antimalarials from nature. *Bioorganic & Medicinal Chemistry*, 17, 3229-3256. ISSN: 09680896.

Krane, B. D., Fagbule, M. O., Shamma, M. (1984). The Benzophenanthridine Alkaloids. *Journal of Natural Products*, 47, 1-43. ISSN: 0163-3864.

Kuetea, V., Krusche, B., Youns, M., Voukeng, I., Fankama, A. G., Tankeo, S., Lacmata, S., Efferth, T. (2011). Cytotoxicity of some Cameroonian spices and selected medicinal plant extracts. *Journal of Ethnopharmacology*, 134, 803-812. ISSN: 0378-8741.

Lalitharani, S., Mohan, V. R., Regini, G. S. (2010). GC-MS analysis of ethanolic extract of *Zanthoxylum rhetsa* (ROXB.) DC spines. *Journal of Herbal Medicine and Toxicology* 4, 1, 191-192, ISSN : 0973-4643.

Lee, S-J., Lim K-T. (2008). Glycoprotein of *Zanthoxylum piperitum* DC has a hepatoprotective effect via anti-oxidative character *in vivo* and *in vitro*. *Toxicology in Vitro*, 22, 376-385. ISSN: 0887-2333.

Ling, K.-H., Wang, Y., Poon, W.-S., Shaw, P.-S., But, P. P.-H. (2009). The Relationship of *Fagaropsis* and *Luvunga* in Rutaceae. *Taiwania*, 54, 338-342. ISSN: 0372333X.

Liu, S.-L., Tsai, I.-L., Ishikawa, T., Harayama, T, Chen, I. S. (2000) .Bishordeninyl Terpene Alkaloids from *Zanthoxylum integrifoliolum*. *Journal of Chinese Chemical Society*, 47, 571-574. ISSN: 0009- 4536.

Maiti, M., Kumar, G. S. (2007). Molecular Aspects on the Interaction of Protoberberine, Benzophenanthridine, and Aristolochia Group of Alkaloids with Nucleic Acid Structures and Biological Perspectives. *Medical Care Research and Review*, 27, 649-695. ISSN: 1552-6801.

Maiti, M., Kumar, G. S. (2009). Biophysical Aspects and Biological Implications of the Interaction of Benzophenanthridine Alkaloids with DNA. *Biophysical Reviews and Letters*, 1, 119-129. ISSN: 1793-0480.

Márquez, L., Agüero, J., Hernández, I., Garrido, G., Martínez, I., Diéguez, R., Prieto, S., Rivas, Y., Molina-Torres, J., Curini, M., Delgado, R. (2005). Anti-inflammatory Evaluation and Phytochemical Characterization of some Plants of the *Zanthoxylum* genus. *Acta Farmaceutica Bonaerense*, 24 (3), 325-330. ISSN: 03262383.

Marr, K. L., Tang, C. S. (1992). Volatile Insecticidal Compounds and Chemical Variability of Hawaiian *Zanthoxylum* Rutaceae Species. *Biochemical Systematic and Ecology*, 20, 209-217. ISSN: 0305-1978.

Matsuhashi, R., Satou, T., Koike, K., Yokosuka, A., Mimaki, Y., Sashida, Y., Nikaido, T. (2002). Nematocidal Activity of Isoquinoline Alkaloids Against a Species of Diplogastridae. *Planta Medica*, 68, 169-171. ISSN: 0032-0943.

Matu, E. N., Staden, J. (2003). Antibacterial and anti-inflamatory activities of some plants used for medicinal purposes in Kenya. *Journal of Ethnopharmacology*, 87, 35-41. ISSN: 0378-8741.

Mbaze, L. M., Poumale, H. M. P., Wansi, J. D., Lado, J. A., Khan, S. N., Iqbal, M. C., Ngadjui, B. T., Laatsch, H. (2007). α-Glucosidase inhibitory pentacyclic triterpenes from the stem bark of *Fagara tessmannii* (Rutaceae). *Phytochemistry*, 68, 591-595. ISSN: 0031-9422.

McManus, H. A., Fleming, M. J., Lautens, M. (2007). Enantioselective Total Synthesis of (+)-Homochelidonine by a Pd^{II}-Catalyzed Asymmetric Ring-Opening Reaction of a *meso*-Azabicyclic Alkene with an Aryl Boronic Acid. *Angewandte Chemie International Edition*, 46, 433-436. ISSN: 1521-3773.

Melo, M. F. F., Zickel, C. S. (2004). Os Gêneros *Zanthoxylum* L. e *Esenbeckia* Kunth (Rutaceae) no Estado de Pernambuco, Brasil. *Acta Botanica Brasilica*, 18, 73-90. ISSN: 0102-3306.

Moccelini, S. K., da Silva, V. C., Ndiaye, E. A., de Sousa, P. T., Vieira, P. C. (2009). Estudo Fitoquímico das Cascas das Raízes de *Zanthoxylum rigidum* Humb. & Bonpl. Ex Willd (Rutaceae). *Quimica Nova*, 32 (1), 131-133. ISSN: 0100-4042.

Murray, R.D.H., Méndez, J., Brown, S.A. (1982). The *Natural Coumarins. Ocurrence, Chemistry and Biochemistry*. John Wiley & Sons LTD. pp. 343-345. ISBN: 0471280577, Chichester.

Nanyingi, M. O., Mbaria, J. M., Lanyasunya, A. L., Wagate, C. G., Koros, K. B., Kaburia, H. F., Munenge, R. W., Ogara, W. O. (2008). Ethnopharmacological survey of Samburu district, Kenya. *Journal of Ethnobiology and Ethnomedicine*, 4, 1-12. ISSN: 1746-4269.

Navarrete, A., Hong. E. (1996). Anthelmintic Properties of α-Sanshool from *Zanthoxylum liebmannianum*. *Planta Medica*, 62, 250-251. ISSN: 0032-0943.

Newman, D. J., Cragg, G. M. (2007). Natural Products as Sources of New Drugs over the Last 25 Years. *Journal of Natural Products*, 70, 461–477. ISSN: 0163-3864.

Ngane, A. N., Biyiti, L., Amvam, P. H., Bouchet, Ph. (2000). Evaluation of antifungal activity of extracts of two Cameroonian Rutaceae: *Zanthoxylum leprieurii* Guill. et Perr. and *Zanthoxylum xanthoxyloides* Waterm. *Journal of Ethnopharmacology*, 70, 335-342. ISSN: 0378-8741.

Ngassoum, M. B., Essia-Ngang, J. J., Tatsadjieu, L. N., Jirovetz, L., Buchbauer, G., Adjoudji, O. (2003). Antimicrobial study of essential oils of *Ocimum gratissimum* leaves and *Zanthoxylum xanthoxyloides* fruits from Cameroon. *Fitoterapia*, 74, 284-287. ISSN: 0367-326X.

Ngoumfo, R. M., Jouda, J-B., Mouafo, F.T., Komguem, J., Mbazoa, C. D., Shiao, T. C., Choudhary, M. I., Laatsch, H., Legault, J., Pichette, A., Roy, R. (2010). In vitro cytotoxic activity of isolated acridones alkaloids from *Zanthoxylum leprieurii* Guill. et Perr. *Bioorganic & Medicinal Chemistry*, 18, 3601-3605. ISSN: 0960-894X.

Nguta, J. M., Mbaira, J. M., Gakuya, D. W., Gathumbi, P. K., Kiama, S. G. (2010). Antimalarial herbal remedies of Msambweni, Kenya. *Journal of Ethnopharmacology*, 128, 424-432. ISSN: 0378-8741.

Nissanka, A. P., Karunaratne, V., Bandara, B. M. R., Kumar, V., Nakanishi, T., Nishi, M., Inada, A., Tillekeratne, L. M., Wijesundara, D. S. A., Gunatilaka, A. A. (2001). Antimicrobial Alkaloids from *Zanthoxylum tetraspermum* and *caudatum*. *Phytochemistry*, 56, 857-861. ISSN: 0031-9422.

Nwaka, S., Hudson, A. (2006). Innovative Lead Discovery Strategies for Tropical Diseases. *Nature Reviews Drug Discovery*, 5, 941-955. ISSN: 1474-1784.

Nyangulu, J. M., Hargreaves, S. L., Sharples, S. L., Mackay, S. P., Waigh, R. D., Duval, O., Mberu, E. K., Watkins, W. M. (2005). Antimalarial Benzo[*c*]phenanthridines. *Bioorganic & Medicinal Chemistry Letters*, 15, 2007-2010. ISSN: 0960-894X.

Pan, L, Chay, H., Kinghorn, A. D. (2010). The Continuing Search for Antitumor Agents from Higher Plants. *Phytochemistry Letters*, 3 (1), 1-8. ISSN: 1874-3900.

Panthi, M. P., Chaudhary, R. P. (2006). Antibacterial Activity of Some Selected Folklore Medicinal Plants from West Nepal. *Scientific World*, 4 (4), 16-21. ISSN 1996-8949.

Patiño, O. J. (2004). *Estudio Fitoquímico Parcial de Zanthoxylum quinduensis (Rutaceae)*. Tesis de grado, Departamento de Química, Universidad Nacional de Colombia, pp. 2-56, Bogotá.

Patiño, O. J., Cuca, L. E. (2010). Isoquinoline Alkaloids of *Zanthoxylum quinduense* (Rutaceae). *Biochemical Systematic and Ecology*, 38, 853-856. ISSN: 0305-1978.

Patiño, O. J., Cuca, L. E. (2011). Monophyllidin, a New Alkaloid *L*-Proline Derivative from *Zanthoxylum monophyllum* (Rutaceae). *Phytochemistry Letters*, 4, 22-25. ISSN: 1874-3900.

Patiño, O. J., Prieto, J. A., Lozano, J. M., Lesmes, L., Cuca, L. E. (2011). Propiedades antibacterianas *in vitro* de metabolitos secundarios aislados de dos especies del género *Zanthoxylum* (Rutaceae). *Revista Cubana de Framacia*, 45 (3). In press. ISSN: 0034-7515.

Pereira, S. S., Lopes, L. S., Marques, R. B., Figueiredo, K. A., Costa, D. A., Chaves, M. H., Almeida, F. R. C. (2010). Antinociceptive effect of *Zanthoxylum rhoifolium* Lam. (Rutaceae) in models acute pain in rodents. *Journal of Ethnopharmacology*, 129, 227-231. ISSN: 0378-8741.

Pérez, R. M., Vargas, R., Martínez, F. J., García, E. V., Hernández, B. (2003). Actividad Antioxidante de los Alcaloides de *Bocconia arborea*. Estudio Sobre Seis Métodos de Análisis. *Ars Pharmaceutica*, 44, 5-21. ISSN: 0004-2927.

Prempeh, A. B. A., Mensah-Attipoe, J. (2008). Analgesic Activity of Crude Aqueous Extract of the Root Bark of *Zanthoxylum xanthoxyloides*. *General Medical Journal*, 42 (2), 79-84.

Prieto, J. A., Patiño, O. J., Delgado, W. A., Moreno, J. P., Cuca, L. E. (2011). Chemical Composition, Insecticide and Antifungal Activities of the Essential Oils of Fruits of three *Zanthoxylum* Species from Colombia. *Chilean Journal of Agricultural Research*, 71, 73-82. ISSN: 0718-5820.

Queiroz, E. F., Hay, A.-E., Chaaib, F., Diemen, D., Diallo, D., Hostettmann, K. (2006). New and Bioactive Aromatic Compouns from *Zanthoxylum xanthoxyloides*. *Planta Medica*, 72, 746-750. ISSN: 0032-0943.

Rahman, M. M., Islam, M. A., Khondkar, P., Gray, A. I. (2005). Alkaloids and Lignans from *Zanthoxylum budrunga* (Rutaceae). *Biochemical Systematic and Ecology*, 33, 91-96. ISSN: 0305-1978.

Ramanujan, S. N., Ratha, B. K. (2008). Effect of alcohol extract of a natural piscicide - Fruits of *Zanthoxylum armatum* DC. on Mg^{2+} - and Na^{+}, K^{+}-ATPase activity in various tissues of a freshwater air-breathing fish, *Heteropneustes fossilis*. *Aquaculture*, 283, 77-82. ISSN: 0044-8486.

Ranawat, L., Bhatt, J. Patel, J. (2010). Hepatoprotective activity of ethanolic extracts of bark of *Zanthoxylum armatum* DC in CCl_4 induced hepatic damage in rats. *Journal of Ethnopharmacology*, 127, 77-780. ISSN: 0378-8741.

Reddy, L. J., Jose, B. (2011). Statistical analysis of the antibacterial activity of *Zanthoxylum rhetsa* seed essential oil. *Journal of Chemical and Pharmaceutical Research*, 3 (1), 440-444. ISSN: 0975-7384.

Ribeiro, C.V.C., Kaplan, M.A.C. (2002). Tendências Evolutivas de Famílias Produtoras de Cumarinas em Angiospermae. *Quimica Nova*, 25, 533-538. ISSN: 0100-4042.

Ross, S. A., Al-Azeib, M. A., Krishnavei, K. S., Fronczek, F. R., Burandt, C. L. (2005). Alkamides from the Leaves of *Zanthoxylum syncarpum*. *Journal of Natural Products*, 68, 1297-1299. ISSN: 0163-3864.

Ross, S. A., Sultana, G. N. N., Burandt, C. L., ElSohly, M. A., Marais, J. P. J., Ferreira, D. (2004). Syncaparmide, a New Antiplasmodial (+)-Norepinephrine Derivative from *Zanthoxylum syncarpum*. *Journal of Natural Products*, 67, 88-90. ISSN: 0163-3864.

Saleem, M. (2099). Lupeol, a novel anti-inflammatory and anti-cancer dietary triterpene. *Cancer Letters*, 285, 109-115. ISSN: 0304-3835.

Saquib, Q. N., Hui, Y.-H., Anderson, J. E., Mclaughlin, J. L. (1990). Bioactive Furanocoumarins from the Berries of *Zanthoxylum americanum*. *Phytotherapy Research*, 4, 216-219. ISSN: 1099-1573.

Schnee, L. (1984). *Plantas comunes de Venezuela* (3 Edition). Ediciones de la biblioteca. Caracas: Universidad Central de Venezuela (UCV).

Segal, E., Elad, D. (2006). Fungal Vaccines and Immunotherapy. *Journal de Mycologie Médicale*, 16, 134-151. ISSN: 1156-5233.

Seidemann, J. (2005). *World Spice Plants: Economic Usage, Botany, Taxonomy*. Springer-Verlag, p. 399-402, ISBN: 3540222790, Berlin.

Sen, R., Chatterjee, M. (2011). Plant derived therapeutics for the treatment of Leishmaniasis. *Phytomedicine*, in press, doi:10.1016/j.phymed.2011.03.004. ISSN: 0944-7113.

Sheen, W.-S., Tsai, I.-L., Teng, C.-M., Chen, I.-S. (1994). Nor-neolignan and Phenyl Propanoid from *Zanthoxylum ailanthoides*. *Phytochemistry*, 36, 213-215. ISSN: 0031-9422.

Sheen, W.-S., Tsai, I.-L., Teng, C.-M., Ko, F.-N., Chen, I.-S. (1996). Indolopyridoquinazoline Alkaloids with Antiplatelet Aggregation Activity from *Zanthoxylum integrifoliolum*. *Planta Medica*, 62, 175-176. ISSN: 0032-0943.

Silva, L. L., Paoli, A. A. S. (2000). Caracterizacaò Morfo-Anatômica da Semente de *Zanthoxylum rhoifolium* Lam.-Rutaceae. *Revista Brasileira de Sementes*, 22, 250-256. ISSN: 0101-3122.

Simeón, S., Rios, J. L., Villar, A. (1989). Pharmacological Activities of Benzophenanthridine and Phenanthrene Alkaloids. *Pharmazie*, 44, 593-597. ISSN: 0031-7144.

Slaninová, I., Táborská, E., Bochořáková H., Slanina, J. (2001). Interaction of Benzo[*c*]phenanthridine and Protoberberine Alkaloids with Animal and Yeast Cells. *Cell Biology and Toxicology*, 17, 51-63. ISSN: 1573-6822.

Somanabandhu, A-O., Ruangrungsi, N., Lance, G. L., Organ, M. G. (1992). Constituents of Steam Bark of *Zanthoxylum limonella*. *Journal of the Science Society of Thailand*, 18, 181-185. ISSN: 0303-8122.

Song, J-H., Chae, S. W., Yoon, K-A., Park, J-S., Choi, H-J. (2010). Antiviral Activity of *Zanthoxylum* Species against Porcine Epidemic Diarrhea Virus. *Journal of Cosmetics and Public Health*, 6 (2), 42-44.

Strand, J. F. (2000). Some Agrometeorological Aspects of Pest and Disease Management for the 21st Century. *Agricultural and Forest Meteorology*, 103, 73-82. ISSN: 0168-1923.

Suryanto, E., Sastrohamidjojo, H., Raharjo, S., Trangongo. (2004). Antiradical Activity of Analiman (*Zanthoxylum achanthopodium* DC) Fruit Extract. *Indonesian Food and Nutrition Progress*, 11 (1), 15-19.

Taborda, M. E., Cuca, L. E. (2007). Un Nuevo Alcaloide Carbazolico de *Zanthoxylum rhoifolium*. *Scientia et Technica*, 13, 191-192. ISSN 0122-1701.

Tang, W., Hemm, I., Bertram, B. (2003). Recent Development of Antitumor Agents from Chinese Herbal Medicines, Part I. Low Molecular Compounds. *Planta Medica, 69*, 97-108. ISSN: 0032-0943.

Tarus, P. K., Coombes, P. H., Crouch, N. R., Mulholland, D. A. (2006). Benzo[c]phenanthridine alkaloids from stem bark of the Forest Knobwood,

Zanthoxylum davyi (Rutaceae). *South African Journal of Botany*, 72, 555-558. ISSN: 0254-6299.

Tatsadjieu, L. N., Essia Ngang, J. J., Ngassoum, M. B., Etoa, F-X. (2003). Antibacterial and antifungal activity of *Xylopia aethiopica, Monodora myristica, Zanthoxylum xanthoxyloides* and *Zanthoxylum leprieurii* from Cameroon. *Fitoterapia*, 74, 469-472. ISSN 0367-326X.

Tillequin, F. (2007). Rutaceous Alkaloids as Models for the Design of Novel Antitumor Drugs. *Phytochemical Reviews*, 6, 65-70. ISSN: 1572-980X.

Tringali, C. (2001). *Bioactive Compounds from Natural Sources: Isolation, Characterization and Biological Properties*. Taylor & Francis, pp. ix-x, ISBN: 0748408908, London.

Tringali, C., Spatafora, C., Calì, V., Simmonds, M. S. J. (2001). Antifeedant constituents from *Fagara macrophylla*. *Fitoterapia*, 72, 538-543. ISSN 0367-326X.

Tsai, I.-L., Lin, W.-Y., Teng, C.-M., Ishikawa, T., Doong, S.-L., Huang, M.-W., Chen, Y-C., Chen, I.-S. (2000). "Coumarins and Antiplatelet Constituents from the Root Bark of *Zanthoxylum schinifolium*". *Planta Medica*, 66, 618-623. ISSN: 0032-0943.

Thuy, T. T., Porzel, A., Ripperger, H., Van Sung, T., Adam, G. (1999). Bishordeninyl Terpene Alkaloids from *Zanthoxylum avicennae*. *Phytochemistry*, 50, 903-907. ISSN: 0031-9422.

Verma, N., Khosa, R. L. (2010). Hepatoprotective activity of leaves of *Zanthoxylum armatum* DC in CCl_4 induced hepatotoxicity in rats. *Indian Journal of Biochemistry & Biophysics*, 47, 124-127. ISSN: 0301-1208.

Villalba, M. A., Carmo, M. I., Leite, M. N., Sousa, O. V. (2007). Atividades farmacológicas dos extratos de *Zanthoxylum chiloperone* (Rutaceae). *Revista Brasileira de Farmacognosia*, 17 (2), 236-241. ISSN: 1981-528X.

Waldvogel, F. (2004). Infectious Diseases in the 21st Century: Old Challenges and New Opportunities. *International Journal of Infectious Diseases*, 8, 5-12. ISSN: 1201-9712.

Waterman, P. G., Grundon, M. F. (1983). *Chemistry and Chemical Taxonomy of the Rutales*. Academic Press, ISBN: 0127376801 London.

Waterman, P. G. (2007). The Current Status of Chemical Systematics. *Phytochemistry*, 68, 2896-2903. ISSN: 0031-9422.

Were, P. S., Kinyanjui, P., Gicheru, M. M., Mwangi, E., Ozwara, H. S. (2010). Prophylactic and curative activities of extracts from Warburgia ugandensis Sprague (Canellaceae) and *Zanthoxylum usambarense* (Engl.) Kokwaro (Rutaceae) against *Plasmodium knowlesi* and *Plasmodium berghei*. *Journal of Ethnopharmacology*, 130, 158-162. ISSN: 0378-8741.

Xia, L., You, J., Li, G., Sun, Z., Suo, Y. Compositional and Antioxidant Analysis of *Zanthoxylum bungeanum* Seed Oil Obtained by Supercritical CO_2 Fluid Extraction. *Journal of the American Oil Chemists' Society*, 88 (7), 1029-1036. ISSN: 1558-9331.

Xiong, Q. B., Shi, D. W. (1991). Morphological and Histological Studies of Chinese Traditional Drug Hua Jiao Pericarpium-Zanthoxili and its Allied Drugs. *Acta Pharmaceutica Sinica*, 26, 938-947. ISSN: 05134870.

Yamazaki, E., Inagaki, M., Kurita, O., Inoue, T. (2007). Antioxidant activity of Japanese pepper (*Zanthoxylum piperitum* DC.) fruit. *Food Chemistry*, 100, 171-177. ISSN: 0308-8146.

Yang, X. (2008). Aroma Constituents and Alkylamides of Red and Green Huajiao (*Zanthoxylum bungeanum* and *Zanthoxylum schinifolium*). *Journal of Agricultural and Food Chemistry*, 56, 1689-1696. ISSN: 0021-8561.

Zirihi, G. N., N'guessan, K., Etien, D. T., Serikouassi B. (2009). Evaluation in vitro of antiplasmodial activity of ethanolic extracts of *Funtumia elastica* , *Rauvolfia vomitoria* and *Zanthoxylum gilletii* on *Plasmodium falciparum* isolates from Côted'Ivoire. *Journal of Animal & Plant Sciences*, 5 (1), 406-413. ISSN: 2071 - 7024.